Mechanisms

of VIRUS INFECTION

Mechanisms
of VIRUS INFECTION

Edited by

WILSON SMITH
Microbiological Research Establishment,
Porton, Wiltshire, England

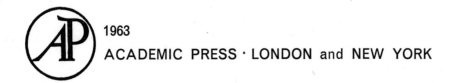

1963
ACADEMIC PRESS · LONDON and NEW YORK

ADADEMIC PRESS INC. (LONDON) LTD.
BERKELEY SQUARE HOUSE
BERKELEY SQUARE
LONDON, W.1.

U.S. Edition published by
ACADEMIC PRESS INC.
111 FIFTH AVENUE
NEW YORK 3, NEW YORK

Library of Congress Catalog Card Number: 63-16559

Printed in Great Britain by Willmer Brothers and Haram Limited, 62-68 Chester Street, Birkenhead.

List of Contributors

G. BELYAVIN, *Department of Bacteriology, University College Hospital Medical School, London, England* (p. 309).

A. COHEN, *Department of Bacteriology, University College Hospital Medical School, London, England* (p. 153).

A. W. DOWNIE, *Department of Bacteriology, The University, Liverpool, England* (p. 101).

W. HAYES, *Medical Research Council, Microbial Genetics Research Unit, Hammersmith Hospital, London, England* (p. 35).

A. ISAACS, *National Institute for Medical Research, Mill Hill, London, England* (p. 191).

W. SMITH, *Microbiological Research Establishment, Experimental Station, Porton, Nr. Salisbury, Wiltshire, England* (p. 1).

D. A. J. TYRRELL, *Harvard Hospital, Salisbury, Wiltshire, England* (p. 225).

J. C. N. WESTWOOD, *Microbiological Research Establishment, Experimental Station, Porton, Nr. Salisbury, Wiltshire, England* (p. 255).

Preface

Research workers in all the various branches of virology are served by a spate of scientific publications, many of which are so highly technical that they are fully comprehensible only to the experts in particular fields of research. At the other end of the scale the student can obtain an elementary knowledge of the viruses and of virus behaviour from the numerous text books now available. Unfortunately, text books even when designed to meet special needs, such as those of the medical undergraduate or the student of botany, are limited as a rule to the presentation of firmly established facts.

The present volume is intended neither as a text book nor as a work of reference for the expert, although it is hoped that both student and research worker may find in it something of use and much of interest. Its subject, "Mechanisms of Virus Infection", represents the central theme of virology, linking all its many branches together and having, moreover, important implications for several other biological sciences. Particular aspects of the subject, especially those pertaining to intracellular virus replication, have received much attention from both scientific and popular writers, but other aspects have been somewhat neglected and there have been few attempts at comprehensive treatment of the virus-host relationship as a whole. This is not because of lack of knowledge; a good deal is known about each phase of the cycle of infection, although much more remains to be discovered and the unsolved problems are full of exciting possibilities. The book therefore aims at the presentation of a balanced picture of the present state of knowledge and of the evidence on which current concepts are founded, together with free speculations and discussions about much that remains to be discovered.

The editor bears sole responsibility for the scope and general plan of the book as a whole, but each contributor was given a free hand to deal with his particular aspect of the main subject in any way he thought fit. Such freedom militates against any uniformity of literary style or methods of approach and also results in some degree of repetition and overlapping. These features, however, are not necessarily wholly undesirable and confer one important advantage, namely that the various chapters can be read either as closely interconnected parts of a general theme or independently as separate accounts of the particular aspects with which they are primarily concerned. The bibliography is not meant to be exhaustive but has been made sufficiently comprehensive to afford a ready means of access to the voluminous literature now available on every facet of the main subject.

April, 1963   Wilson Smith,
                                                        Salisbury.

Contents

CHAPTER 1

Mechanisms of Virus Infection
General Considerations

WILSON SMITH

Microbiological Research Establishment
Porton, Wiltshire, England

I. Introduction

This book is concerned with the series of events which comprise the infection of a host organism with a virus parasite. Although there is a very broad, basic common pattern underlying all virus infections, irrespective of the class of host and the type of virus involved, the anatomical and physiological differences between animals, plants and bacteria determine certain fundamental differences in their interactions with the viruses which parasitize them. Adequate treatment of the subject in relation to each of these major branches of virology is not possible within the scope of a single volume; while, therefore, frequent references to plant viruses are unavoidable, the book in the main is limited to consideration of the animal viruses, except for a single chapter which summarizes present knowledge and ideas pertaining to the bacterial viruses. This latter is included because so much of the experimental evidence, on which any intelligent discussion of virus infectivity mechanisms must be based, derives from bacteriophage research. Thus, the observable phenomena of infections of bacteria with viruses, and the mechanistic interpretations which have now been firmly established, provide a useful model with which the behaviour of animal viruses can be compared and the relevant hypotheses evaluated. Even with such a limitation of the field of enquiry the variability of structure, chemical constitution and biological behaviour of the animal viruses present a gallimaufry of bewildering complexity. Too few viruses have, as yet, been studied in sufficient detail to validate generalizations except for a few of the broadest character. Unfortunately, this has not always been sufficiently appreciated by virologists, with the result that phenomena experimentally demonstrable in one particular system are sometimes accepted as pertaining to viruses in general. Caution is especially called for in extrapolation from bacteriophage research. Undoubtedly, the elucidation of infectivity mechanisms utilized by some of the bacterial viruses has been a potent stimulus to investigations of animal viruses; but a critical approach is still necessary whenever the concepts of virus eclipse, the intracellular dominance of viral nucleic acid, virus latency and so forth are under consideration.

There is little need to stress the importance of the subject from the practical standpoint of man's health and well-being. In human medicine the viruses have usurped the place of the bacteria as the most important class of disease-producing agents, largely because they are not yet amenable to antibiotic therapy and chemotherapy. Viruses, highly specific for man, cause devastating pandemics (influenza), cyclical epidemics (measles) and persistent endemic infections (common cold). Viruses infecting lower animals may also affect man in either of two ways. Some, like the Arbor viruses, which can infect man as an alternate host species, create reservoirs of infection in animals, from which man is constantly liable to attack. Others, though unable to infect human beings, may yet cause enormous economic loss and malnutrition by infection of domestic livestock; outstanding examples are the viruses of foot-and-mouth disease, rinderpest and Newcastle disease of fowls. In spite of the efficacy of certain specific prophylactic measures within the limited ranges in which their application is practicable, it is becoming increasingly clear that control on a scale comparable with that achieved for many bacterial infections must await a fuller understanding of the long chain of host–virus interactions which constitute the infective process.

On a long-term view the scientific implications of virological research may be even more important than any practical measures of disease control which constitute the more immediate objectives. The means by which heritable characters are transmitted, with a nice balance between their conservation and continuous modification, is one of the central mysteries of life. Another such mystery is the mechanism of protein synthesis, and yet a third is the determination and control of morphogenesis. In all of these such slight insight as we now possess has been gained partly from studies of the viruses and the processes involved in their intracellular replication. There can thus be no doubt that further elucidation of these virological processes will contribute to the final solution of the fundamental problems mentioned and others of like nature. The magnitude of the research effort still needed to fill the enormous gaps in our present knowledge of the various aspects of the host–virus relationship will, however, be all too clearly apparent in the chapters which follow.

II. The Evolution of Virology

Appreciation of the present status of virology and evaluation of the significance of recent advances must depend largely upon knowledge of past effort and achievement. In contrast to the beautiful precision of much present-day experimentation, facilitated in many cases by the availability of elaborate and costly apparatus, the probings of the early pioneers may seem crude, but it is to their efforts that we owe much of the basic information on which current concepts are founded.

The story of virus research is the story of the discovery of a class of disease-producing agents quite unlike any known previously, the gradual recognition of their importance and of the magnitude of the new field of investigation opened up by their discovery, and the subsequent exploration of the field on an ever increasing scale and at an ever increasing tempo. The result is that virology today is a major research activity of university departments and research institutes all over the world. From time to time there have been shifts of the major effort from one part of the field to another, so that virology as a whole has passed through various phases, each phase being characterized by its particular interest and the type of approach adopted for the investigation of outstanding problems. However, while the recognition of such phases may have some use in reviewing the evolution of current knowledge and concepts, any suggestion that different aspects of virus research fall into well-defined periods would be both misleading and mischievous. The growth of virology, like that of an individual, has been sometimes fast, sometimes slow, and the emphasis at times has rested on the development of particular aspects; yet withal it has been a continuous process of unfolding and expansion with synchronous development on many fronts.

A. Initial Discoveries and Pioneer Investigations

The birth of virology was heralded by Ivanowski's discovery that a mosaic disease of the tobacco plant is due to infection with an invisible, filterable agent, the virus we now refer to as tobacco mosaic virus (TMV) (Ivanowski, 1892). His discovery was soon followed by the isolation of other viruses. Foot-and-mouth disease of cattle was the first animal disease for which a viral aetiology was definitely proved (Loeffler and Frosch, 1898). Within a few years certain human ailments, notably yellow fever, poliomyelitis and vaccinia were similarly characterized.

At that time the only means of detection of such agents was by their gross pathological effects on their hosts, while their differentiation from pathogenic micro-organisms rested solely on their filtrability through bacterial filters and their invisibility by high-power microscopy. It was inevitable, therefore, that for some time virus research centred round clinical, pathological and epidemiological studies of those diseases in which, although obviously caused by some transmissible infective agent, no visible bacterial or protozoal organism could be incriminated. Even so, some outstanding experimental work was done by the early virologists with results which impinge directly on the problems of virus infectivity. For example, the nontransmissibility of yellow fever by even the closest contact between sick and healthy persons was firmly established and, *per contra*, the essential participation of a mosquito vector in the chain of transmission from man to man was proved (Reed *et al.*, 1901). From this work, and the subsequent research which stemmed from it, many problems arise which still await solution. Why are most blood-sucking insects, including mites, fleas, lice and ticks, unable to transmit yellow fever infection from man to man? Why are some species of mosquitoes unable to transmit the virus in spite of the fact that virus multiplies in their tissues after ingestion of infected blood? Why the necessity for virus multiplication in the vector species? These and similar questions are a salutary reminder, in the face of the impressive corpus of knowledge presented in later chapters, that innumerable problems remain to be elucidated.

Another example of the far-reaching significance of very early experimental work is the transmission of paralytic poliomyelitis to monkeys (Landsteiner and Popper, 1909). Apart from its immediate importance in the poliomyelitis research then in progress, it was a pointer to the necessity for adaptations of viruses to laboratory animals if experimental investigations were to be rationally planned and continuously pursued. Such adaptations have indeed played a major role in making possible the kind of experiments needed for the analysis of host–virus interactions.

Two other outstanding discoveries of this opening phase of virology, which lasted roughly up to the end of World War I, must be mentioned. The first was that bacteria are themselves subject to fatal infections with filtrable and transmissible agents (Twort, 1915). The nature of these agents, originally called bacteriophages, was for long a subject of violent controversy, but today they are universally accepted as bacterial viruses. Their supreme importance lies in the fact, well exemplified in Chapter 2, that they provide the most suitable material for the investigation of many facets of virus–host cell interactions.

The second discovery of special importance was that certain sarcomata of fowls could be transmitted by means of cell-free, and bacteria-free, filtrates (Rous, 1911). The idea of a virus aetiology of tumours was so revolutionary that for a long time many orthodox pathologists refused to accept the fowl sarcomata as true neoplasms; a position which finally had to be abandoned in the face of accumulating evidence from tumours of various other kinds. Without begging the question of the complete aetiological pattern of neoplasms, which may of course involve the interplay of more than one factor, it is fairly safe to say that the virus-induced tumours reflect a type of cell–virus association different from that obtaining in acute virus diseases. One suspects that this type of association may represent an intermediate stage in the evolution of virus parasitism from a totally destructive process to the symbiotic relationship of virus latency.

B. Development of Organized Laboratory Research

Considerable expansion of virus research would have occurred after the end of World War I in any case, but the process was probably greatly accelerated by the emotional impact of the great influenza pandemics of 1918 and 1919. Experimental evidence, derived largely from the pandemics, clearly pointed to a viral aetiology of this disease, though several years had to elapse before this was definitely proved (Smith, Andrewes and Laidlaw, 1933). Many other highly contagious and dangerous diseases, both of man and lower animals, were likewise suspected as being virus infections on the basis of the purely negative evidence that no visible microbes could be incriminated. Progress demanded positive evidence: the isolation of the causative agents and rigorous proof of their causal relationship with the diseases in question. The end of the war therefore ushered in a new phase of virus research with its major emphasis on experimental investigations in the laboratory.

The studies of the preceding phase had shown clearly that, in their overt clinical and pathological manifestations, there are no essential differences between viral and bacterial infections. Indeed, it is still not possible to distinguish between some bacterial and viral illnesses without recourse to laboratory aids. It is not surprising, therefore, that at this early stage of organized laboratory research virology was regarded as constituting a minor branch of bacteriology, with the result that it passed chiefly into the hands of bacteriologists and pathologists, more especially those with medical qualifications and experience. This in turn meant that the techniques used were the classical techniques of bacteriology, pathology and immunology which past experience had shown to be such powerful tools for the conquest of microbial diseases. They were, however, quite inadequate for probing into the constitution and essential nature of the viruses themselves; indeed they were not even adequate for obtaining viruses in a state approaching the degree of purity required for chemical and physical analysis. Moreover, the main driving force was the urgent need for practical measures of control over diseases such as influenza, man's helplessness against which had so recently and dramatically been demonstrated. These were the factors which channelled research for a number of years into explorations of what viruses do to their animal hosts rather than what viruses are in themselves. Such explorations tended to follow a common pattern, the sequential steps of which were usually somewhat as follows:

1. Transmission of the disease of unknown aetiology to an experimental animal by the inoculation of material from a clinical case.
2. Serial transmission in the experimental animal species.
3. Exclusion of microbial aetiology by infections with bacteriologically sterile filtrates.
4. Accumulation of evidence of causal relationship of the isolated virus with the naturally occurring disease, e.g. by infection of volunteers, serological evidence, etc.
5. Studies of the clinical and pathological manifestations of the natural and experimental infections.
6. Investigations of the immunological responses to infection.
7. Applications in diagnosis and prophylaxis.

In this way several diseases of man and lower animals were firmly characterized as virus infections and the main features of the interplay between the isolated viruses and their experimental animal hosts were established. From this stemmed some notable successes in disease control, but of more interest in the present context is the influence which this phase of research had upon the course of later developments and the relation of the solid body of knowledge acquired by such means to modern concepts of infectivity mechanisms. It is obvious, of course, that the pattern of virus research at any given time is influenced by what has been done previously, but special significance attaches to some of the achievements of what might be called the pathological era of virus research. A few of the more notable of these merit brief discussion.

1. Obligate cell parasitism

The recognition that all viruses must parasitize living cells for their replication came slowly from numerous abortive attempts to grow them on lifeless media, coupled with their successful cultivation outside the animal body provided only that the medium contained living tissue cells. In passing, it may be suggested, purely as a speculation, that this situation may be altered in the near future, for the production of synthetic DNA and RNA from pools of their constituent nucleotides and the synthesis of protein-like molecules from pools of amino acids by means of synthetic RNA have revolutionized our ideas of what may soon become possible in the synthesis of biological agents (Grünberg-Manago and Ochoa, 1955; Hurwitz and Furth, 1962; Nirenberg and Matthaei, 1961). Be that as it may, however, it is beyond question that the concept of obligate cell parasitism was firmly established largely by the laborious efforts of many early workers to disprove it, since when it has remained unchallenged up to the present time and has been the axis round which all hypotheses of infectivity mechanisms have been constructed.

2. The particulate nature of viruses

It is scarcely an exaggeration to say that the designs of all experiments aimed at clarification of virus infectivity mechanisms are based on the belief that all viruses are particulate entities, each with its own peculiar physical, chemical and biological characteristics. The younger modern virologist, accustomed to pictorial representations of viruses of diverse shapes and sizes by electron micrographs, may find it difficult to believe that for many years this was a highly controversial issue. Nevertheless, it was out of this controversy, at a time when microscopic resolution of even the largest viruses was impossible, that ingenious experimentation not only settled the question but in the process of doing so established many of the classical techniques of virus purification, concentration and assay. Moreover, from this contribution of earlier workers stem current concepts of virus maturation as a final stage of replication, the production of incomplete virus from lack of co-ordination of intracellular synthetic processes, the multiparticle content of pock-forming and plaque-forming units and so forth.

3. Host and tissue specificity

The proof of causal relationship of newly isolated viruses with the natural diseases in question, and the study of distinguishing viral characteristics, usually involved detailed investigation of the spread, localization and excretion of the viruses in experimental animals. With some viruses the difficulty of achieving serial experimental transmission necessitated the testing of every possible route of inoculation in an extensive range of experimental animal species. From investigations of this kind the concept of tissue tropism of viruses arose, which for many years afforded the best basis of classification. Although tissue tropisms are seldom if ever absolute, and the terms dermotropic, neurotropic, pneumotropic, etc., have largely gone out of use, tissue specificity remains a very important and little understood viral characteristic. It is not difficult to accept that fine biochemical differences in the metabolism of different types of cell within the same host probably account for the fact that one type will support virus replication while another type fails to do so. It is also well known that cell susceptibility to infection may depend upon the chemical constitution or the configuration of some of its surface components. For example, the susceptibility or non-susceptibility of certain Salmonella species and types to a particular phage is determined by their possession or lack of particular somatic surface antigens (Burnet, 1927), and the susceptibility of respiratory mucosal cells to invasion by the myxoviruses depends on the integrity of the mucopolysaccharide cell receptors. Eventually the tissue tropisms of several other viruses may be expected to find similar explanations. But there remain puzzling phenomena for which it is difficult to suggest convincing hypotheses. Tissues may be completely non-susceptible in the intact animal host, yet when explanted into culture media may support virus growth readily. One suspects that herein may lie a valuable clue for the understanding of certain aspects of virus behaviour at both the host organism and the cellular levels.

4. Antigenic constitution

Long before the discovery of the viruses themselves, diseases now known to be of virus aetiology (for example, smallpox) were known to confer resistance against subsequent attack. The immunogenicity of viruses was therefore never in question. For a long time, however, it was questioned whether the viruses could be antigenic and whether the immunity resulting from viral and bacterial infections could possibly be of the same essential nature. Eventually transmission of various virus infections to laboratory animals made it possible to test the virus-neutralizing potencies of sera and then to demonstrate the association of acquired resistance and the presence of virus-neutralizing antibodies in the blood-stream. But most early attempts to elicit the *in vitro* serum reactions of agglutination and precipitation failed completely, and although complement fixation reactions were frequently reported their specificity was doubted because of the crude nature of the virus material used as antigens. The pioneer work in this field was done with vaccinia virus and led eventually to the unequivocal demonstration of the applicability and specificity of the serum reactions in this case. By their aid the antigenic complexity of the virus was unravelled and the way opened for those later antigenic analyses of many other viruses which have contributed much to our knowledge of host–virus relationships.

5. Susceptibility of embryonic tissue

The peculiar susceptibility to infection of certain cells of non-susceptible tissues when they are removed from the restraints of the intact host organism has already been mentioned. A point of great interest is whether this has any connection with the fact that embryonic tissues are in many instances much more susceptible than are the adult tissues to which they give rise. The first inkling of this differential susceptibility came from the discovery of Goodpasture, Woodruff and Buddingh (1931) that the chorioallantoic membrane of the chicken embryo can be infected with the viruses of vaccinia and herpes simplex, to which hatched chicks are totally resistant. This led to the development of an extensive range of chick embryo techniques which have not only served practical purposes such as the isolation of new viruses and the preparation of virus vaccines but have also had extremely fruitful applications in the study of various host–virus interactions and especially in the analysis of growth cycle phenomena. The chick embryo and de-embryonated egg techniques (Beveridge and Burnet, 1946) represent a transitional phase between limitation to adult animal hosts for the investigation of virus behaviour and the development of the present-day methods of cell culture which allow even firmer control of complicating, extraneous variables. In addition to its remarkable susceptibility to so many different viruses, the chick embryo has the great advantage that it lacks the immunological response mechanisms which so profoundly affect the course of animal infections. From the pointer of chick embryo susceptibility came the subsequent exploitation of mammalian embryos and sucklings for the isolation and study of recalcitrant viruses such as those of the Coxsackie group.

C. NATURE OF VIRUSES

The dependence of experimental design, in the investigation of virus infectivity mechanisms, upon recognition of the particulate nature of viruses has already been mentioned. A further consequence of this recognition was an extension of interest from what viruses do in the hosts they parasitize to what viruses are in themselves. The problem is largely a physical and chemical one, so that chemists and physicists were inevitably attracted to this field of enquiry and, since about the early nineteen-thirties, have played an ever increasing part in virological research.

Much early effort was directed to the characterization of viruses in physical terms. Prior to the development of electron microscopy, this meant in effect the estimation of the size and shape of virus elementary particles by indirect means. Of the many physical methods employed, involving centrifugation, diffusion, viscosity determinations, etc., filtration was especially productive. The development of membrane filters of graded pore size (Elford, 1931) made it possible to arrange most of the known viruses in an order of descending magnitude from about 300 mμ to about 20 mμ. It is indeed remarkable how little correction of the early figures has been necessary in the light of the more direct measurements now possible.

Among the animal viruses, vaccinia remained for a long time the only one amenable to chemical analysis. The prime requisite for this kind of investigation is an adequate supply of material in a state at least approaching chemical purity. This was quite unachievable for all except the largest viruses until the more powerful techniques of the modern phase of virological research had been developed. Vaccinia virus, however, could be obtained in large amounts from scarified rabbit skin and was found to be sedimentable by centrifugation speeds of only a few thousand revolutions per minute (MacCallum and Oppenheimer, 1922). Its purification and concentration were therefore accomplished by a number of independent workers to a degree which allowed chemical, physical and serological analyses with results which are still accepted as valid. In one respect the fact that so much of the early work had to be confined to vaccinia was unfortunate, for this virus is exceptionally complex both chemically and antigenically. The elementary bodies were found to contain, in addition to protein and nucleic acids, carbohydrates, lipids including neutral fat cholesterol and phospholipid, and copper. Moreover, several biologically active substances were found, such as phosphatase, catalase, lipase, biotin and flavin. Such findings, together with the demonstration of numerous antigens both at the surface and within the deeper structure of the elementary particle, tended towards an exaggerated view of virus complexity and a reluctance to admit the possibility that some animal viruses might be comparable in simplicity of construction with certain plant viruses being investigated at about the same period. Subsequent work has, of course, shown this to be the case with several of the very small animal viruses such as poliomyelitis virus.

Nevertheless, the impact of plant virus research on animal virologists was startling when tobacco mosaic virus, the first virus to be discovered, was found to be obtainable in paracrystalline form (Stanley, 1935). Previously the dominant view was that viruses were micro-organisms restricted in some of the properties traditionally associated with living entities because of their small size. The crystallization of other plant viruses in the form of true three-dimensional crystals made this view untenable in respect of viruses in general and led many virologists to assume that there was a basic line of cleavage between plant and animal viruses, the latter being not only more complex and highly organized but also of essentially different nature. However, the line of cleavage, if such exists, between relatively simple crystallizable viruses and complex ones with well-differentiated morphological components, does not lie at this point but rather at some point in the ascending order of magnitude of the animal viruses, the smallest of which can now be obtained in true crystalline form. A more modern dilemma is the difficulty of attributing functions to the morphologically defined substructures of large viruses whose basic pattern of replication appears to be no different from that of the smallest and simplest.

III. Major Facets of the Host–Virus Relationship

A. The Infection Cycle

The most important virus characteristic, and possibly the only one shared by all viruses, is obligate cell parasitism. Although individual virus particles survive for variable periods in extracellular environments, species survival is wholly dependent upon intracellular replication and hence upon recurrent cycles of association with some higher host organism. This statement may possibly need qualification in respect of bacterial lysogeny, but it is questionable whether the viral genome, integrated, in this condition, with the host genome, can properly be regarded as a virus (Lwoff, 1957). It may be trite to say that, in order to infect a cell, an animal virus must first gain entry into the body of the animal host, but the reminder may serve to focus attention on the fact that animal virologists have been so fascinated by the results of pioneer bacteriophage researches that they have tended to neglect those aspects of virus infections which pertain solely to metazoan hosts. For all viruses the infection cycle comprises entry into the host, intracellular replication and subsequent escape into the external environment; but for bacterial viruses this cycle is relatively simple because of the unicellular nature of the host organism, and it is not surprising that most of the pioneer work on infectivity mechanisms was done with phage–bacteria systems. In the case of animal viruses the situation is more complicated. In order to find cells suitable for its replication, the virus must first penetrate the outer defence barriers of the animal body, and, having done so, it may then have to travel to sites far removed from the portal of entry. Moreover, release from the infected cell after completion of intracellular replication does not complete the cycle; subsequent escape from the body of the animal host is an essential prerequisite for the initiation of a new cycle in a fresh host.

This more complicated cycle of infection is not, of course, peculiar to the animal viruses. Plant viruses, too, must gain entry into highly organized, multicellular hosts and be subsequently released into the external environment. There are, however, certain aspects of the virus–host relationship which pertain solely to the animal viruses, more especially to those for which man is the only natural host species. In the transfer of plant viruses from one plant to another the host plays a purely passive role, the transport being effected by external agencies, chiefly air currents and insect vectors. But in animal diseases the activities and habits of the host populations determine to a considerable extent the pattern of virus behaviour and the kind of transfer mechanism best suited to ensure virus survival.

Thus, the animal viruses present three main facets of the host–parasite relationship, namely the interactions of the viruses with the host organism as a whole, with the host cell and with the host community. These, although interdependent and sequentially related, need to be considered separately, for their investigation demands different techniques. The sequence of subsequent chapters and their respective contents have, in fact, been planned in accordance with this general line of approach.

B. Interaction between Viruses and Host Organisms

It is obvious that different mechanisms are needed by different viruses to cope with the extracellular phases of their association with host organisms. The problems facing one of the highly neurotropic Arbor viruses are much more complex than those of a respiratory virus which gains immediate contact with susceptible cells on simple inspiration and after replication within, and release from the cells, is expired direct into the external environment. Each individual case is governed by a large number of factors, many of them unknown, but among which may be cited the size of the virus particle, its chemical constitution and the configuration of its surface components, the localization of susceptible cells within the host body and the cytopathic effects of cell infection. These and numerous other factors must invariably affect the course of events in any virus invasion of a normal animal; that is to say, of an animal without any previous contact with the particular virus in question. Whenever invasion occurs in an animal with some degree of acquired specific immunity, additional potent factors come into play. The presence of specific, virus-neutralizing antibodies in the blood stream and tissue fluids constitutes a formidable obstacle to the spread of virus within the body and extension of the infection from cell to cell. One imagines that the latency of some viruses and the direct cell-to-cell passage of others via intercellular bridges may represent successful evolutionary counters to the challenge of immunological barriers.

It will be evident from the discussions in Chapter 3 of the pathways of spread of viruses within the host and the specific localization of infections in various organs and tissues that little is known about the exact mechanisms underlying such variations of behaviour. This is especially true of the so-called neurotropic viruses. In many cases alternative mechanisms seem to be available, the choice of which must rest on variable factors in both the internal and external host environment. The interest and importance of this lies, of course, in the fact that the final outcome in clinical and pathological terms may be very different, according to which alternative has been operative. A striking example is poliomyelitis virus infection, which can present itself as an inapparent infection, a localized infection, a generalized infection without neurological involvement or a disease chiefly characterized by virus attack upon the central nervous system.

Everyone with extensive experience of animal experimentation has encountered the difficulties which arise from individual variation of susceptibility. Our ignorance of the determining factors is exemplified by the general adoption of the 50% end-point, based upon statistical analysis of results from large numbers of animals, in assays of biological agents. The degree of variability is sometimes truly astonishing, as, for example, when occasional animals survive the infection of a thousand or more LD50's, and clinical observation suggests that in the epidemiology of human diseases individual non-susceptibility may play a role of considerable importance. There is, of course, no doubt that susceptibility to infection is affected by age, sex and physiological factors such as malnutrition, hormonal imbalance and so forth; this, however, tells us nothing about the basic mechanisms involved, which offer a challenge to future research.

C. Virus Host–Cell Interactions

1. The cycle of cell infection

The dominant phenomenon of virus infection is intracellular replication; this is the event to which all other host–virus interactions are subservient, for without it they would in themselves be meaningless. It is not surprising, therefore, that the replication process has engaged the attention of virologists to the relative neglect of other phases of the cell infection cycle. The cycle comprises attachment of virus particle to the cell wall, penetration of the particle into the cell interior, replication of both the viral genome and other viral constituents, maturation of the complete particle and finally release of new virus from the cell. One of the most outstanding landmarks of virology, with an influence upon conceptual developments and the orientation of research comparable to that which resulted from the demonstration of virus crystallizability, was the astonishing discovery that the RNA of tobacco mosaic virus, freed from the viral protein, is by itself infective (Gierer and Schramm, 1956). Subsequent investigation has led to claims of infectivity of the extracted nucleic acids of about a score of animal viruses, including both RNA and DNA viruses. Some of these claims are supported by evidence which is wellnigh incontrovertible, but several have been made on the basis of experiments which are wide open to criticism. Moreover, it should not be forgotten that the infective efficiency of extracted nucleic acids is invariably much lower than that of the intact virus particle on a weight for weight basis of the nucleic acid involved; also that persistent efforts to demonstrate the infectivity of nucleic acids of many viruses have been abortive. While it is impossible, therefore, to exaggerate the importance of the dominant role which the viral nucleic acid plays in the infectious process, the recognition of its dominance has perhaps resulted in some neglect of the possible functions of other constituents. It may be true that many plant viruses, and even some of the smallest animal viruses, consist of a core of infective RNA, with a protein coat whose only function is to protect the vital nucleic acid in extracellular environments, but the validity of extending the concept to embrace all small viruses, as Crick and Watson (1956) have suggested, may be doubted, and in the case of some larger viruses it is certainly not applicable. In this connection it is surely significant that the phage DNA of the bacterial virus ϕX 174 may be infective for the protoplasts of bacteria although the bacteria themselves are resistant both to the intact phage particles and extracted DNA. Similarly, the RNA of several animal viruses will infect cells which are not susceptible to the viruses themselves (Holland, McLaren and Syverton, 1959a,b). Nonsusceptibility, therefore, is not necessarily due to intracellular conditions which are unsuitable for initiation of replication by the viral nucleic acid.

Research on the phases of the virus–host cell association other than those which occur intracellularly has been limited to a very few viruses, mostly to the myxoviruses. The latter are, of course, pre-eminently suited for experimental investigation of the processes of attachment, penetration and release because of their possession of specific receptor sites complementary to cell receptors, and of the enzyme neuraminidaze which destroys cell receptor substrate. This very fact, however, enjoins caution against uncritical acceptance of generalizations until many other viruses have been studied with the same thoroughness.

2. Cytopathogenicity

Most of our knowledge about viral cytopathogenicity is derived from investigations of virus–cell interactions under the abnormal conditions of *in vitro* cell culture, and, as will be evident from the chapter on virus toxicity, extrapolations from the results of such investigations to the phenomena of natural infections of animals are not yet possible. The changes producible in one type of cell may not occur in cells of another type and the dependence of cytopathic effects upon various environmental conditions is easily demonstrable in many cases. For instance, there are several viruses which give rise to clear plaques in cell monolayers maintained under an agar overlay but which show no demonstrable cytopathic effects on the same cells in fluid media (Henderson and Taylor, 1959, 1960; Hsiung, 1959; Porterfield, 1959). Indeed, cells which are susceptible to infection *in vitro* may be resistant *in vivo* and, conversely, those susceptible *in vivo* may be wholly resistant *in vitro*.

All this, however, does not detract from the importance of cytopathogenicity studies for the understanding of natural virus infections. Any interference with the integrated synthetic processes of the normal healthy cell is bound to cause pathological change of some sort and degree, though this may not always be detectable with the cytological techniques now available. Whenever the infection leads to the synthesis of relatively large amounts of foreign viral material, the degree of interference is likely to result in complete disorganization of the normal cellular metabolism, culminating in cell death and disintegration. This was virtually the only type of cytopathic effect recognized by the early virologists, but technological advances, especially in methods of cell culture, have led to the recognition of other types such as rounding of the cell, vacuolation of the cytoplasm, increase or decrease of granularity, abnormal distribution of nuclear chromatin, giant cell and syncytial formation, etc. Some of these are common to many, or even most, virus infections but others are more or less specific and hence have diagnostic significance of some practical importance. Much more important, however, are the causal relationships between intra-cellular biochemical reactions and cytopathic changes which charac-terize different virus infections and different stages of the infection process. For example, one would like to know what changes in the chemical constitution of the cell wall lead to fusion of contiguous cells into syncytial masses and what particular metabolic changes are responsible for the altered chemical constitution. Certain cell abnor-malities attributable to the focal synthesis of viral antigens can indeed be recognized by means of fluorescent-antibody staining, but prac-tically nothing is yet known about the effects of virus penetration, maturation and release upon the constitution and architecture of the cell.

It is usual to draw a distinction between cytopathic effects associated with true infection and consequent virus multiplication and those due to the cytotoxicity of certain viruses whether they be living or dead. It is questionable how far such differentiation is justifiable, for cyto-toxic effects produced by inactivated virus may be associated with the synthesis of viral material although maturation of new infective virus particles fails to occur. Thus, irreversible cell changes may occur at quite early stages of the virus replication process. Nevertheless, there is evidence that in some cases cytopathic effects can be produced by viruses, or by factors separable from the virus particles, in the complete absence of any demonstrable synthesis of viral material (Everett and Ginsberg, 1958; Pereira, 1958; Rowe et al., 1958b). The complexity of cytopathic and cytotoxic mechanisms is further emphasized by the demonstration in polio-infected cells of a "non-viral toxin" which is antigenically related, not to a viral, but to a cellular component (Ackermann, Payne and Kurtz, 1958). It is extremely unlikely that any of the factors necessary for the production of cytotoxic effects would ever occur naturally in the animal body in the absence of a progressive infection with virus multiplication, but investigations of cytotoxicity as distinct from cytopathogenicity are likely to throw further light on infectivity mechanisms.

3. Virus latency

The lack of general agreement on the precise meaning to be attached to the term "virus latency" is a source of confusion. It is frequently used to embrace virus persistence and symbiosis as well as true virus latency. The terms, however, are not strictly synonymous, and the following definitions, representing the writer's personal views, are suggested as an aid to clear thinking on the subject.

Virus persistence: the continuing presence of a pathogenic virus in the body after recovery of the host from a clinical or subclinical infection.

Virus symbiosis: an association between a nonpathogenic virus and a host organism which is of mutual benefit.

Virus latency: an association between a potentially pathogenic virus and a host organism which gives rise to signs of infection only if, and when, some trigger mechanism comes into play.

In the context of these definitions, pathogenicity and non-pathogenicity relate, of course, only to the particular host species under consideration; thus, a virus symbiont may be highly pathogenic for some other species of animal and it may even be cytopathic for the cells of the symbiont host if these are cultivated *in vitro*.

Virus persistence has been shown to occur in very many virus infections and may be either short or of long duration; it may even last throughout the remainder of the host's life. There are instances, as, for example, in blue tongue of sheep and African horse sickness, where it appears to be linked with attenuation of the virus, a phenomenon which invites the speculation that it may represent an intermediate stage in the progressive evolution of viruses from full virulence to their ultimate goal of symbiosis. It differs, however, from both symbiosis and some states of latency in its dependence upon the immunological responses of the host for its initiation and subsequent maintenance. Apart from its practical importance as a factor affecting the epidemiological patterns of certain diseases, the chief interest of virus persistence lies in its connection with the mechanisms whereby viruses may evade the immunological clearing processes of mammalian hosts.

Some early virologists postulated the existence of symbiont viruses on purely philosophical grounds without having the technical resources needed to attack the problem experimentally. Whether true virus symbiosis exists at all, in the defined sense of a relationship conferring benefits on both parasite and host, still remains doubtful, though there is good evidence that it is of widespread occurrence in the more restricted sense of parasitism devoid of harmful effects on the host. If a rise of lactic dehydrogenase in the plasma is of any advantage to the mouse, the Riley virus could probably be regarded as a true symbiont, for it establishes a permanent association with the mouse without any other detectable sign of "infection" and moreover it is non-antigenic (Riley *et al.*, 1960).

True latency undoubtedly occurs in nature, the classical example being herpes simplex virus infection of man. At present one can only speculate about the basic mechanisms of its natural occurrence in the light of phenomena observed and experimentally induced for the most part in cell culture systems. In such systems the carrier state, not necessarily true latency, may be either induced or shown to be dependent upon several quite different conditioning factors, including virus inhibitors (Ackermann and Kurtz, 1955), the nutritional state of the cells (Morgan, 1956), cell genetic factors (Vogt and Dulbecco, 1958; Takemoto and Habel, 1959), virus interference (Chambers, 1957; Henle *et al.*, 1958) and immunological incompetence (Hotchin and Clinits, 1958). To what extent these factors operate in naturally occurring latency is quite unknown, but there is little doubt that genetic constitution and immunological incompetence are determinants in some instances. Very little also is known about the trigger mechanisms which activate latent viruses to assume their pathogenic role as incitants of disease. The viruses of diseases of fowls seem to be especially prone to occur in normal birds in a latent state until unknown additional factors operate to activate them, and the Bittner virus (milk factor) provides a striking example of virus latency in a mammalian host which may or may not be the prologue to tumour formation under the stimulus of some activator governed by genetic factors.

The perfect example of virus latency is bacterial lysogeny, and speculation about the occurrence of a similar association between animal viruses and their host cells is almost inevitable whenever the subject is under discussion. As yet we have no definite evidence in the field of animal virology of the sort of association between the viral genome and the cell genome which is held to account for the lysogenic state, but it seems unlikely that such genetic interaction will prove to be strictly limited to bacterial viruses. Indeed, evidence is now accumulated from studies of the carrier state with Rous sarcoma virus (Prince, 1960), with NDV and HeLa cells (Puck, 1958) and with other virus–cell systems which points in this direction, while Dulbecco (1961) in an analysis of the neoplastic conversion of hamster and mouse embryo cells by infection with polyoma virus is left with two hypotheses which can reasonably account for the change, one of which is alteration of the cell genome by direct action of the virus by a process akin to a bacterial lysogeny. At any rate, genetic modification of some sort must occur in animal cells as a result of infection with tumour viruses, though the nature of the modification remains a mystery. It is at least reasonable to expect that the role of viruses as aetiological agents of neoplastic diseases will become much clearer when the cell–virus interactions involved in the initiation and maintenance of virus latency have been further elucidated.

4. Cellular immunity

The controversy whether acquired specific immunity to infective agents is wholly dependent upon humoral factors or is partly based on an increased cell resistance independent of those factors, is a very old one. Until fairly recently the consensus of opinion had hardened against the development of any cellular immunity apart from the conferring of antibody-producing function on certain specialized cells. This position is no longer tenable. The discovery of virus interference (Hoskins, 1935; Findlay and MacCallum, 1937) provided the first clear indication of the existence of immunological responses at the cellular level, and the subsequent discovery of "Interferon" (Isaacs and Lindenmann, 1957) was an important advance towards elucidation of the underlying mechanisms. This aspect of the virus–cell association is considered in detail in Chapter 4.

D. VIRUSES IN RELATION TO HOST COMMUNITIES

The behaviour of viruses in relation to host communities conforms in general to the basic ecological and epidemiological patterns of pathogenic bacteria. Such features as do pertain especially or exclusively to viruses are merely variations on the general theme which have been evolved to compensate for the limitations imposed by obligate cell parasitism. The virus must find a new host very soon after its excretion from the animal body, for not only is extracellular replication impossible but also extra-host survival is precarious and usually of short duration. Obligate cell parasitism would seem to call for the evolution of a resistance mechanism to ensure long survival in the external environment, but, so far as we know, viruses have failed signally to evolve anything comparable with the highly efficient resistance mechanisms of many bacteria. The virus protein which may serve as a protective coating for the nucleic acid is itself very vulnerable to the inimical physical conditions of the external world and, in view of its other possible functions, discussed above, would seem to merit a protection which is lacking.

Within a large, closely knit community the introduction of a "new" virus from outside results characteristically in its rapid dissemination, dependent upon direct transfer from one susceptible individual to another. More complicated relationships between virus and host community develop with the passage of time. Long-continued association results in a build-up of herd immunity, and this constitutes a formidable barrier to virus survival. With antigenically stable viruses, it is only by constant introduction of fresh susceptibles, chiefly by new births, that the association is maintained. Less stable viruses, however, overcome this immunological barrier in another way, namely by the constant production of mutants and variants with the increased survival value demanded by the particular circumstances. The classical example of frequent changes of dominant antigenic type is provided by the influenza viruses, though the multiplicity of antigenic types of many other viruses indicates that this kind of lability may be one of the most important mechanisms for survival.

In the wider context of transmission from community to community and from country to country, epidemiological behaviour is closely linked with the mechanisms of persistence and latency already discussed, about which far too little is yet known. The geographical distributions of various diseases, the sudden inexplicable appearances of viruses in areas far removed from endemic foci of infection, the sweep of pandemics round the world, the simultaneous outbreaks in several centres of population, etc., all present puzzles which demand for their solution further exploration of virus behaviour at the levels of individual host and susceptible cells.

IV. Modern Approaches to the Study of Virus Infectivity

In Section II above it was emphasized that virology has evolved by a continuous process of expansion so that any chronological systematization is bound to be, to some extent, artificial. There is nevertheless some justification for special comment on certain aspects of the virological research carried out since the end of World War II. In all countries, except U.S.A., the war caused an interruption of virus research almost amounting to its complete cessation, but on the conclusion of hostilities there was a re-awakening of interest in the biological sciences in general and virology in particular. In the virological field chief interest during the last decade has centred on the intracellular phenomena of infection, somewhat to the neglect of other and broader aspects of the virus–host relationship which no doubt eventually will come to claim renewed attention. There were good reasons for this channelling of research into its modern pattern. Both the direction and tempo of basic researches are determined, to some extent, by the technical resources available. By the time general conditions favourable for the resumption of basic research had returned after the war, various new powerful tools and techniques had become available which opened up new approaches to the exploration of biological phenomena at the molecular level. The applicability of these to the investigation of intracellular virus replication was obvious, but there was also a general recognition by workers in several different disciplines that viruses could be used as probes to penetrate the mysteries of normal life processes. A classical method of approach to investigation of the normal is the introduction of extraneous factors which cause abnormalities, and, whatever changes may be imposed on the cell by virus invasion, the basic mechanisms of nucleic acid and protein synthesis remain the same whether the end-products are destined for incorporation in a normal cell or in a virus particle. Thus, virology in some of its aspects has become one branch of a new science of molecular biology to which cytologists, cytogeneticists, biochemists, physicists and others make essential contributions.

A. Technical Developments

The technological developments which have influenced the direction and scope of modern virus research are numerous and most of them have had wide application outside the field of virology, or even of biology in general. A few merit special mention because of their particularly important bearing on the work to be discussed in subsequent chapters.

1. Electron microscopy

In the early stages of its development the electron microscope could do little more than differentiate between viruses of different sizes and of grossly dissimilar outline images. Even this, though of little importance in the case of the animal viruses, led to a reorientation of bacteriophage research through the discovery of the tailed bacterial viruses. (Ruska, 1941; Luria and Anderson, 1942). The later production of instruments with greatly increased powers of magnification and resolution has now brought the animal viruses, even the smallest, within the scope of detailed morphological analysis, and, equally important, has revealed the fine structure and complex architecture of animal tissue cells.

2. Cell cultures

In investigations of the reactions which occur between tissue cells and animal viruses, certain kinds of experiment would have been impossible without the exclusion of the many extraneous factors which complicate the situation in the body of the infected host. The bacterial viruses together with pure suspensions of susceptible host bacteria provided ideal systems for this type of controlled experiment long before the development of *in vitro* cell culture techniques made it possible to carry out comparable studies with animal viruses.·It is not surprising therefore that pioneer work was done chiefly in the field of bacteriophage research and that the corpus of knowledge thus acquired still dominates general virological concepts. Bacteriophage research has, moreover, supplied models on which a great deal of subsequent experimentation with the animal viruses has been based. Many cell lines can now be used, either in free suspension or in monolayer culture, with almost the same facility as can suspensions and plate cultures of bacteria, and this has brought within the scope of animal virology many of the classical approaches which were so fruitful in the study of bacteriophage phenomena. A good example is the application of the technique of agar overlay (Dulbecco, 1952) for the production of discrete plaques in cell monolayers by the cytopathic viruses.

There are, however, certain important differences between bacterial and tissue cell systems which tend to be overlooked. The bacterial cell is the entire, intact, host organism so that all the factors which are operative in natural infections are still present in artificial *in vitro* experiments. The animal tissue cell either in suspension or culture is, on the contrary, divorced from the cell-regulating mechanisms of the intact host. In some instances, at least, this divorce results in the cell becoming something quite other than what it was *in vivo*, and the fact that the change may modify its responses to virus invasion is beyond question.

3. Specific staining methods

The resolving power of the modern electron microscope extends down to particles of macromolecular size, but electron microscopy nevertheless has serious limitations in the analysis of cellular changes induced by virus infection. While it may permit the recognition of mature virus elementary bodies within the cell, or even of incomplete virus components if they are of distinctive shape, it is of no help in differentiating viral precursor materials from other cell contents of the same order of particle size. For this purpose specific staining techniques are essential. Feulgen staining for DNA and acridine orange for RNA, though not specific for viral, as distinct from cellular, nucleic acids, do reveal increases, decreases and redistributions which are often highly significant. For the visual detection of viral antigenic material fluorescent-antibody staining is, at present, the only available technique, but this can be made so highly specific that it is likely to have extended application in future research. Unfortunately, the impermeability of the living cell to antibody globulins prevents the continuous observation of intracellular antigen synthesis as a dynamic process.

4. Isotope labelling, radioactive tracers and autoradiography

Such knowledge as we now possess concerning the mechanisms of nucleic acid replication and protein synthesis has been largely derived from experiments with cell–virus systems in which isotopic labelling made it possible to define the functions and to follow the activities of particular components of the system. The isotopes commonly employed are, heavy nitrogen ^{15}N, heavy carbon ^{14}C, radioactive phosphorus ^{32}P, and radioactive sulphur ^{35}S. These are used to replace the normal isotopes in various essential nutrients of the medium in which host cells are grown and viruses produced. A switch from labelled to unlabelled medium or vice versa can be made at any desired stage of the infection process and previously labelled cells or virus can be used in a system otherwise completely normal. Separation of virus particles from cells, and the extraction from both of them of constituents such as DNA, RNA, and ribosomes are achieved by standard physical and chemical techniques, after which labelled components are differentiated from unlabelled ones of like nature either by their radio–activity or by their abnormal weight as determined by centrifugation in sucrose density gradients.

By a combination of autoradiography, suitable staining and photography, carried out on one and the same preparation from an infected culture, it is sometimes possible to establish both the utilization of a radio–actively labelled substance for the production of a particular viral or cellular component and also the intracellular locus at which the synthesis is effected.

B. VIRUS AND CELL MORPHOLOGY

One approach to the elucidation of virus–cell interactions is the direct visualization of the deviations from the normal which result from infection. Before the advent of the electron microscope such deviations as could be observed by light microscopy were far too crude to yield much information about the mechanisms involved in their production, though some of them, such as the inclusion bodies of various types, were distinctive enough to have diagnostic significance. Appreciation of the significance of intracellular abnormalities depends upon the accumulation of data concerning both the viruses as such and the architecture of the normal cell, the latter representing the extremely important contributions of cytologists and histologists to virology. Morphological analysis of virus structure is based primarily upon the study of purified suspensions of the elementary particles. This is a formidable undertaking bedevilled by the readiness with which the particles become distorted under the conditions imposed by electron microscopy. Not only must preparations be dried and fixed, for examination *in vacuo*, but also, in order to obtain information additional to the outline shape of the elementary bodies and the presence of particularly electron-dense material, various special techniques must be employed. The introduction of metal shadowing opened up the possibility of three-dimensional visualization, and the technique of "negative staining" developed by Brenner and Horne (1959) has proved to be invaluable for the revelation of fine surface structure.

It is probable that all viruses contain an inner core of nucleic acid disposed as a coiled helical strand or strands and that this serves as a scaffolding for the symmetrical arrangement of the outer layers, consisting of proteins, lipoproteins, mucoproteins, etc. But studies on a number of viruses belonging to different groups have shown that, within this common framework, there is room for a surprisingly wide range of architectural patterns and a surprising structural complexity of some of the larger viruses. For example, several myxoviruses are reported to be characterized by a well-defined outer membrane enclosing an inner whorled component and a series of projections from the outer membrane (Horne *et al.*, 1960), while in adenoviruses the inner core is enclosed within a so-called capsid, consisting of many sub-units (capsomeres) whose geometrical configuration and fixed number determine the size and shape of the entire particle. While the resolution of virus structure, in terms of sub-units of various kinds, is interesting in itself, its great importance lies in its applicability to correlations of structure and function as a means of interpreting the specific behaviour patterns of different viruses. It must be admitted that, as yet, animal virologists have touched only the fringe of problems of this nature. When electron microscopy is used for observations on the infected cell the difficulties are greatly increased. The morphological differentiation of viral material from constituents of the normal cell becomes possible only when its organization has proceeded to a stage at which morphological characteristics specific for the virus are recognizable and the necessity of using ultra-thin sections makes such recognition uncertain unless relatively large amounts of the virus precursor structures have been formed. Even so, much valuable information about the various phases of virus attachment, penetration, maturation and release has been obtained by such means.

A major limiting factor at present is the inapplicability of electron microscopy to cells in the living state. When this becomes possible, continuous observation coupled with time-lapse cinematography will undoubtedly clarify some of the intracellular phenomena associated with virus infection which at present can have only inferential and hypothetical interpretations.

C. Viral Nucleic Acids

It is quite beyond the scope of this book to include a detailed account of the nucleic acids, but a brief outline in the simplest terms, of present-day concepts regarding their constitution, functions, replication and genetic coding, may be helpful by way of introduction to some of the discussions presented in subsequent chapters.

1. Constitution

The nucleic acids found in tissue cells, bacteria and viruses are of two kinds, ribose nucleic acid (RNA) and deoxyribose nucleic acid (DNA). The molecules of both consist of long chains of nucleotides, each of which is a combination of a pentose sugar linked to a phosphate group and to either a purine or pyrimidine base. The sugar and phosphate groups alternate to form a sort of backbone from which the bases, attached to the sugar groups, project. The DNA bases are the two purines adenine and guanine, and the two pyramidines cytosine and thymine; those of RNA are the same except that uracil replaces thymine. Two other important differences distinguish the two kinds of nucleic acids: first, the pentose sugar of RNA is ribose, while that of DNA is deoxyribose; second, RNA molecules always consist of a single strand, whereas DNA molecules are nearly always double-stranded, though they do occur in the form of single strands in at least two of the known bacterial viruses.

The sequence of nucleotide bases along the molecular strands differs in different species, though in one and the same species they are of course identical in every molecule. The nucleic acids from two different sources may therefore, in some cases, be distinguishable by the relative proportions of the four bases in each of them. In double-stranded DNA, however, although the ratio adenine + thymine to guanine + cytosine varies from species to species, there is always a one to one ratio of adenine to thymine and of guanine to cytosine. This is because the nucleotide base sequences of the two strands are invariably complementary to each other, in that adenine is always cross-linked to thymine and guanine to cytosine. The simplest pictorial representation of the molecule is a ladder in which chains of alternating sugar and phosphate groups form the sides, which are tied together by rungs, each rung consisting of a complementary pair of bases. The ladder is then twisted spirally to form a double helix. Single-stranded DNA is constructed just like each of the strands of the double-stranded form except that the ends are joined together to produce a closed loop. RNA molecules are similar but are open-ended.

One exception to the position as just stated should be mentioned because of its unique value as an experimental probe. The DNA of one group of bacterial viruses, the T-even group, is of an unusual kind in that, instead of cytosine, 5–hydroxymethylcytosine is incorporated. This makes it readily distinguishable from the DNA of the host cell, *Escherichia coli*, and for this reason the system has been exceptionally useful for investigating the usurpation of the host cell's metabolic machinery by the infecting virus.

2. Functions

It is now believed that in tissue cells all the information needed for the transmission of heritable characters to daughter cells resides in the DNA of the nuclear chromosomes. Recognition of the supreme importance of DNA as the repository of genetic information stemmed from the discovery of pneumococcal-type transformation by Griffith (1928), and the subsequent demonstration that transformation could be effected by DNA extracted from bacteria of the transforming type. (Avery, MacLeod and McCarty, 1944). Tissue cells and bacteria contain also RNA which, under the ultimate control of the DNA, directs the synthesis of proteins, including the cellular enzymes on which the metabolic processes and growth of the entire organism depend. The viruses, too, contain these nucleic acids, but with few exceptions possess one or other type but not both together. For instance, the nucleic acids of all the known plant viruses are RNA's, those of nearly all bacterial viruses are DNA's, while there are many animal viruses representative of each type. The nucleic acids are linked to protein, the exact mode of linkage being still controversial, and many of the smallest viruses consist solely of nucleoprotein, though larger ones may have several other constituents. It is not surprising, therefore, that the proportions of nucleic acids to other constituents of the virus particle vary greatly in different viruses. The RNA content of influenza virus has been estimated to be approximately 1% of the dry weight, while that of poliomyelitis viruses is from 20% to 30%; the DNA content of vaccinia virus is from 5% to 6% and that of phage T2. about 40%.

The fact that the viral nucleic acids subserve the same purposes as those of tissue cells is beyond question. The classical experiments of Hershey and Chase (1952) first showed that the DNA of the bacterial virus T2 is the genetic determinant of all the phenotypic characters of the mature virus particle. Subsequently, DNA extracted from phage $\phi \times 174$ was found to be infective for bacterial protoplasts and to give rise to the production of mature virus particles, identical in every respect with those produced by the infection of normal bacteria with intact virus. The stimulus of these findings led to successful attempts to infect animal tissue cells with the DNA or RNA extracted from various animal viruses; again with the result that the progeny virus was found always to be indistinguishable from the virus from which the infective nucleic acid had been derived.

The functions of cellular DNA are therefore twofold: first, to set in train the process of self-replication in order to ensure transmission of genetic information to daughter cells; second, to pass this information over to the synthesizing machinery of the cell so that the right materials will be manufactured. This second purpose is effected by imprinting coded instructions on RNA molecules which themselves participate actively in protein synthesis. Viral nucleic acid, be it DNA or RNA, has precisely the same functions but needs to borrow the machinery of the host cell for the purpose. A point of great interest is how the nucleic acid of RNA viruses manages to assume the functions of both cellular DNA and cellular RNA by carrying the genetic code, ensuring its own replication and passing into the synthesizing machinery of the cell the information required for the production of all the other viral components. The natural assumption would be that it makes use of the cellular DNA, but of this there is no direct evidence.

3. Replication, genetic coding and control of protein synthesis

The evidence that all the information needed for the hereditary transmission of the specific characters of self-replicating entities can be enshrined in DNA is incontrovertible; the experiments with the T-even phages, already mentioned, provided the first formal proof of this fact. Whether the DNA is invariably the sole repository of this information in organisms which contain both kinds of nucleic acids, DNA and RNA, is perhaps still open to doubt. What is certain is that RNA must also be capable of carrying and transmitting a full genetic code, because it is the only kind of nucleic acid in many viruses, some of which have apparently retained their specific characteristics virtually unchanged through centuries of passage through their natural hosts. This, together with the fact that in both DNA and RNA the molecule consists of a long chain of nucleotides which, though only four in kind, can be arranged in sequences of almost infinite variety, points to the sequences as coded instructions for the regulation of synthetic processes. Recent researches have not only confirmed that this is so but have actually taken the first steps in the formidable task of decoding. In these nucleic acid codes the four nucleotide bases represent different letters; sequences of three or four of them represent words signifying the various substances used as building stones in biosynthesis; and longer sequences represent sentences which carry instructions as to how the building stones must be assembled in order to produce the required end-products.

For preservation of a specific code the fundamental synthetic process is the production of more nucleic acid with exactly the same nucleotide sequence along a molecular strand of exactly the same length as the parent molecule. Replication of the complete entity, be it virus, bacterium or tissue cell, entails also the synthesis of all other components, and finally their assembly in the right order and arrangement. Before outlining the currently accepted view of these processes, three sources of the experimental evidence on which the hypotheses are largely based should be mentioned, namely the synthesis of RNA, of DNA, and of protein in cell-free media in the test tube. These remarkable achievements stemmed from the original discovery by Grünberg-Manago and Ochoa (1955) of an enzyme polynucleotide phosphorylase, capable of coupling ribonucleoside diphosphates together in a random manner to form synthetic polynucleotides; a discovery which led to concerted attacks on the problems of biosynthesis by many workers. As a result certain salient points have now been firmly established.

1. By means of certain polymerases either DNA or RNA can be artificially synthesized from mixtures of their respective nucleoside triphosphates but the synthesis depends upon the presence of a little preformed DNA which acts as a primer of the reaction. (Kornberg, 1957; Weiss and Nakamoto, 1961).

2. The proportions of the bases in synthetic DNA parallels the base composition of the primer DNA, and the same is true of synthetic RNA with uracil substituting for thymine.

3. Synthetic DNA polymers can themselves be used as primers for RNA synthesis in which case the RNA always has a base sequence complementary to that of the primer. For example, if a primer with the sequence G–T–A–A were to be used, the RNA formed would have the sequence C–A–U–U. (Letters represent the names of the nucleotide bases.)

4. The in vitro synthesis of polypeptide chains from a pool of amino acids requires the presence of RNA and the amino acid sequence is determined by the RNA nucleotide base sequence. Nirenberg and Matthaei (1961) showed that with a synthetic RNA consisting of repeating units of uridine the polypeptide formed consisted solely of repeating units of the amino acid phenylalanine. This can only mean that the base sequence adenine–adenine–adenine of DNA is transcribed as uracil–uracil–uracil in RNA and this is the RNA code word for phenylalanine.

The current concepts of normal intracellular nucleic acid replication and protein synthesis suppose that each strand of the nuclear DNA molecule serves as a template. Nucleotides drawn from the cellular pool of metabolites are lined up on the templates in the order dictated by the principle of selective base-pairing and are coupled together by enzymic activation. New complete molecules of DNA are formed by the linking together of complementary strands. RNA is produced in the same way, receiving the species-specific code, at least in the first instance, from the DNA template. RNA molecules, however, are not all identical. Some are long chains of high molecular weight and constitute template RNA; others are short chains of relatively low molecular weight and function as transfer RNA. The latter carry only a very small part of the genetic code. Both kinds of RNA are directly involved in protein synthesis which occurs largely in the cell cytoplasm on the ribosomes, which may be regarded as machines capable of functioning only when provided with an RNA template. The task of the transfer RNA molecules is to attach to themselves the particular amino acids for which they are coded and carry them to the ribosomes. Here once again complementary base-pairing of the transfer RNA against a small section of the template is the mechanism which ensures correct alignment of amino acids for the production of the specific polypeptides required.

The production of intermediate metabolites from the nutrients which enter the cell by diffusion, and also each subsequent step in their assembly to form nucleic acids, proteins and other cell components, requires both the transference of energy and enzymic activation. The enzymes themselves are proteins and have to be synthesized under DNA instruction. The viruses, however, possess neither the enzymes required nor the means of providing energy for synthetic reactions; hence their obligate cell parasitism. Viral infection of the cell means the introduction of a foreign genetic code and the whole future course of events is an expression of competition between the cellular and viral nucleic acids for control of the cell's metabolic machinery. With a double-stranded DNA virus it is believed that virus entry is followed immediately by release of its DNA, unwinding of the helix and separation of the strands so that each may function as a template for synthesis of its complement. RNA of viral type, that is to say with base ratios corresponding to the virus DNA and carrying the viral code, is formed from the cellular pool of preformed nucleotides and using the cell's preformed enzymes and energy transfer mechanism for the purpose. This RNA then proceeds to organize the synthesis of viral protein on the cell ribosomes, from the cellular amino acid pool. In the case of single-strand DNA virus, the closed loop opens and the same sequence of events follows. The nature of the link uniting the two ends of the DNA molecule, the mechanism by which it is broken on entry into the cell and the reason why its artificial rupture extracellularly renders the DNA non-infective are still unknown. With RNA viruses the first essential step is replication of the viral RNA. It is not known whether this occurs directly by synthesis of new RNA on the viral template or whether preliminary production of viral type DNA is involved. There would seem to be no compelling reason why RNA, having once been endowed with a specific base sequence, should not be able to replicate in the same way as single-strand DNA.

Although the picture just presented is widely accepted, at least in its main features, it should be emphasized that in many of its facets it is purely hypothetical. If this is kept in mind, however, it does provide a useful basis for the evaluation of new experimental phenomena as these are met with in the course of further research.

D. Viral Genetics

Before World War II any suggestion that viruses could possess genetic machinery closely similar in many respects to that of man himself would have been regarded as utterly fantastic. Today, not only are the nucleic acids of both viruses and tissue cells recognized as the repositories of genetic information and governors of hereditary transmission of characters, but the viral nucleic acid molecule has been shown to have a gene structure similar to that of the mammalian chromosomes, with linkage groups at fixed loci on the molecular strand. It is this which makes possible experimental investigations of virus behaviour at the genetic level. The researches of what may be regarded as the modern phase of virology have brought to light a number of phenomena which are explicable only on the basis of interactions between the genomes of a virus and a host cell. Some of these phenomena occur perhaps only under artificial experimental conditions and thus have little or no relevance to what occurs in nature, but others undoubtedly are pertinent to the mechanisms of natural virus infection, not only in so far as these relate to intracellular events but also in the broader context of virus behaviour in the animal host and in host populations.

1. Virus mutation

The most potent factor in the evolution of living organisms is genetic mutation with subsequent selection of mutant forms better fitted to survive than the parent forms. There is ample evidence from controlled laboratory experiments that new virus forms can arise as a result of this process. In the laboratory mutants can be produced with great ease by the use of mutagenic agents such as X-rays or nitrogen mustard, coupled with the provision of a selective environment which is weighted against the parental type, as for example by inclusion of specific antibodies in the growth medium. In nature, although spontaneous mutation probably occurs regularly at a fairly constant rate, only an extremely small percentage of the mutants produced have the increased survival value needed for their emergence as new virus types. The stability of some viruses, such as those of measles and mumps, extending as far as can be judged from the available evidence over very long periods, is remarkable; but equally remarkable is the lability of others, such as the influenza viruses, which results in the periodic replacement of one dominant strain after another. This mutational diversity accounts for some of the epidemiological features of various diseases discussed in later chapters; here it may be pointed out that its underlying cause is as yet unknown and presents an intriguing problem for future research.

2. Recombination and reactivation phenomena

Under experimental conditions host cells may be infected with two different viruses which, although related to each other, can be distinguished by certain marker characters such as infectivity or noninfectivity for a particular animal species. Progeny virus will then be of three kinds, two of them identical with the parental forms and the third representing a hybrid with marker characters derived from each parent. If the hybrids, on segregation, breed true to type, it is a legitimate assumption that the mixed phenotypic characters reflect the incorporation of genetic elements from both parental forms in the genome of the new entity. The phenomenon is referred to as viral recombination, for it is believed that the genetic mixing occurs at the time when sub-units of the nucleic acid molecule combine together to form the complete molecular strands. First observed with bacterial viruses (Delbrück and Bailey, 1946; Hershey and Rotman, 1948, 1949), recombination was later demonstrated with animal viruses (Burnet and Lind, 1942). It has proved to be one of the most useful probes for the analysis of viral genetic constitution, but whether, or to what extent, it occurs in nature is not known. It would seem to offer an efficient mechanism for the evolution of new viruses, but the conditions for its operation, involving simultaneous infection with related but different viruses, must be rare under natural circumstances. The importance of an event, however, is not necessarily related to the frequency of its occurrence.

Similarly, the various methods of reactivating viruses which have been rendered non-infective by one or other means have been usefully

applied in genetic studies but are as yet demonstrable only under
artificial conditions, possibly because we lack the means for their
detection otherwise. There would certainly seem to be every opportunity for the natural occurrence of photoreactivation, a process in
which virus inactivated by ultra-violet light irradiation becomes
infective again on exposure to visible light of certain wavelengths
(Dulbecco, 1949b, 1950). Opportunities must also exist for the natural
occurrence of the type of reactivation in which heat-inactivated viruses
of the pox group replicate in cells which are infected with a related but
different virus (Fenner *et al.*, 1959). If these processes do in fact occur
under natural conditions, it is not difficult to imagine various ways in
which they could affect both the course of an infection in the individual
host and the spread, persistence and variable characters of epidemics
in host communities.

3. Lysogeny, transduction and cell-transformation

The fact that interactions between viral and host cell genomes can
occur has been known to workers in the field of bacteriophage research
for several years, but for some reason or other the suggestion that
similar interactions might take place between animal viruses and
animal tissue cells is only now coming to be accepted as a reasonable
hypothesis for the explanation of certain natural occurrences. Two
phenomena which undoubtedly involve this kind of host–virus association in the case of some bacterial viruses are lysogeny and transduction
(Zinder, 1953), full descriptions of which are given in Chapter 2. One
aspect, however, pertaining to both of them calls for brief mention
here. This is the vitally important fact that transduction always, and
lysogeny sometimes, result in a permanent change in the phenotypic
characters of the host. The best example of lysogenic conversion is
transformation of a non-toxinogenic strain of *Corynebacterium diphtheriae* into a toxinogenic strain when the former is infected with a
temperate phage (Freeman, 1951). The conversion is not effected by
infection with virulent phage, and, as far as is known, the ability to
produce diphtheria toxin is invariably associated with the lysogenic
state, being dependent upon the integration of prophage within the
bacterial genome. Another fact of significance in any attempt at
speculative extrapolation to the field of animal virology is that mutation
of a prophage may render it incapable of initiating the production of
mature vegetative phage particles while leaving it still transmissible as
part of the bacterial genome, and in some cases still capable of inducing
bacterial cell lysis. It is obvious that, should such a mutation be
associated with lysogenic conversion, the new phenotypic character of

the host would inevitably be ascribed to a spontaneous mutation of the host genome without participation of a virus being suspected.

The possible occurrence of a phenomenon analogous to bacterial lysogeny as the basis of some of the states of virus latency in animals has already been mentioned, but the implications of lysogenic conversion and transduction go further than this. Is it possible that these mechanisms may operate to alter the genetically controlled characters of animal tissue cells? Some experimental findings, especially from work with polyoma virus, are very suggestive. Transformations of cell morphology and growth characteristics due to infections with this virus *in vitro* have been reported by several workers (Vogt and Dulbecco, 1960; Dulbecco and Vogt, 1960; Sachs and Medina, 1961). In some cases the transformed cells are oncogenic when inoculated into animals of the homologous species. For example, polyoma virus infection of mouse embryo cells results in cell destruction, but some cells may survive and thereafter show altered morphology. Infection of hamster cells fails to produce the cytocidal effect, but after an interval of time foci of altered cells appear which eventually replace the original type. These, on inoculation into hamsters, give rise to tumours. Often it is not possible to demonstrate the presence of virus in either the transformed cells or in the induced tumours. Dulbecco (1961), in reviewing the available evidence, suggested two alternative explanations: first, that the virus infection converts the cell into a malignant cell by destruction of some cell regulator; second, that the cell genome is altered directly by the viral DNA by a process akin to bacterial lysogeny.

As far as the author is aware, transduction has never been suggested as a possible mechanism of viral carcinogenesis. Yet it might only require the transfer of a growth-regulating factor from one type of tissue cell to another type with slower growth potential in order to release the latter from the normal restraints of the particular tissue of which it forms a unit.

In order to change the hereditary characters of a mammalian host, a virus would, of course, have to interact with the genome of the germinal cells. Although this is a possibility, we have no present evidence that it ever occurs.

V. Future Outlook

Some of the likely short-term developments of future virological research are not difficult to foresee. In the near future notable advances in the field of molecular biology are to be expected, and these will stem, as in the past, very largely from virological investigations because of the relative simplicity of the constitution and structure of some viruses and the ease with which they can be manipulated in *in vitro* systems. Now that a break has been made into the nucleic acid coding mechanism, decoding of the genomes of the simpler viruses will proceed apace; so also will the *in vitro* synthesis of nucleotide polymers and protein polypeptide chains of increasing length and complexity. In assessing the claims for artificial virus synthesis, however, it is necessary to realize how far removed anything which has been accomplished so far, or is likely to be accomplished in the foreseeable future, is from the biosynthesis occurring within the host cell. The production of nucleotide polymers and polypeptides in the test tube requires not only a supply of preformed building blocks but also the presence of enzymes and other constituents extracted from living cells. Biosynthesis poses the old problem of the chicken and the egg; every synthetic reaction requires enzymic activation and every enzyme is a product of biosynthesis. The fact that viruses borrow cell enzymes for their replication does not make solution of this fundamental problem any easier.

Concurrently with such work at the molecular level, accumulation of new knowledge about virus behaviour in naturally infected hosts and in host communities will proceed at an increased tempo because of the continued expansion of technical resources. The isolation of many more symbiont viruses should lead to elucidation of the mechanisms involved in the various types of virus persistence and latency. As intimated above, this might well turn out to be a milestone in the long search for the intrinsic cause of neoplasia.

How far these developments of basic virological research are likely to lead to new and better methods of disease control it is impossible to forecast. It is probable that specific prophylaxis and therapy will long continue to be based on standard immunological procedures, as employed to-day, but eventually more effective measures may be evolved, based upon the rapidly expanding knowledge of interference phenomena and the underlying factors concerned.

Long-term developments can never be forecast with any degree of certainty. There are some who look to virology to explain the evolution of life from inorganic matter, some who envisage the total elimination of human infectious diseases, some who prophesy the artificial production of new viruses which could be used for the benefit of man, and so on. The recent advances in virology as in other branches of science should surely prevent us from holding that anything is impossible; but speculations devoid of some measure of supporting evidence, while entertaining on occasion, serve no very useful purpose.

CHAPTER 2

The Bacteriophage Model

WILLIAM HAYES

Medical Research Council, Microbial Genetics Research Unit,
Hammersmith Hospital, London, England

I. Introduction

The inclusion of a chapter on bacteriophage in a book otherwise devoted exclusively to animal viruses demands the initial justification that bacteriophages (or phages, as we shall call them) are indeed viruses. The category of infectious agents known as viruses embraces entities displaying such widely different characteristics with respect to morphology, chemical constitution and infective behaviour that it is difficult to find among them the basis for a common definition. Size, and its associated property of filtrability, is not a valid criterion since we must be able clearly to distinguish viruses from very small bacteria, for example; nor is pathogenicity, for it is easy to conceive (though often difficult to demonstrate) the mutational loss of this property by a virus particle without affecting its fundamental viral nature in any way. The two most widely agreed features that are common to all viruses are that they are infectious and have no capacity for autonomous multiplication. This definition has been extended in detail by Lwoff (1959) to include such additional features as the possession of only one type of nucleic acid from which, alone, the virus particle is reproduced, and the absence of a built-in metabolic system. This means, in effect, that virus particles are quite distinct from either cells or cell organelles; as Lwoff says, "A virus is a virus." In all these respects, as we shall see, phages qualify as viruses. In fact, the real justification for this chapter is that many of the more precise ideas about the nature of viruses and their origin have stemmed from the study of phages.

During the last two decades the mechanisms of phage infection and reproduction have been the subject of an immense amount of detailed study. The prolific and successful outcome of these researches is a consequence of a number of more or less unique features of many phage–bacterium systems. (a) The efficiency of phage infection is such that every phage particle has a probability approaching 1.0 of causing infection; (b) infectious phage particles can be counted simply and accurately, so that experimental results can be expressed quantitatively; (c) the bacterial host can not only be cultivated and manipulated under well controlled conditions, either as large homogeneous populations or as single cells, but is also amenable to various kinds of physical and chemical analysis during the course of infection; (d) the genetic constitution of both phage and bacterial host can be studied in detail by means of genetic crosses.

As a result of these advantages, our knowledge of all aspects of phage infection is more advanced than that of any other virus, so that there has been considerable incentive to regard phage as a model virus and to try to adapt phage technology to the investigation of animal and plant viruses. This is a perfectly reasonable attitude to take, provided that we bear in mind the likelihood that phage may represent a unique adaptation of the basic viral principle. Little or nothing is known for certain about how viruses originated or evolved, but the discovery of "episomes" in bacteria (see Jacob, Schaeffer and Wollman, 1960) and the genetic homology that has recently been found to exist between certain phages and their host cells (Section V, C and D) lends plausibility to the idea that phages may have evolved by a sequence of mutational steps from normal bacterial constituents. If this is so, each phage strain would have an independent origin and, far from being related to other viruses, would have no phylogenetic link even to other strains of phage; the features common to different phages would be a consequence of independent adaptations to a similar type of environment, the bacterial cell, and not to a common ancestry. According to this view, viruses in general would be expected to display wide dissimilarities, depending on the particular cellular entities from which they arose and the particular types of cellular environment that controlled their evolution.

A. The Classification of Phages

Until recently virtually all phage isolates examined appeared to conform to a rather specific stereotype in being constructed of a somewhat tadpole-shaped protein sheath enclosing deoxyribonucleic acid (DNA). Unlike viruses in general, therefore, no meaningful classification of phages was possible on the basis either of morphology or of the type of nucleic acid they contain. It was only with respect to their mode of interaction with host bacteria that clearcut categories of phage could be recognized. The primary distinction is between *virulent* and *temperate* phages.

Virulent phages may be defined as those producing an infection which is invariably followed by lysis of the host bacterium and liberation of progeny phage particles. Virulent phages can, in turn, be subdivided into *autonomous virulent* and *dependent virulent* types (Whitfield, 1962). Infection by an autonomous virulent particle results in rapid destruction of the nucleus of the host bacterium, which thus plays no role in phage development, and immediate cessation of the synthesis of bacterial substance. In the case of dependent virulent phage, on the other hand, not only does specific bacterial metabolism continue during most of the lytic cycle, but the phage appears to depend for its development on the integrity of the bacterial nucleus.

Temperate phages are distinguished by having the alternative of either lysing or *lysogenizing* the bacteria they infect. Lysogenized bacteria are termed *lysogenic*; they carry the phage in a "latent" state known as *prophage* and transmit it indefinitely to their progeny as if it were a normal bacterial constituent. The decision as to whether infection by a temperate phage is followed by the lytic or the lysogenic response, depends largely on the physiological state of the bacteria and can be profoundly modified by the environmental conditions.

It so happens that, mainly for arbitrary reasons, most research into the nature of phage and the mechanism of phage infection has employed a particular set of seven virulent phages, known as the T series (T1–T7), which infect *Escherichia coli*. Of these, T2, T4 and T6 ("T-even") and T5 are autonomous virulent, while T1, T3 and T7 are dependent virulent phages. Apart from Section V, most of the work we shall describe here was done with phages T2 and T4.

Very recently the possible categories of phage have been extended by the discovery that minute bacterial viruses exist which, morphologically, appear to resemble the small animal viruses rather than normal bacteriophage. Moreover, one group of these viruses contains ribonucleic acid (RNA) instead of DNA (see Section VII C 2 and 3). These viruses should prove of great interest to virologists in general, but at the moment little is known about the details of their behaviour.

II. General Description of Methods

A full account of the methods used in phage research would encompass not only biochemistry and genetics, which have made the basic contribution, but also such diverse topics as electron microscopy, serology, radiobiology, and the physico-chemical techniques concerned with analysis of the structure of nucleic acids and proteins. All this we will take for granted, merely giving the results and their interpretation, and will here describe only those elementary procedures upon which the design of nearly all phage experiments rests, and some knowledge of which is necessary for an understanding of current concepts about the nature of phage and its association with its host. The reader interested in more detail can find it in the original papers or, more easily, in the many excellent and comprehensive reviews that have appeared in recent years, to which reference will be made under the appropriate headings.

The Enumeration of Phage Particles

A suitable dilution of a phage suspension is mixed with a few drops of concentrated culture of a sensitive bacterium, in a small volume of molten "soft" agar, cooled to 45°C. The mixture is then poured over the surface of nutrient agar in a Petri dish, forming a thin "top layer" which is allowed to harden before incubation at 37°C. (Adams, 1959). After incubation, the growth of uninfected bacteria yields a confluent turbidity throughout the surface layer, except at the site of infection of a bacterium by a phage particle, where a small area of clearing is found. This area of clearing is termed a *plaque* and results from the serial transmission of the progeny phage particles, emerging from lysis of the initially infected bacterium, through adjacent cells until a visible area of lysis is produced; this "chain reaction" is ultimately brought to a halt by the slowing and cessation of host-cell metabolism upon which phage multiplication depends.

By counting the number of plaques which result from plating a given volume and dilution of phage suspension with a sensitive bacterial culture, the number of *plaque-forming units*, or particles in the suspension which actually infected and lysed individual bacteria, i.e. the *plaque titre*, can be assessed. The proportion of total phage particles which are capable of forming plaques, termed the *efficiency of plating* (EOP), is found by comparing the plaque titre with the actual number of phage particles in the suspension as estimated, for example, by electron microscopy. The EOP of phages on their hosts is high, and is usually found to lie between 0·5 and 1·0 under optimal plating conditions (Luria, Williams and Backus, 1951; Kellenberger and Arber, 1957). The plaque titre of a given suspension, however, is dependent on many factors such as the ionic and nutritive constitution of the medium in the plates and the physiological state of the bacteria with which the plate is seeded, as well as on the temperature of incubation. Moreover, the EOP of a given phage for a particular host may be profoundly modified by procedures designed to purify the phage, by mutations arising in either phage or bacterium, or by a single passage of the phage through another host strain which is equally sensitive to it (phenotypic modification; Section VIIB4). Since estimation of the EOP usually involves electron microscopy, when working with virulent phage it is generally assumed to be approximately unity; optimal experimental conditions are employed and standardized as rigorously as possible, and the number of phage particles then inferred directly from the plaque titre.

B. The Recognition of Phages

A number of diverse methods and criteria are available for the recognition and identification of different strains and mutant types of phage. The most important of these are: (a) plaque morphology; (b) host range, i.e. the ability of the phage to plaque, or not to plaque, on a series of different bacterial hosts which may comprise naturally distinct strains or species of bacteria, or else be mutants of the same bacterial strain, selected for specific resistance to infection by a particular strain of phage (Sections IIIC and VIA); (c) serological specificity, which is usually assessed by the ability of a specific antiserum to neutralize the infective capacity of the phage (Section IIIC); (d) the shape and dimensions of the phage particles as seen by electron microscopy (Section III, A and D.). Since all these criteria will be dealt with in later sections in so far as they are involved in the analysis of phage structure and function, we will here consider only the more general and methodical aspects of plaque morphology which illustrate some of the experimental variables arising in phage experiments.

1. Plaque size

The mean plaque diameter is one of the characteristic features of particular phage–bacterium combinations. Nevertheless, considerable variation in size may be found between individual plaques on the same plate, or between the mean plaque size obtained under different experimental conditions. Many factors can influence plaque size :

(a) The size of the phage particle itself, which largely determines its rate of diffusion through the medium; in general, small phages tend to produce large plaques and *vice versa*, although this correlation is by no means complete. Similarly, increasing the concentration of agar in the medium will reduce plaque size by slowing diffusion.

(b) The rate of adsorption of the phage to its host. This may be an inherent property of the phage–host relationship or may be conditioned by such environmental factors as the population density of the host bacteria, as is shown by the greater uniformity of plaque size when adsorption is allowed to occur in a fluid medium, unadsorbed particles then being neutralized by antiserum prior to dilution and plating. Delay in adsorption will extend the duration of each wave of infection so that growth of the surrounding bacteria becomes restrictive while the plaque is still small.

(c) The number of particles liberated per infected bacterium (*burst size*). The burst size may vary from only a few to many hundreds of particles, depending on the particular strain of phage and host employed as well as on the physiological state of the infected bacteria and the nutrients available for their growth; the burst size is markedly reduced as the nutritional content of the medium becomes depleted, and this, as we have seen, is one of the normal factors limiting plaque size.

2. Plaque morphology

Plaques are much more than mere circumscribed areas of clearing in a "lawn" of bacterial growth; they show reproducible individualities of structure which are of value in the identification of phage strains and may be used as genetic markers in phage crosses. Thus plaques may have clear or turbid floors; their edges may be clearcut or fuzzy; their walls may be abrupt or shelving; they may or may not be surrounded by halos of partial clearing. These differences reflect physiological differences in the phage–bacterium relationship which can sometimes be defined in terms of phage function. For example, temperate phages tend to yield plaques which are turbid owing to growth of lysogenized bacteria on their floors. From large populations of temperate phage, mutants may be isolated which have lost, wholly or in part, the ability to lysogenize. These will tend to lyse all the bacteria and so, like virulent phages, yield plaques which are either clear or much less turbid than the wild-type when plated on sensitive bacteria.

Wild-type (r^+) virulent phages T2, T4 and T6, plated on their host *E. coli* B, produce small plaques with a turbid halo, owing to a phenomenon called *lysis inhibition*, whereby the adsorption of phage particles to previously infected bacteria greatly extends the time these bacteria require to burst (Doermann, 1948). Mutants of these phages, termed r (for rapid lysis), which do not show lysis inhibition can readily be isolated, and these give rise to larger, clear plaques easily distinguishable from the r^+ type (Hershey, 1946) (See Plate 1). When independently isolated r mutants are mated by mixed infection of *E. coli* B, wild-type, r^+ recombinant particles are found among the progeny. This is therefore a clear case of a change in plaque morphology which is genetically determined in the phage and is of particular importance as one of the character differences most widely used in the genetic study of phage. Other genetically determined, distinct differences from wild-type plaque morphology are exemplified by *tu* mutants of phage T4 which yield plaques circumscribed by a turbid ring (Doerman and Hill, 1953), the *m* mutants of phages T2 and T4, which produce minute plaques (Hershey and Rotman 1949), and the "star" mutants described by Symonds (1958), which produce fuzzy plaques. Comparable varieties of plaque-type mutants are found among temperate phages (Jacob and Wollman, 1954; see Section V D).

Plaques surrounded by halos of partial lysis which extend beyond the region of phage diffusion have been reported (see Adams and Park, 1956) and are probably due to production by the infected cells of lytic enzymes whose synthesis is genetically determined by the phage. This is certainly so in the case of certain mutants of phage T4 which are unable to produce the temperature-stable, lysozyme-like enzyme required for their liberation from infected cells at 37°C. Plating such infected cells on sensitive bacteria *in the presence of egg-white lysozyme* is followed by release of the imprisoned mutant phage particles and the formation of secondary plaques. If the surrounding bacteria on the plate are now killed by chloroform vapour, a halo of lysis develops beyond the plaque perimeter in the case of the majority of mutants; this zone is caused by modified lysozyme, and its appearance differs with different mutants (Streisinger *et al.*, 1961).

C. The One-step Growth Experiment

This experiment, devised by Ellis and Delbrück (1939), remains the standard procedure for studying the kinetics of phage multiplication in infected bacteria. To a young culture of sensitive bacteria is added a suitable dilution of phage suspension. The mixture is left for a few minutes to allow adsorption of the phage; phage antiserum is then added to neutralize unadsorbed particles, and the mixture highly diluted in warm broth and incubated at 37°C. At intervals of a few minutes thereafter, samples are removed and plaque counts performed to assess the number of plaque-forming units present. In the case of the virulent phage T2 and its host, *E. coli* B, it is found that the plaque count remains constant until about 25 minutes from the beginning of the experiment (the so-called *latent period*), when it begins to rise sharply until a plateau is reached about 10–20 minutes later. The latent period represents the shortest time that elapses between infection and the bursting of the bacteria with liberation of progeny phage particles. During this period free phage particles are absent from the mixture, owing to the previous addition of antiserum and to dilution; thus, the plaques which are counted arise from the bursting of isolated infected cells on the assay plate and not from single phage particles, i.e. they indicate only the number of *infected cells* plated. The rise in plaque titre, however, is brought about by the progressive bursting of infected cells in the growth tube and the liberation from them of free phage particles; these particles are prevented from adsorbing to other bacteria by the low population density of the latter in the diluted mixture. The plateau is achieved when all the infected cells have burst and all the progeny of the single cycle of phage multiplication have been liberated. The rise period represents not only the scatter between the true latent periods of individual phage–bacterium complexes, but is also a function of variation in adsorption time leading to asynchrony in the onset of phage multiplication. Since phage growth is dependent on bacterial metabolism, this latter factor may largely be obviated by allowing adsorption to take place in the presence of cyanide (Benzer and Jacob, 1953) or chloramphenicol (Hershey and Melechen, 1957) and then removing the drug by dilution. (For technical details see Adams, 1959, pp. 473–481.)

The ratio of the plaque titre at the plateau to that during the latent period indicates the mean number of phage particles liberated per infected bacterium and is known as the *burst size*. In the case of phage T2 this is usually 100–200 under optimal conditions. Both the latent period and the burst size differ widely with different strains of both phage and bacterium, as well as with variations in the physiological and nutritional state of the host. Although the burst size is obviously dependent on what happens during the latent period, the two are not necessarily correlated in a direct way. For example, under poor nutritional conditions or when lag phase bacteria are used, an increased latent period may be followed by a reduced burst size (Delbrück, 1940b; Hedén, 1951). On the other hand, the phenomenon of lysis inhibition, which occurs in undiluted mixtures of wild-type phage T2, T4 or T6 with *E. coli* B (see Section II B 2, above), increases both latent period and burst size (Doermann, 1948), as do inhibitors of protein synthesis (such as 5-methyl tryptophan and chloramphenicol) if added about the middle of the latent period and subsequently diluted out (Hershey and Melechen, 1957). Despite the susceptibility of latent period and burst size to such a complex range of environmental influences, it transpires that the number of infecting phage particles per bacterium, i.e. the *multiplicity of infection*, has no significant effect on either. This is not due to exclusion of all save one of the infecting particles from the infective process, since genetic analysis of the phage progeny issuing from single bacteria, multiply infected with genetically marked particles, indicates that many particles may participate in the recombination process which occurs during phage growth (Dulbecco, 1949a; see Section VII B 2).

D. The Single-burst Experiment

One-step growth experiments yield information about the minimum latent period and average burst size of phage particles in large *populations* of infected cells during a single cycle of development. The single-burst experiment was designed by Burnet (1929) and developed by Ellis and Delbrück (1939) to reveal the phage output from *individual* infected bacteria. Phage and bacteria are mixed and, after allowing time for adsorption, the mixture is greatly diluted so that small aliquots have rather a low probability of containing a single infected bacterium. A large number of such aliquots is then dispensed into separate tubes of broth at 37°C. When it is judged that every infected bacterium will certainly have burst, the entire contents of each tube are plated for plaques. From the number of tubes which are found to contain no phage particles, the proportion of the remainder of the tubes which received only one infected bacterium can be calculated from Poisson's formula. Provided that this proportion is high, the range of burst sizes issuing from single bacteria can be assessed from the range of variation of plaque counts on the individual plates; this is found to be very wide and significantly greater than the variation in size of the bacteria involved (Delbrück, 1945a).

By combining the methods of the one-step growth experiment with the single-burst experiment, it has been found that there is no correlation between the latent period and the burst size for individual infected bacteria (Ellis and Delbrück, 1939). The single-burst experiment has proved a valuable tool for investigating problems in phage genetics; whether, for example, the reciprocal recombinant types found among the progeny particles, emerging from a bacterial population mixedly infected with genetically different parental phages, are likely to have arisen from the same, or different, recombination events (see Section VII B 2).

III. Structure and Chemical Constitution of Phages

In all biological research nowadays, use tends to be made of every new method or technique, from whatever field, that promises to unravel various aspects of the complicated systems that underlie the processes of life. In examining the structure of phage the methods of chemical, serological and genetic analysis have proved vital accessories to the basic method of high-resolution electron microscopy.

A primary requirement for structural analysis is to obtain phage preparations of high purity. This is usually accomplished by cultivation to high titre in aerated, liquid synthetic media; the phage particles are then separated and concentrated from the complex bacterial debris in the lysate, first by removal of bacterial nucleic acids by enzymatic attack, and then by such methods as filtration, precipitation and differential centrifugation (see Herriot and Barlow, 1952; also Adams, 1959, pp. 454–460). Virtually pure preparations of phage particles can be achieved by the single procedure of centrifugation in a caesium chloride density gradient (Meselson, Stahl and Viuograd, 1957; Weigle, Meselson and Paigeu, 1959) which separates them from other components and concentrates them into a band at their specific buoyant density in the gradient; however, only relatively small numbers of particles can be isolated in this way. Since at least half of the particles emerging from the usual purification procedures are also plaque formers (Luria *et al.*, 1951), it may be assumed that the analytical results to be described refer to actual infective particles. Most of these results have been obtained from the virulent phage T2, grown on its host, *E. coli* B; although this phage is known to differ from some others in certain respects which will be indicated later, there is reason to believe that the broad features it displays are widely shared.

A. The Anatomy of Phage

Electron microscopy has shown that, with very few exceptions (see Section VII,C2 and C3), all the strains of phage so far examined possess the same broad anatomical features, although considerable variation in detail is found. The basic design resembles that of a tadpole, comprising a polyhedral head attached to a cylindrical tail. Phages T2, T4 and T6, which have been investigated in most detail, are identical in appearance in addition to being closely related serologically and genetically; their heads have the form of a bipyramidal, hexagonal prism 65 mμ wide and 100 mμ long, and to them is attached a 25×100 mμ tail (Plate 2(a)). Their volume is thus roughly one thousandth that of the bacteria they infect. Phages T1 and T5 have longer but more slender tails, while phages T3 and T7, once thought to be tailless, have, in fact, rudimentary tails (10×15 mμ) (Anderson, 1953; Williams, 1953; Williams and Frazer, 1953). The morphological features of some well-known strains of virulent and temperate phages may be compared in Plates II and III (see also Bradley and Kay, 1960).

Phage particles become attached to bacteria by means of their tails (Anderson, 1953). Kellenberger and Arber (1955; see also Kozloff and Henderson, 1955; Williams and Frazer, 1956; Brenner et al., 1959) demonstrated that adsorption of phages T2 and T4 to isolated cell-wall material resulted in a striking alteration of their tail structures; the upper part of the tail, known as the *sheath*, became contracted and thickened, revealing an inner *core* 10 mμ wide and extending the full length of the tail (Plate 2(b)). Using various techniques to separate components of the phage particle, these authors demonstrated the presence of a number of long fibres attached to the core. The beautiful electron microphotographs of Brenner et al., (1959) reveal very clearly that in T2 there are six of these *tail fibres* which appear to be attached to a *base plate* located at the tip of the core (see Plate 2(b)). We will return, in Section IIID, to these various anatomical components and their presumptive functions. For the moment we may note that, unlike most of the plant and animal viruses which have been morphologically defined, phages have a complicated and very sophisticated structure.

B. Chemical Analysis

Chemical analysis of highly purified preparations of phage, including all the virulent coliphages T1–T7 as well as the temperate phages λ (from *E. coli* K-12) and P22 (from Salmonella), have shown that they are composed of approximately equal amounts of deoxyribonucleic acid (DNA) and protein (see Stent, 1958). These phages contain neither ribonucleic acid (RNA) nor lipoid in appreciable amounts. Recently, however, a phage has been discovered which contains RNA but no DNA and which specifically infects male strains of *E. coli* K-12 (Loeb and Zinder, 1961).

Insight into the structural organization of the protein and nucleic acid in phage particles first emerged from study of the effects of osmotic shock on the T–even phages. If these phages are rapidly transferred from high salt concentrations to distilled water, they lose their infectivity; at the same time the DNA dissociates from the protein and becomes sensitive to the action of DNAase. Electron microphotographs of osmotically damaged particles shows that their basic anatomical features are preserved, except that their heads appear collapsed and empty—the so-called phage "ghosts" (Anderson, Rappaport and Muscatine, 1953; see Plate 3(a)); outside the "ghosts" can be seen a tangle of DNA threads, 20Å in diameter (Williams, 1953). Since "ghost" particles which have been separated from their discharged DNA not only retain nearly all the phage protein but are still able to adsorb to sensitive bacteria (Hershey, 1955), it became clear that it is the phage head that is susceptible to osmotic shock and that it comprises a protein sheath which encloses and protects the DNA. In addition to DNA, osmotically shocked T2 particles release into the environment about two per cent of phage protein, as well as a small amount of acid-soluble peptide (containing only aspartic acid, glutamic acid and lysine), spermidine and putrescine (Hershey, 1955, 1957a; Ames, Dubin and Rosenthal, 1958).

C. SEROLOGICAL and GENETIC ANALYSIS

The protein coat of phages is antigenic and generates antisera whose action on homologous phage suspensions may be recognized by neutralization of infectivity as well as by *in vitro* reactions. It is possible, by various chemical treatments, to separate or selectively destroy various components of the phage particles so that serological analysis can be related to structure. Thus, in the case of phage T2, antisera prepared against phage heads have no ability to neutralize infectivity, while neutralizing antisera do not react *in vitro* with head preparations; thus, neutralizing antibody acts on the tail (Lanni and Lanni, 1953). T2 particles which have lost their tail fibres and tail tips no longer react with neutralizing antibody (Kozloff, Luce and Henderson, 1957); nevertheless, intact T2 particles neutralized by antiserum, although unable to infect, can still adsorb to host cells (Nagano and Oda, 1955).

It follows that distinct components are responsible for adsorption and for triggering infection and that these reside at the distal end of the tail.

Genetic analysis has permitted the resolution of the adsorption structure into at least two protein components. The phages T2 and T4 are closely related genetically, since recombinant particles inheriting characters from each are found among the progeny of mixed infection of *E. coli* B. Bacterial mutants can be isolated which are resistant to either T2 (mutant B/2) or T4 (mutant B/4) owing to specific alterations in cell-wall structure, so that T2 cannot adsorb to mutant B/2 but plaques normally on mutant B/4, and *vice versa*. Thus, the two phages possess different tail structures, i.e. have a different *host range*, and can be distinguished from one another by plating them on B/2 and B/4 bacteria. When wild-type *E. coli* B is mixedly infected with both phages, some of the progeny particles plaque only on mutant B/2 and others only on B/4. Unexpectedly, however, about half the particles which infect, say, B/2 bacteria give rise to "second generation" progeny which can no longer infect B/2 but only B/4. This indicates that although these particles initially possessed the protein tail structure (*phenotype*) of phage T2, their genetic constitution (*genotype*) was that of phage T4, since the progeny of single infection by them were of pure T4 type. This phenomenon is called *phenotypic mixing* and shows that, in mixed infection where protein coats of both specificities are synthesized together in the cell, the genetic material of individual phages becomes coated with either homologous or heterologous protein in a random way (Delbrück and Bailey, 1946; Novick and Szilard, 1951). Phenotypic mixing is important with respect to the process of phage maturation and will be discussed further in Section IV C 6. In the present context, the significant point is that when *E. coli* B is mixedly infected with phages T2 and T4, half the total progeny do not resemble either parent in phenotype but can infect both B/2 and B/4 bacteria; the "second generation" progeny of these particles, however, are either pure T2 or pure T4 in type. This can only be explained by the existence in the phage tail of two regions, each of which can be constructed of either T2– or T4–specific protein in a random manner when the tail is being assembled (Streisinger, 1956; Brenner, 1957).

D. Microscopic Resolution of Structural Components

As has been mentioned, there are several methods for dissociating the morphological components of phage; these include treatment with cadmium cyanide (Kozloff and Henderson, 1955), hydrogen peroxide (Kellenberger and Arber, 1955) and freezing and thawing (Williams and Frazer, 1956). The most successful results, however, have come

from the methods of Brenner *et al.* (1959), which enable pure preparations of T2 tail fibres and sheaths to be made (the original article should
be consulted for details). These preparations have been examined
microscopically, using the method of negative staining by "embedding"
in phosphotungstic acid (developed by Brenner and Horne, 1959), and
have also been defined chemically. The earlier finding that the tail
comprises a core surrounded by a contractile sheath has been confirmed. The architecture of the sheath is that of a hollow cylinder, built
up from a number of helically arranged sub-units, which conserves a
constant volume on contraction; chemically, the sheath comprises
about 200 repeating protein sub-units, each of about 50,000 molecular
weight. The core is a hollow cylinder, 800 Å long and 70 Å in diameter,
with a central hole of 25 Å diameter, fitted proximally to the hexagonal
head; at its distal extremity is a hexagonal plate to which are attached
six tail fibres, each 1300 Å long and 20 Å wide, with a characteristic
kink in the middle. Chemical analysis shows that the tail fibres have a
protein sub-unit of molecular weight not less than 100,000. The head
membrane is composed of a large number of repeated protein sub-units
of 80,000 molecular weight. Most of the morphological features
described can be seen in Plate 2.

IV. The Mechanism of Infection

A. Adsorption of the Phage

The first step in infection must clearly be random collision between a
phage particle and a bacterium, followed by attachment of the phage
tail in such a way that infection supervenes. There has been some
controversy as to whether this irreversible attachment is necessarily
preceded by a stage of reversible adsorption, or whether reversible
adsorption (which undoubtedly occurs) is merely a non-specific event
which does not involve the machinery of infection. Since the question
remains open (review: Hershey, 1957, b) we shall not discuss it further.

The process of adsorption involves the cell surface, the phage particle,
the environment, and the interactions which occur between them.

1. The cell surface

The bacterial cell is contained by two structures, an outer, rigid *wall*
and an inner, semipermeable *membrane*. When the outer cell wall is
removed from intact, living bacteria by treatment with lysozyme
(Weibull, 1953; Zinder and Arndt, 1956) or with penicillin, which acts
by preventing new cell wall formation (Lederberg, J., 1957), the cells
are transformed into spherical structures called *protoplasts* which lyse
osmotically when suspended in water, leaving empty cell membranes

which can be purified. Suspensions of cell walls, which preserve the shape of the bacteria, may be prepared by mechanical rupture or chemical lysis. The membranes and walls of cells are chemically very different. When phage is mixed with cell walls isolated from sensitive bacteria, the phage adsorbs to them and is inactivated (Weidel, Koch and Lohss, 1954; Kellenberger and Arber, 1955); on the other hand, protoplasts are not infected by phage, although they are able to support phage growth if infected prior to removal of the cell wall (Weibull, 1953); nor can protoplast membranes bind phage (Zinder and Arndt, 1956). The site of attachment of phage is, therefore, the cell wall.

The specificity and rapidity of adsorption of most phages, together with the large number of particles which the bacterial cell can generally accommodate (a single $E.$ $coli$ B bacterium can adsorb up to 200 T2 particles), suggest that the chemical groupings on the cell wall which are specific for a particular phage are both numerous and widespread. Despite this, bacteria saturated with one phage type usually retain the capacity to adsorb others (Weidel, 1953a). The most precise information on the biochemical architecture of the cell wall with respect to phage adsorption has come from the isolation of the bacterial receptors and their chemical and serological analysis; (reviews: Garen and Kozloff, 1959; Fisher, 1959).

$Shigella$ $sonnei$ in phase I is sensitive to coliphages T2 and T6; from phase I cultures, phase II mutant strains can be isolated which have become sensitive to phages T3, T4 and T7, in addition to T2 and T6. The two phases are serologically different. Goebel and his colleagues (Baker, Goebel and Perlman, 1949; Jesaitus and Goebel, 1952) isolated and purified the somatic antigens of both phases and showed that they were lipopolysaccharide–protein complexes which specifically inactivated only those phages to which the initial cultures were susceptible. Removal of the protein from the purified phase II antigen destroyed its ability to inactivate phages T2 and T6, but not T3, T4 or T7. The two groups of phages therefore adsorb to different bacterial receptors. More recent studies, by Weidel and his colleagues, of $E.$ $coli$ B receptors for these phages have considerably extended this work. It appears that the cell wall consists of two layers. One is composed of lipoprotein soluble in 90% phenol, the protein moiety being characterized by a wide spectrum of amino acids but devoid of diaminopimelic acid. The other layer, remaining after phenol extraction, is of lipopolysaccharide nature and appears to constitute the rigid framework of the wall; it can be resolved into a network consisting of (a) large units containing phospholipid material, glucose, glucosamine and L–gala–D–mannoheptose, which are linked together by (b) smaller units made up of glucosamine, muramic acid, alanine, glutamic acid and diaminopimelic acid (Weidel et al.

1954; Weidel and Primosigh, 1958). The arrangement of these layers, and some insight into their receptor activity, can be inferred from their interaction with phages T2, T6 and T3, T4, T7, all of which adsorb to, and are inactivated by, the unfractionated cell walls. Phenol extraction completely removes receptor activity for T2 and T6 which must therefore reside in the lipoprotein layer; at the same time the rate of adsorption of T4 is increased, so that its receptor is presumably located in the lipopolysaccharide layer which underlies the lipoprotein. The receptors for T3 and T7 likewise reside in the lipopolysaccharide layer.

E. coli B yields mutants which are singly resistant to phages T3, T4 or T7; in addition, however, mutants can be isolated which have acquired simultaneous resistance to all three phages (B/3, 4, 7). Chemical analysis of the lipopolysaccharide fraction of cell walls from these triply resistant strains has revealed a complete absence of the sugar L–gala–D–mannoheptose (Weidel *et al.* 1954), which is thus defined as a common and essential receptor component for all three phages, although the existence of singly resistant mutants indicates that it is not the only one. Receptors for phage T5 appear to lie in the outer lipoprotein layer but are distinct from those for T2 and T6 since they can be selectively extracted by dilute caustic soda (Weidel, 1953a).

2. The environment

The irreversible attachment of phage to sensitive bacteria depends on many environmental factors of which temperature, the ionic content of the medium and the presence or absence of required *adsorption cofactors* are the most important. The conditions requisite for infection differ for different phages and have been best defined for the T series. All these phages are as rapidly adsorbed at $0°$ as at $37°C$, but whereas the attachment of T1 and T7 remains reversible at $0°$, that of T2 is irreversible, since infective phage particles cannot be recovered at this temperature, although the bacteria are neither killed nor infected (see Garen and Kozloff, 1959). Adsorption does not occur at all in distilled water but requires the addition of an inorganic salt which probably facilitates the initial contact by neutralizing the net negative charge on bacterium and phage. In some cases, however, particular phages show a specific cation requirement; thus, phage T2 will adsorb only in the presence of monovalent cations, some strains of T4 are Ca^{++} –dependent, although independent mutants can be isolated from them (Delbrück, 1948), while the temperate phage, λ, requires Mg^{++} for adsorption.

In addition to such inorganic cofactors, several strains of phages T4 and T6 have been described which must be sensitized by L–tryptophan before adsorption can occur in synthetic medium (see Anderson,

1948b; Delbrück, 1948). This sensitization is temperature-dependent and reversible by dilution or the addition of indole; it is also remarkably specific, since anthranilic acid, indole and D–tryptophan, for example, are ineffective. The activating function appears to reside in the amino and carboxyl groups of the tryptophan molecule. Mutations to trypto-phan-independence occur, showing that the requirement for tryptophan is genetically determined. Brenner (review, 1959) carried out genetic studies of a number of independently isolated strains of phage T4 which required tryptophan and found that the determinants of the cofactor requirement are all located in a single gene, distinct from that which specifies the host-range protein. Moreover, when requiring and non-requiring strains were crossed, the cofactor requirement showed phenotypic mixing; about 75% of the initial progeny particles were of non-requiring $(C+)$ phenotype, but among these the c^+ and c genotypes were equally distributed, as shown by the behaviour of the "second generation" progeny (see Section III C). This suggests that the site of cofactor activation is a protein distinct from those determining host-range specifity and presumably located in the phage tail. The mechanism of the activation is unknown, but may be connected with protein denaturation and associated with unwinding of the tail fibres (see below) (Sato, 1956).

3. Interaction of phage and host following adsorption

Infection of the bacterium is triggered by the irreversible attachment of the phage tail to the cell wall. It is therefore important to find out (a) what component of the phage tail is responsible for the attachment, and (b) what is the nature of the mechanism that is triggered by it.

It has already been mentioned that various methods are available for fractionating the various morphological components of phage (Section III,B and D). The ability of a number of these components to adsorb to sensitive bacteria has been assessed. Complete tails and isolated tail fibres were found to attach, but heads did not (Williams and Frazer, 1956). In another investigation in which tail cores (rods) were tested, some were found to attach, while others did not; the fraction which did attach appeared to consist of cores that had retained their tail fibres (Kellenberger and Séchaud, 1957). The DNA liberated by osmotic shock of phage T2 particles does not absorb, while the empty protein "ghosts" do (Hershey and Chase, 1952). The evidence therefore points to the tail fibres as the organs of attachment.

The triggering mechanism presents a more complex problem. The interaction of phage T2 (or T4) particles with isolated cell-wall material is followed by unwinding and disappearance of the tail fibres, which seem to be wrapped around the tip of the tail in intact phage, as well as by contraction of the sheath and protusion of the tail core (Kellenberger and Arber, 1955; Brown and Kozloff, 1957). This change is shown in Plates 2 (a), (b) and 3 (a). Unwinding of the tail fibres is also brought about by treatment with alkali, but contraction of the sheath does not supervene unless the pH is lowered to below neutrality. This dependence of sheath contraction on pH suggested an analogy with myosin. This was strikingly confirmed by the similarity of the effects of EDTA (ethylenediaminetetraacetic acid), in conjunction with various monovalent cations, on myosin ATPase activity on the one hand, and on the morphology and infective capacity of phage T2 on the other (Garen and Kozloff, 1959).

It had long been known that treatment of sensitive bacteria with a high multiplicity of the T–even phages is followed by prompt and non-infective lysis of the cells—the so-called "lysis from without" (Delbrück, 1940b)—even though the phage was previously inactivated by irradiation. Weidel (1951) showed that this phenomenon was associated with structural changes in the cell walls and the release of material from them, and suggested that these changes might be due to the presence of an enzyme in the phage particles. Such an enzyme was subsequently demonstrated in phages T2, T4 and T6 (Barrington and Kozloff, 1954; Koch and Weidel, 1956; Weidel and Primosigh, 1958), as well as in the temperate phage λ (Fisher, 1959); the enzyme can be released from the phage by freezing and thawing. It transpires that T2, T4 and T6 enzymes all act on the underlying liposaccharide layer of the cell wall, with the liberation of large amounts of alanine, glutamic acid and diaminopimelic acid which, it will be remembered, are the principal constituents of the links holding together the receptor sites, in this layer, for phages T3, T4 and T7 (Section IV A1). Conversely, it has been shown that the specific phage receptors are unaffected by the phage enzyme. Thus, the enzymes of these three phages act on molecular groupings in the cell wall which are distinct from those to which the phages attach; the action of the enzymes is to break down the bridges which preserve the rigidity of the cell wall, thus opening a gate for infection (Weidel and Primosigh, 1958).

Of the considerable number of organic and inorganic agents which have been tested for their effects on the morphology of phage T2, only certain organic complexes of zinc appeared to mimic the action of cell walls (Kozloff and Henderson, 1955). Further investigation of the possible role of zinc in phage–bacterium interactions showed that this metal, tightly bound to the cell wall, is essential for the unwinding of the tail fibres as well as for the liberation of the phage enzyme (Kozloff and Lute, 1957).

The current model of the mechanism of infection may be summarized as follows. The tail of the phage particle adheres, perhaps non-specifically, to the cell wall. The tail is thus brought into contact with zinc complexes which activate the unwinding of the tail fibres. These fibres then attach specifically to certain molecular groupings in the cell wall; at the same time, the phage enzyme is released and bores a hole through the rigid layer of the wall. The significance of contraction of the sheath will be discussed in the following section.

B. PENETRATION BY THE PHAGE

We have seen, from chemical analysis and osmotic shock experiments (Section III, A and D), that phage is made up almost exclusively of DNA and protein; from the anatomical point of view, the DNA (together with a little protein) is enclosed within a protein envelope to form the head of the phage. To the head is attached a structurally complicated protein tail which is primarily involved in initiating infection. The question as to whether infection follows penetration of the cell by the whole or only part of the phage particle was answered by the famous and definitive "blendor" experiment of Hershey and Chase (1952).

Preparations of phage T2 were made in which the particles were labelled either with radioactive phosphorus (^{32}P) incorporated exclusively into the DNA, or with radioactive sulphur (^{35}S) present only in the protein. After infection of an $E.$ $coli$ B culture with one or the other preparation of phage, and removal of unadsorbed phage by centrifugation, the cells were violently agitated in a blendor for various times to shear off the adsorbed particles; this treatment did not reduce the plaque-forming ability of the infected bacteria. The distribution of ^{32}P or of ^{35}S between the cells and the extraneous medium was then assayed. It was found that the blendor treatment removed from the infected cells about 80% of the sulphur but only about 20% of the phosphorus of the infecting particles. Moreover, nearly all of the 20% of phage sulphur which remained bound to the cells could be accounted for by failure of the treatment to remove all the attached phage coats (Hershey, 1953); similarly, most of the 20% of phage DNA found in the medium was present in intact phage particles which had not infected the bacteria (Hershey and Burgi, 1956). Essentially the same results have been obtained with phage T5 (Luria and Steiner, 1954; Lanni, 1954). It is therefore evident that the phage DNA is injected into the infected bacterium while its protein coat remains outside. This is borne out by electron microphotographs of infected cells which show that the heads of many of the attached particles appear empty, like those of the phage "ghosts" obtained from osmotic shock. In addition, as high as

50% of the ^{32}P label (i.e. the DNA) of the infecting phage may be found in the progeny particles, while less than 1% of the protein label is so transferred.

It is now apparent that a small amount of protein, amounting to not more than 3% of the total phage protein, *is* injected along with the DNA (Hershey, 1955), but most of this comprises the acid-soluble peptide, containing mainly lysine and glutamic and aspartic acids, which is contained within the head and is liberated by osmotic shock (Section IIIB); some polyamines are likewise injected (Ames *et al.*, 1958) and are passed on directly to the progeny particles.

The mechanism of injection is not yet clear, although some plausible interpretations of the known data have been suggested. For example, there is morphological evidence that the core of the tail penetrates into the cell during infection; thus, the phage particle may really behave like the "micro-syringe" model suggested by Hershey, contraction of the sheath providing the motive force to drive the core through the small region of cell wall previously softened by the phage enzyme. Kozloff and Henderson (1955) found that treatment of suspensions of T2 particles, altered by cadmium cyanide, with compounds containing primary amino groups, such as glucosamine and some amino acids, lead to discharge of the phage DNA in the absence of host cells; since such substances are liberated from the cell wall by the phage enzyme (Weidel and Primosigh, 1958; see Section IVA1), they might well act as the trigger for DNA injection (Garen and Kozloff, 1959).

Apart from the mechano-chemical aspects of injection, the nature of the physical forces which propel the DNA presents a difficult problem which is not understood at all. The head of a phage particle contains about $2 \cdot 5 \times 10^{-16}$ grams of DNA of molecular weight about $1 \cdot 3 \times 10^8$. If, as is almost certainly the case (see Section VIIC1), this DNA is in the form of a single double-helix, composed of twin polynucleotide strands (Watson and Crick, 1953a; see Section VIIA, Fig. 2), then it contains about 2×10^5 nucleotide pairs; according to the Watson–Crick model, the diameter of the double helix is 20 Å, while the distance between nucleotide pairs is $3 \cdot 4$ Å, so that what is transferred from phage to bacterium during infection is a viscous thread about $6 \cdot 8 \times 10^5$ Å long and 20 Å in diameter. In the case of phage T2, the kinetics of infection and electron microscopic measurement show that this thread is transferred in a minute or so through a tube 800 Å long and 25 Å in diameter.

C. THE INTRACELLULAR DEVELOPMENT OF PHAGE

1. The eclipse period and the kinetics of phage growth

A one-step growth experiment (Section IIC), performed at low multiplicity of infection with one of the T-even phages, shows that an average

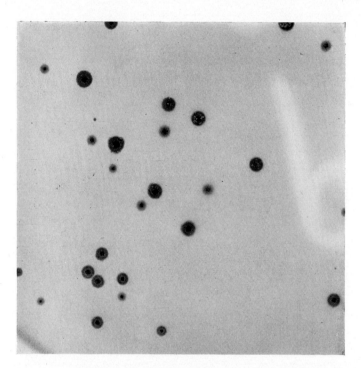

PLATE 1. Plaques produced by wild type and mutant particles of phage T4 on *E. coli* strain B. The small, poorly defined plaques arise from wild-type (r^+) particles which are susceptible to lysis inhibition. The larger, clearer plaques with well-defined edges arise from mutant r (rapid lysis) particles which are not susceptible to lysis inhibition. The white background against which the plaques are seen comprises a confluent growth of the host bacteria.

(Kindly provided by Dr. N. D. Symonds.)

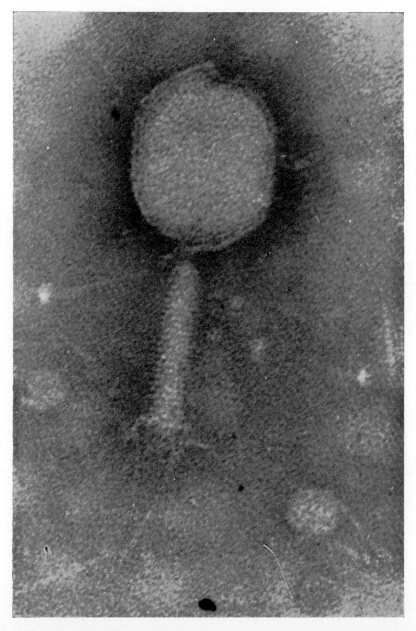

PLATE 2. Electron-microphotographs of the virulent phage T2 (PTA embedded, × 550,000).

(a) Intact particle showing head and tail. The suggestion of a base-plate can be seen at the tip of the tail. The cross-striations along the length of the tail are spaced at approximately 30 Å.

(From Brenner *et al.*, 1959; reproduced by kind permission of the authors and publishers.)

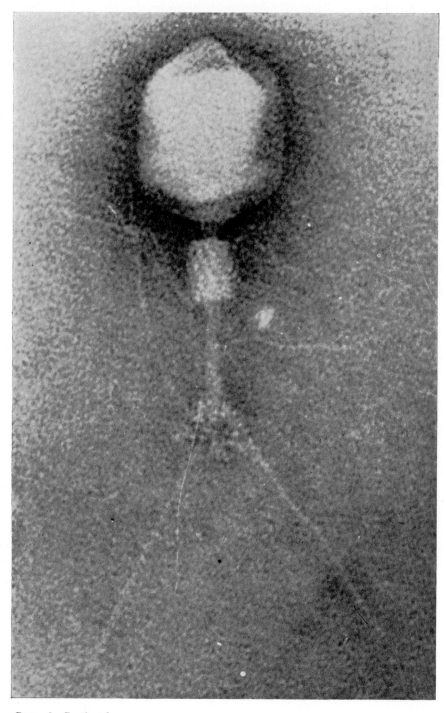

PLATE 2—Continued.
    (b) Particle treated with hydrogen peroxide, showing the relations of the filled head, contracted sheath, core and tail fibres.

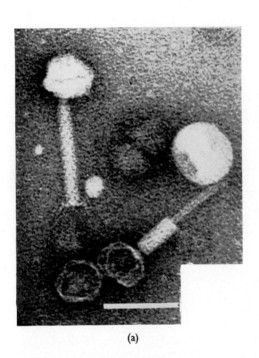

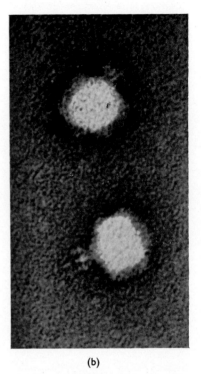

(a)   (b)

PLATE 3. Electron-microphotographs of the temperate phages, P2 and P22 (PTA embedded).

(a) Particles of phage P2, which infects and lysogenizes Shigella and *E. coli*. An intact particle is seen at top left. At bottom right is a particle with contracted sheath and collapsed, empty head which has discharged its DNA ($\times$ 200,000).

(b) Particles of phage P22 which infects and lysogenizes Salmonella. The particles are intact, have an hexagonal head and only a rudimentary tail; the base-plate can be clearly seen ($\times$ 300,000).

(Kindly provided by Dr. T. F. Anderson.)

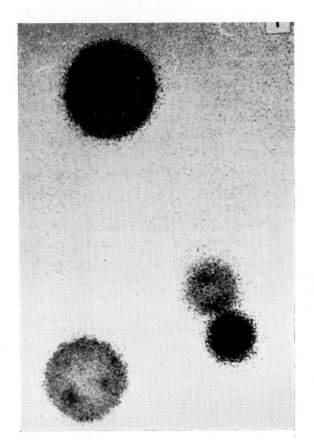

PLATE 4. Showing the four types of plaque which arise when the progeny of a cross between wild-type (h^+r^+) and doubly mutant (hr) T2 phages is plated on a mixture of host bacteria, comprising *E. coli* B (sensitive to both phages) and *E. coli* B/2 (sensitive only to phages carrying the h (host range) mutation). The h character determines whether the plaques are turbid (h^+) or clear (h); the r character determines whether the plaques are small (r^+) or large (r). The plaque morphology reflects the phage genotype as follows: *Top:* clear, large plaques indicate doubly mutant parental type (hr). *Right upper:* turbid, small plaques indicate the wild parental type (h^+r^+). *Right lower:* clear, small plaques indicate the recombinant type hr^+. *Bottom left:* turbid, large plaques indicate the reciprocal recombinant type, h^+r.

(From Hershey and Chase, 1951; reproduced by kind permission of the authors and publishers.)

period of some 25 minutes intervenes between the initial infection by a single particle and the bursting of the cell to liberate several hundred progeny particles. In phage terminology, this period is known as the latent period. A direct approach to the nature of the intracellular events occuring during this period is to break open the infected bacteria at intervals and to study the kinetics of growth of the phage particles being produced within them. This was first done by Doerman (1952), who lysed samples of infected cells, throughout the course of a one-step growth experiment with phage T4, by treating them with cyanide and an excess of phage T6 (lysis from without). These premature lysates were then assayed for the presence of infective phage by plating on indicator bacteria sensitive to T4 but resistant to T6. The outcome of the experiment was that no infective particles were found until about 12 minutes after infection, i.e. about half-way through the period required for natural lysis. Thereafter, however, infective particles began to appear and then increased at a constant rate until the normal plateau titre was achieved (see Fig. 1). These results have been unequi vocally confirmed, using other phages and such different methods of dis rupting the infected bacteria as by sonic oscillation (Anderson and Doermann, 1952), chloroform (Séchaud and Kellenberger, 1956), streptomycin (Symonds, 1957), or by forming protoplasts from pre viously infected cells and then lysing them by osmotic shock (Brenner and Stent, 1955).

The significance of the premature lysis experiment is twofold. First, the existence of an *eclipse period* shows that the intracellular state of the phage during the early stages of infection is different from that of the initial infective particle; this, in fact, is to be expected from the fact that only the DNA and a small fraction of the protein of the infective particle is injected. This non-infective form of phage is called *vegetative phage* (Hershey, 1952). Secondly, following the eclipse phase, the rate of increase in the number of infective phages is constant, i.e. *linear with time*, and does not follow the exponential course expected of regularly dividing particles. At the time these findings came to light they appeared to be more compatible with the growing idea that phage proliferation might be due to the independent synthesis and later assembly of its component parts, rather than to successive replications of a complete structure. This idea sprang from various sources. For example, the basic discovery that the genetic material of *Pneumococcus* (transforming principle) was composed of virtually pure DNA (Avery, MacLeod and McCarty, 1944) suggested that phage infection might also be genetic, the role of the infecting DNA being to determine the cellular synthesis of new phage DNA and protein. Again, Luria (1947) had found that irradiated phage particles which, singly, could not infect, were nevertheless capable of yielding normal progeny on multiple infection (*multiplicity reactivation*) and proposed that the phage genetic material is dispersed into sub-units in the host cell and then replicated independently in a sub-unit "pool" from which intact genomes could ultimately be reconstituted (Section VII D2). Finally, Visconti and Delbrück (1953) found, from a mathematical analysis of the results of phage crosses, that the recombination data could best be explained by assuming a complete mixing of the intact genetic structures of the parental particles in a DNA "pool," accompanied by multiple rounds of pairwise mating. An experimental test of this concept required the availability of specific methods for the recognition and estimation of phage DNA and protein against the background of bacterial metabolism.

2. The synthesis of phage DNA

Study of the kinetics of phage DNA synthesis in a one-step growth experiment was made possible by the discovery that the DNA of the T-even series of phages is unique in possessing the pyrimidine base 5–hydroxymethylcytosine (HMC) in place of the cytosine of *E. coli* DNA (Wyatt and Cohen, 1953). *E. coli* was mixed with phage T2 under conditions leading to infection of all the bacteria with maximal synchrony. At intervals during the latent period, samples were prematurely lysed and assayed for infective particles, as well as for total DNA and its content of HMC and cytosine; from the relative amount of HMC in the DNA of intact phage particles, the phage DNA fraction could be assessed in terms of phage equivalents (Hershey, Dixon and Chase, 1953; Vidaver and Kozloff, 1957). The results showed that synthesis of phage DNA commences at about six minutes after infection and then rises sharply, so that by the time the first infective particles appear at 12 minutes the cell contains about 50–80 phage equivalents of HMC-containing DNA. Thereafter the number of phage equivalents of DNA and of infective particles increase linearly at the same rate until the cells burst (Fig. 1). If lysis of the cells is delayed, both curves continue to rise at the same rate as before (Hershey and Melechen, 1957). Thus, when the phage DNA pool reaches a certain size, infective particles begin to form and, thereafter, a steady state is maintained. The implication is that the phage DNA is irreversibly withdrawn from the pool and incorporated into phage heads at the same rate as it is synthesized. Hershey (1953) confirmed this by showing that a pulse of ^{32}P label taken up by the pool DNA *early* in the latent period is very efficiently transferred to intracellular phage, but it is not returned again to the pool.

It might be thought that the proliferating phage T2 DNA would be built up primarily from precursors present in the bacterial cell at the time of infection. Cohen (1948) demonstrated that this was not so by infecting ³²P-containing bacteria immediately after transfer to a non-radioactive medium, and then examining the progeny phage particles, after purification, for their content of radioactive and non-radioactive

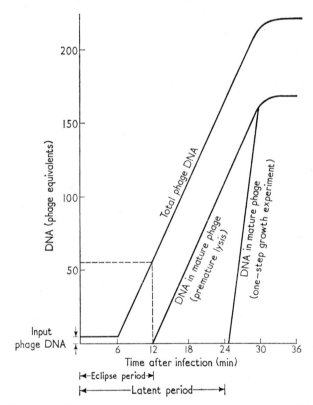

Fig. 1. Idealized curves illustrating the kinetics of synthesis of phage DNA in bacteria infected with one of the T-even phages. The phage equivalents of DNA in mature particles, whether derived from premature lysis or from a one-step growth experiment, correspond, of course, to the actual number of phage particles found, so that the figure also shows the kinetics of phage growth (Section IV,C1).

phosphorus. It was found that the phosphorus in their DNA was predominantly (2/3) non-radioactive, i.e. that their DNA originated primarily from precursors in the medium rather than in the infected bacterium. The same finding emerged from the reciprocal experiment where non-radioactive bacteria were infected immediately after transfer to a ^{32}P-containing medium; in this case the progeny particles showed a predominance of ^{32}P. Later experiments utilizing bacteria labelled specifically in the thymine of their DNA, showed that most of the host contribution came from the bacterial DNA (Hershey et al., 1954) and was incorporated mainly into those particles formed early in the latent period (Stent and Maaløe, 1953). Since the phage DNA cannot incorporate cytosine, this means that the bacterial DNA must be broken down before being built up again into phage DNA. In fact, much of the host DNA disappears on infection with the T-even phages to reappear again in the progeny phages, the host cytosine having been converted into HMC (Cohen, 1953). A cytological corollary to these findings is the rapid disappearance of the bacterial nucleus following infection with the T-even phages, as well as with phage T5 whose nucleic acid bases are similar to those of the host (Luria and Human, 1950).

3. The synthesis of phage protein

Phage protein can readily be recognized and separated from bacterial protein by its specific interactions with phage antisera and its ability to adsorb to the cell walls of sensitive bacteria. By combining these properties with tracer studies employing radioactive sulphur, ^{35}S, which is incorporated into the protein but not into the DNA of phage, the intracellular synthesis of phage protein can be followed, during one-step growth experiments, in much the same way as has been described for phage DNA. Moreover, the total amount of phage protein detected can be expressed in phage equivalents, by dividing it by the average protein content of a single phage particle. Phage protein first appears in the infected cell about nine minutes after infection, i.e. after the commencement of DNA synthesis but a few minutes prior to the appearance of infective particles, and then rises to 30–40 phage equivalents. Thereafter the rate of increase parallels that of the phage DNA. This protein is less sedimentable, and therefore smaller, than intact particles; experiments employing pulses of ^{35}S show that part of it, at least, is later incorporated into infective phage and is, therefore, precursor material (Maaløe and Symonds, 1953; Hershey et al., 1955). Experiments in which the infected bacteria were exposed to short pulses of ^{35}S, injected into the medium at various times, indicated that the rate of uptake of ^{35}S into the total intracellular protein was constant throughout the latent period, about one half being transferred at a uniform rate to phage particles from the tenth minute onwards. During the first five minutes of infection, however, very little of the assimilated ^{35}S found its way into phage (Hershey et al., 1954). This seemed to indicate that, at the very beginning of the infection, a class of proteins different from the precursors of the phage coat is formed. The significance of this finding is discussed in the next section. The constituents of phage protein are derived almost exclusively from the medium; for example, when phage was grown, in an unlabelled medium, in bacteria whose protein had previously been isotopically labelled in one of its amino acids, virtually none of the label appeared later in the phage progeny (Kozloff et al., 1951).

4. The nature of non-precursor protein

As was mentioned above, the first few minutes of infection by the T-even phages is characterized by the appearance of protein distinct from the phage coat-precursor protein. Two lines of evidence suggest that this is not normal bacterial protein, but is synthesized de novo following injection of the phage DNA. First, although protein continues to be made after phage infection at about the same rate as before, the synthesis of specifically bacterial protein, such as inducible enzymes like β–galactosidase, ceases abruptly (Benzer, 1953), as might be expected from the rapid breakdown of the bacterial nucleus. Secondly, host cells treated with inhibitors of protein synthesis, such as chloramphenicol or 5-methyltryptophan, either before or up to five minutes after infection, fail to synthesize either phage protein or DNA; on the other hand, inhibition of protein synthesis later in the latent period, at about the time when precursor protein starts to appear, has no effect on the synthesis of phage DNA, although, of course, no protein is produced until the inhibitor is removed (Burton, 1955; Tomizawa and Sunakawa, 1956; Hershey and Melechen, 1957). Since the phage DNA contains HMC while the bacterial DNA does not, it seemed plausible that the early protein comprised new enzymes, specified by the infecting phage genome and required for the building of HMC–DNA replicas of it. A considerable range of such enzymes, synthesized within the first few minutes of infection, has been defined. The more important of these include: (a) an enzyme which hydroxymethylates deoxycytidine 5'–phosphate as an essential step in HMC synthesis (Flaks and Cohen, 1957, 1958); (b) an enzyme which phosphorylates hydroxymethyldeoxycytidine (HMC) 5'–phosphate, leading to synthesis of the triphosphate; (c) an enzyme which breaks down deoxycytidine triphosphate, thus preventing the incorporation of cytosine into the phage DNA; (d) an enzyme involved in the direct glucosylation of the HMC–DNA which is characteristic of the T-even phages (Kornberg et al., 1959). These enzymes were not found in uninfected or phage T5 – infected bacteria.

5. RNA synthesis following phage infection

Bacteriophages, with the single exception of that recently reported by Loeb and Zinder (1961), contain no RNA. Following infection with the T-even phages the normal high rate of bacterial RNA synthesis is rapidly arrested and no further overall increase occurs. Nevertheless, study of the incorporation of environmental ^{32}P into the RNA of infected bacteria showed not only that a small amount of new RNA with a high rate of metabolic turnover was being synthesized (Hershey, 1954) but that the rate at which the ^{32}P was taken up individually by the four RNA nucleotide bases was different from that found for normal RNA synthesis, and corresponded roughly to the ratio of the equivalent bases in the phage DNA (Volkin and Astrachan, 1957). It is beyond the scope of this book to discuss in any detail the relevant problem of how the genetic information contained in the DNA "code" is translated into the functional language of protein synthesis; it is enough to indicate here that recent work has provided good evidence for the following hypothesis. The genetic information for specific protein synthesis is coded for by the sequence of the four nucleotide bases along the DNA double helix which constitutes the genetic material of the cell (or phage). Protein synthesis occurs in the cytoplasmic ribosomal particles which contain the bulk of the stable RNA of the cell and provide templates, based on the DNA code, on which the amino acids can be aligned in their correct sequence prior to polymerization into specific protein. Since protein synthesis is strictly dependent on the integrity of the DNA, the templates in the ribosomes must be unstable and have a high turnover, and so cannot be the ribosomal RNA itself (Riley *et al.*, 1961). Recent work by Brenner, Jacob and Meselson (1961a) on *E. coli* infected with phage T2, using isotopic "density" labels to distinguish old ribosomes from new, and ^{35}S and ^{32}P tracers to follow new protein and RNA synthesis, has revealed the following facts:

(a) The synthesis of new phage protein takes place in old ribosomes which, before infection, had been the site of synthesis of bacterial protein.

(b) Synthesis of phage protein is associated with the appearance of a new RNA fraction, termed "messenger" RNA, which has a high turnover as well as an affinity for the ribosomes which is reversible by altering the Mg^{++} concentration. This "messenger" RNA fraction is almost certainly the same as that described by Volkin and Astrachan (1957) as having a base composition equivalent to that of the phage DNA. The role postulated for it is to transcribe the DNA code from the chromosome and carry it to the ribosomes where it becomes the template for protein synthesis. Hall and Spiegelman (1961) have shown that when messenger RNA from T2-infected cells is heated and cooled with T2 DNA, but not with DNA from the *E. coli* host, DNA–RNA complexes are formed, indicating a high degree of homology between the base sequences of the two. RNA fractions analogous to the messenger RNA we have described have also been isolated from normal, uninfected *E. coli* cells (Gros *et al.*, 1961).

6. Assembly of the phage components

We have discussed the way in which phage DNA, after its injection into the host cell, determines first of all the synthesis of enzymes required for its own replication and then the synthesis of the various structural proteins which form the coat of the mature particle. The result is that DNA and protein pools are formed which increase linearly. When these pools reach a certain size, infective phage particles begin to appear and increase in number, but the size of the pools remains constant. The fact that the pools are formed before the appearance of phage, while a proportion at least of the materials in the pools is later incorporated into phage particles, strongly suggests that the components of phage are synthesized separately and are then randomly withdrawn from the pools and assembled into complete particles. This process is known as *maturation* and constitutes a complicated problem in morphogenesis about which virtually nothing is known.

Four further lines of evidence support the maturation concept.

(*a*) Electron microscopy of phage lysates, whether derived from premature or natural lysis, reveals the presence of empty phage heads ("doughnuts") (Levinthal and Fisher, 1952; Anderson *et al.*, 1953) as well as unattached rods which, presumably, are free tail components (Kellenberger and Sechaud, 1957). These structures, which are not infective, only begin to appear a few minutes before the end of the eclipse period and then increase in number at the same rate as the completed particles (Levinthal and Fisher, 1952).

(*b*) In genetic crosses between phages T2 and T4, whose tail proteins have different adsorption specificities, the *genotype* of a proportion of particles initially displaying the adsorption specificity of one parental type subsequently yield only progeny of the other type. This phenomenon means that these particles possess the genetic material of one parental type and the tail protein of the other, and is called *phenotypic mixing* (see Sections III C and IV B 2); the proportion that is found between the two parental types among the progeny of phenotypically mixed particles indicates a random association of genomes and protein-coat components; this can only be interpreted in terms of the random assembly of prefabricated DNA and protein structures (Delbrück and

Bailey, 1946; Novick and Szilard, 1951; Streisinger, 1956; Brenner, 1957, 1959).

(c) The addition of various dyes of the *acridine* series to infected cells during the latent period is followed by lysis, but no infective or morphologically mature particles are released; the synthesis of phage DNA and protein, however, is unaffected by the drug and incomplete phage-coat structures are present in the lysate (Foster, 1948). If the drug is added to infected bacteria after the eclipse period, the lysate may contain infective particles which had been formed before its addition. Different acridines act specifically on certain phage strains, temperate as well as virulent phages may be susceptible, and phage mutations leading to acridine resistance have been reported (review: Adams, 1959, pp. 278–281). Acridine dyes therefore appear to interfere with the final assembly of phage constituents, possibly by inactivating one or more maturation enzymes, or by altering the physical state of precursor DNA (Volkin and Astrachan, 1957).

(d) Mutations affecting the genome of temperate phages in the prophage state (see Section V) have been described, which prevent the production of phage particles (*defective phages*). In the case of inducible systems, the lysogenized bacteria may lyse normally after u.v. induction, but no (or very few) phage particles are found in the lysate. In one such case the mutations appear to involve only the stage of maturation, since all the recognizable materials of the phage are produced normally following induction (Jacob and Wollman, 1956).

In considering the possible mechanisms which might control maturation, the fact that it may be an *automatic* function determined by the physical attributes of the various components, analogous to the *in vitro* reconstitution of tobacco mosaic virus from purified protein and RNA fractions (Fraenkel-Conrat and Williams, 1955), should not be forgotten. Phage, however, is a much more complicated organism than TM virus, whose genetic material consists of a single strand of RNA arranged helically within the long axis of a homogeneous protein rod (see Gierer, 1960). In phage, not only must many different proteins be organized into very specific alignments, but the phage DNA must be tightly and accurately folded to permit its inclusion within the phage head; it has been suggested that the peptide released from the head with the DNA, on osmotic shock (Sections III B and IV B), may form a scaffold for this folding, while the function of the polyamines, spermine and putrescine, is to neutralize the charge on the DNA.

D. Lysis of the Infected Cell

Under standard conditions, lysis supervenes at a standard time after infection. This time, however, does not seem to be necessarily related either to the number of mature phage particles which accumulate or to the size of the DNA and protein pools. For example, the pool size and the burst size may be greatly increased by lysis inhibition (Section II B 2) or reduced by nutritional and physiological factors; conversely, in the case of certain defective phages or on the addition of acridine dyes, lysis occurs at the normal time in the absence of particle formation. Lysis does not occur, however, if protein synthesis is stopped soon after the eclipse period is over, although the size of the DNA pool may continue to increase. The fact that a high multiplicity of T-even phages causes rapid "lysis from without" (Delbrück, 1940b), and the discovery of an enzyme in the phage tail which can break down the cell wall (Barrington and Kozloff, 1954; Section IV A 3), suggested that lysis might be due to synthesis, under the control of the phage genome, of a lytic enzyme in the infected cell. Direct evidence is now available that such enzymes are in fact synthesized and play a primary role in determining the onset of lysis. For example, two types of defective λ prophage have been described. Induction of the K.12 strain of *E. coli*, lysogenized with one of these types, is followed by lysis at the end of the normal latent period, and the lysate is found to contain a lytic factor for chloroform-treated *E. coli* cells; induction of the other type of defectively lysogenic strain is not followed by lysis although the cells are killed, and no lytic factor can be extracted from them (Jacob and Fuerst, 1958). Streisinger *et al.*, (1961) have demonstrated the existence of mutants of phage T4 which can synthesize only a defective lysozyme-like enzyme or no enzyme at all; the mutant phages multiply and mature normally in *E. coli*, but are not liberated from the cells they infect unless these are treated with egg-white lysozyme after the latent period is over (Section II B 2).

V. Temperate Phages and Lysogeny

We have so far discussed bacteriophage almost entirely in terms of the behaviour of virulent phages, and especially of the T series of phages, which have been objects of the most concentrated study during the past 20 years. Virulent phages may be defined as those whose only interaction with sensitive bacteria is to replicate within them, so that the infected bacteria are inevitably lysed and new phage particles liberated. Not very long after the original discovery of bacteriophage it became apparent that some strains of bacteria could themselves act as an initial source of phage which was active against other strains. Cultures of such strains always contained free phage particles, but otherwise appeared normal. These *lysogenic bacteria* appeared to carry the phage as an intracellular entity, since phage-free bacteria could not be obtained by such methods as repeated single colony isolation, by growing the bacteria in the presence of specific antiphage serum or, in the case of lysogenic sporing bacilli, by heating the spores at temperatures which destroyed the free phage. Moreover, when sensitive bacteria were infected by phage derived from a lysogenic strain, some of the bacteria survived and themselves acquired the lysogenic trait. Thus, phages derived from lysogenic strains have alternative interactions with sensitive bacteria which they infect; they may either enter the *lytic cycle* characteristic of infection by virulent phages, or else they may *lysogenize* the infected cells. These phages therefore lack the obligatory virulence of virulent phages and so are called *temperate*. Moreover, because only a proportion of the infected cells are lysed, temperate phages yield *turbid plaques* from the growth of lysogenized bacteria within the lysed area (Section II B 2; historical reviews: Jacob and Wollman, 1959; Stent, 1960).

A. The Recognition of Lysogeny

The two main characteristics of lysogenic bacteria are: (a) they carry the temperate phage (or, rather, the potentiality to produce it) in some intracellular form, and (b) they are specifically immune to superinfection by the carried phage or by mutant variants of it (Section VI B). Thus, the phage released by, and present in cultures of, lysogenic bacteria cannot lyse or form plaques on these bacteria. For this reason, the fact that strains of bacteria are lysogenic may pass unnoticed indefinitely. The recognition of lysogeny therefore depends on the availability of a sensitive "indicator" strain which is not lysogenic for the phage to be tested (although it may be lysogenic for other, unrelated, temperate phages) but on which the phage can form plaques.

In the first instance, an investigation to determine whether or not a particular bacterial strain is lysogenic is usually empirical. The presumptive free phage particles in a culture are freed from viable bacteria, by such means as filtration or treatment of the culture with chloroform or heat, and then plated on a number of different bacterial strains, of the same or related species, to see whether plaques are formed with any of them. When the presumptively lysogenic strain is sensitive to streptomycin, a simple and widely applicable method is to plate the culture directly, with streptomycin-resistant mutant bacteria of the indicator strains, on media containing streptomycin; the growth of the lysogenic bacteria is suppressed without affecting plaque production by free phage particles (Bertani, 1951).

An alternative method of detecting lysogeny is to plate a high dilution of the bacterial strain to be tested with undiluted cultures of the indicator bacteria, so that isolated colonies of the lysogenic cells grow upon a "lawn" of indicator cells. Under these conditions two types of plaque may be found. One is a normal, turbid plaque resulting from infection of the indicator bacteria by free phage particles present in the lysogenic culture; the other consists of a halo of lysis surrounding a colony of the lysogenic strain (*colony-centred plaque*) and is due to liberation of phage particles from the growing lysogenic clone. This simple method usually gives the clearest results when the nutritional or other characters of the indicator bacteria are such that they multiply more slowly than the lysogenic bacteria; otherwise they may enter the stationary phase of growth and become physiologically resistant (Section II B 1) before the phage liberated by the lysogenic clone has had time to initiate a spreading infection.

Since the demonstration of lysogeny depends on the chance availability of sensitive indicator strains, it can never be excluded on the basis of negative findings. Nevertheless, it is now becoming apparent that lysogeny is a very widespread phenomenon. The majority of bacterial genera and species that have been systematically studied have been found to carry temperate phages, while in *Salmonella* and *Staphylococcus*, for example, absence of lysogeny appears to be exceptional. Moreover, single bacteria may carry more than one type of phage; as many as five different phage types have been found to be released by a single strain of *Staphylococcus* (Rountree, 1949).

B. THE NATURE OF PHAGE RELEASE

Burnet and McKie (1929) first demonstrated the absence of infective phage from disrupted lysogenic cells and, about the same time as the elder Wollman (1928), put forward the idea that lysogeny signified the *inheritable potentiality of the bacteria to generate phage*, rather than a continuous leakage of phage particles from parasitized cells. This concept was unequivocally established by Lwoff and Gutman (1950) who found, from studying pedigrees of isolated, lysogenic cells of *B. megatherium*, by means of micromanipulation, that as many as 19 generations could pass without the production of phage; occasionally a cell was seen to disappear, and, when this happened, it was always accompanied by the appearance of phage particles in the observed micro-drop. Thus, every cell of a lysogenic culture inherits the capacity to liberate phage, but this capacity is only expressed by any particular cell with a rather small probability, which may vary with the particular strain of temperate phage from as high as 10^{-2} to as low as 10^{-5} per cell generation. For any given phage strain, the probability of lysis per cell generation remains more or less constant under standard conditions, so that the proportion of free phage particles to bacteria in a growing broth culture tends also to remain constant, the ratio between the two being determined, in addition, by the average burst size and the efficiency with which the released particles become readsorbed to the bacteria. The form, or component, of the phage which carries the hereditary information necessary for the production of infective phage was termed *prophage* by Lwoff and Gutmann (1950).

The next question was the nature of the spontaneous alteration of balance between prophage and bacterium that resulted in lysis and phage liberation. Lwoff and Gutmann (1950) had noticed, during their pedigree studies, that the proportion of bacteria which produced phage might vary as much as sixfold between experiments, and considered that phage production might be induced by external factors. Shortly afterwards it was discovered that exposure of lysogenic bacteria to u.v. light, in doses too small to affect bacterial growth appreciably, was followed, after one or two divisions, by lysis and liberation of phage particles by virtually the entire population (Lwoff, Siminovitch and Kjelgaard, 1950). This *induction* was very dependent on the nutritional state of the bacteria (*B. megatherium*), since lysis did not occur unless they were grown, both before and after irradiation, on a rich medium (Lwoff *et al.*, 1950; Lwoff, 1961). A wide range of other agents, including X-rays (Latarjet, 1951) and γ-rays (Marcovitch, 1956) as well as nitrogen mustards (Jacob, 1952 a), organic peroxides and hydrogen peroxide (Lwoff and Jacob, 1952), have been found to be effective inducers.

The phenomenon of induction enabled a comparison to be made of the kinetics of phage production, within lysogenic cells after induction on the one hand, and following infection of sensitive cells on the other. Both turned out to be very similar with respect both to the length of the latent period and also to the presence of infective phage in premature lysates; it therefore seemed likely that the effect of induction was to shift the prophage from its "latent" condition into the vegetative state (Jacob and Wollman, 1953). Unlike infection by virulent phages of the T–even type, neither induction of lysogenic bacteria nor infection of sensitive (non-lysogenic) bacteria by temperate phage greatly represses the ability of the bacteria to synthesize bacterial enzymes and to multiply up to the end of the latent period.

Not all lysogenic bacteria are inducible by u.v. light. The property of inducibility or non-inducibility appears to be a function of the genetic constitution of the prophage and not of the bacterium, since the same bacterial strain may be inducible when lysogenized by one strain of phage, and non-inducible when lysogenized by another. Conversely, there is evidence that the inducing agent acts primarily on the bacterium. For example, Marcovich (1956) has shown that the X-ray target size for induction is as large as the whole bacterial nucleus, while Jacob (1952b) found that the outcome of inducing bacteria doubly lysogenized with two closely related, inducible prophages was incompatible with a primary effect on the prophages themselves. These somewhat conflicting aspects of the induction process will be reconciled when we come to consider the mechanism of the immunity conferred by prophage on lysogenic bacteria (Section VIB).

C. The Prophage–bacterium Relationship

Lysogeny is a very stable property of lysogenic bacteria, and in general its loss is no more frequent than the mutational loss of normal, genetically controlled characters. If, as one hypothesis proposed, prophage exists in the form of autonomous, cytoplamic particles, then very many particles would have to be present in each bacterium to account for such stability. There is indirect evidence, however, that the number of prophages of one kind per bacterium is no greater than the number of nuclei. For example, if different ratios of two temperate phage mutants are used to mixedly infect sensitive bacteria, equivalent ratios are found among the progeny particles issuing from the infection; when a lysogenic strain carrying a mutant prophage of one type is induced by u.v. light, and at the same time is super-infected with different multiplicities of the other mutant, it is found that a multiplicity of about $\times$ 3 yields equal numbers of the two mutants among the progeny, suggesting that each bacterium carries, on the average, three prophages of each kind which is the same as the mean number of nuclei per bacterium (Jacob and Wollman, 1953).

An alternative hypothesis envisaged that the prophage was replicated and inherited in some form of association with the bacterial chromosome, i.e. that its distribution to daughter bacteria was linked with that of the bacterial genome itself. A test of this hypothesis required a sexual or parasexual system in bacteria whereby the spatial relations between genetic determinants could be studied by means of genetic analysis. Such a system, termed *conjugation*, was discovered in a particular strain of *E. coli* called K–12 by Lederberg and Tatum (1946) and has since been developed into a highly refined, if somewhat complicated genetic tool (reviews: Hayes, 1953, Wollman, Jacob and Hayes, 1956; Jacob and Wollman, 1958; Hayes, 1960, 1962). *E. coli* K–12 is known to possess a single chromosome on which the genes determining a large number of characters have now been "mapped". The discovery that *E. coli* K–12 was lysogenic for an inducible prophage, called λ, and the isolation from it of a non-lysogenic derivative, permitted the determinant of lysogeny to be analysed genetically, just like that of any other character, in crosses between lysogenic and non-lysogenic strains. It was found to occupy a specific location on the bacterial chromosome, very close to a cluster of genes associated with galactose fermentation (*gal* genes) (Lederberg and Lederberg, 1953; Wollman, 1953). When the two parents, instead of being distinguished by lysogeny and non-lysogeny, were differentially marked by lysogenization with recognizably different mutants of λ phage, the progeny of the cross inherited the two types of lysogeny in exactly the same way as they had inherited lysogeny and non-lysogeny in the previous crosses (Appleyard, 1954). Thus, the determinant of lysogeny is the prophage itself and not some bacterial gene which controls it; it occupies a specific site on the bacterial chromosome and is inherited as if it were a bacterial gene. These findings were later confirmed, using an improved system of genetic analysis, by Jacob and Wollman (1957) who also defined the chromosomal locations of 14 other prophages, seven of which were inducible and seven non-inducible. The inducible strains showed no cross-immunity (i.e. lysogenization with one strain did not prevent lytic infection by another), and all were found to have distinct locations distributed over a region of chromosome amounting to about one quarter of its total length. The non-inducible prophages were also situated at specific loci but these were distributed over the remainder of the chromosome and were not interspersed with those of the inducible prophages. It is not yet known whether this distribution has any significance with respect to the process of induction. In addition to this work, genetic studies with strains of *E. coli* doubly and triply lysogenized with mutants of the non-inducible phage P2 (Plate 3(a)), has demonstrated the existence of three alternative locations for this prophage which show a preferential order of occupancy (Bertani, 1956).

D. Interactions of Prophage and Bacterial Chromosome

1. The effects of phage mutations

As with virulent phages, mutations involving such characters as host range, plaque size and plaque morphology are also found in temperate phages. In the case of phage λ, in particular, genetic analysis by means of mixed infections with mutants having multiple marker characters has shown that the genes controlling these characters are arranged linearly on a single chromosome (Jacob and Wollman, 1954; Kaiser, 1955). Among the mutations studied were some which interfere with the ability of the phage to establish the lysogenic state, so that the mutant phages produce clear instead of turbid plaques. Most of these *clear-plaque mutants* are unable to plaque on bacteria lysogenized with the wild-type phage, i.e. they cannot override the immunity conferred by the prophage state; but others, termed *virulant mutants*, can do so. All clear-plaque (c) mutants fall into one or the other of three phenotypic groups which can be distinguished by plaque morphology. Genetic analysis of the sites of these mutations reveals that they are all located on a small region of the phage chromosome, called the C region, within which they are arranged in three clusters, representing separate genetic loci (c_1, c_2 and c_3,), each of which corresponds to one of the three phenotypic groups. Despite the inability of each mutant to lysogenize by itself, pairs of mutants from different groups, but not from the same group, can co-operate in establishing lysogeny at the normal rate following mixed infection of sensitive bacteria. This shows that each of the three mutational groups is blocked in the determinant of a different function, mediated by some diffusible product; thus, two mutant strains which are unable to fulfil different functions can, between them, provide all the products necessary for lysogenization (Kaiser, 1957). The establishment of the prophage state therefore involves at least three functions which are determined by a small region of the phage chromosome. Similar results have been obtained from analysis of clear-plaque mutants of phage A of Salmonella (Levine, 1957).

We have referred above to the seven inducible phages which can lysogenize *E. coli* K–12. Although the prophage of each of these strains occupies a different locus on the bacterial chromosome and produces immunity only against the homologous phage and its mutant derivatives, nevertheless all these phages, including λ, display considerable serological and genetic similarity and can yield phages recombinant for many of their characters in mixed infection. In the case of two of these phages (λ and 434), recombinants could be obtained which were hybrid for all segments of the chromosome except the c_1 locus, which is therefore the only region of the two chromosomes which lacks genetic homology. It was found that both the specific immunity and the prophage location of these hybrid phages was exclusively that of the parent from which it had inherited the c_1 locus, and was independent of any other chromosomal region (Kaiser and Jacob, 1957). Thus, a single functional prophage locus, or *cistron* (Benzer, 1957), determines not only the ability to lysogenize but also the location of the prophage on the bacterial chromosome and the specific immunity it confers.

2. Recombination between prophage and bacterial chromosome

In *E. coli* K–12 lysogenized with the inducible phage λ, the prophage occupies a location on the bacterial chromosome very close to that of a cluster of genes responsible for the fermentation of galactose. If a culture of a galactose-fermenting (gal^+) lysogenic strain is induced to liberate phage by treatment with u.v. light, and the phage so obtained is then used to infect a non-galactose-fermenting (gal^-) strain, a very small proportion of the surviving bacteria acquire the ability to ferment galactose in addition to becoming lysogenic. This phenomenon is known as *transduction;* a small fraction (about 10^{-6}) of the liberated phage particles act as vectors of that region of chromosome to which the λ prophage was linked in the lysogenic bacteria. On the other hand, phage preparations obtained by the *lytic infection* of non-lysogenic gal^+ bacteria have no transducing capacity, which, apparently, can only be acquired by this particular phage when in the prophage state.

Clones of initially gal^- bacteria which have become gal^+ through transduction are unstable with respect to this character, since they continue indefinitely to yield a proportion of stable gal^- progeny. This shows that they must have retained their original gal^- gene after acquiring the gal^+ gene imported by the phage, so that they are really *heterozygous* for the *gal* region and have the genotype λ-gal^+/gal^-. Such transductants are called *heterogenotes*. If, now, a population of heterogenotes is induced by u.v. light, and the phage they liberate is again used to infect gal^- bacteria, instead of the very small number of gal^+ transductants formerly found, very large numbers appear; about half the phage particles now carry the gal^+ gene (Morse, Lederberg and Lederberg, 1956).

It was then found that the transducing phage liberated from hetero-genotic cells is *defective:* first, it is unable to replicate vegetatively and yield progeny on induction without the cooperation of super-infecting wild-type phage; secondly, genetic analysis shows that a specific part of its chromosome is missing (Arber, Kellenberger and Weigle, 1957; Campbell, 1957). The inference is that transducing particles initially arise as a result of a rare recombinational event between the prophage and the adjacent region of bacterial chromosome, with the result that part of the prophage chromosome is substituted by a fragment of bacterial chromosome which includes the *gal* region. Examination of a number of independently isolated strains of λ-defective transducing phage by the density gradient centrifugation method had shown that, unlike wild-type λ, they differ considerably in density owing to a variable DNA content; this suggests that the recombinant event is not a simple, reciprocal exchange, but that a given segment of the prophage can be substituted by variable lengths of bacterial chromosome (Weigle *et al.*, 1959).

Phage λ is the only known phage which mediates *restricted trans-duction* of a single, specific chromosomal region, although a similar type of association has been described for the non-pathogenic sex factor, *F*, of *E. coli* which determines maleness in cells harbouring it and which, like temperate phages and other episomes, can alternate between cytoplasmic and chromosomally attached states (see Jacob *et al.*, 1960); the sex factor, however, can only be transferred from cell to cell by conjugation. On the other hand, *generalized transduction*, whereby any chromosomal region of the donor bacteria can be transferred, is found to occur in many bacterial genera and species, including *E. coli* K–12, and can be mediated by a considerable range of phages (review: Hartman and Goodgal, 1959). There is evidence that generalized transduction may also be performed by defective phage particles and that the mechanism of the two forms of transduction is basically similar (Luria *et al.*, 1958). It is probably significant that, of the many temperate phages which lysogenize *E. coli* K–12, only the one which can carry out generalized transduction (phage Pl: Lennox, 1955; phage 363: Jacob, 1955) does not appear to have a mappable prophage locus on the chromosome (Jacob and Wollman, 1957). It is remarkable that this phage is able jointly to transduce two other prophages together with the linked *gal* region of the donor chromosome (Jacob, 1955). These experiments reveal considerable homology between the genetic material of temperate phages and that of their hosts.

3. The mechanism of prophage attachment

It may be asked whether the prophage chromosome is actually *inserted* into the physical structure of the bacterial chromosome by an event analogous to recombination, or whether it merely *adheres* to the chromosome by the synapsis of homologous regions. There are two main arguments against insertion. One is that a reciprocal recombination event leading to insertion would be followed by replacement of part of the bacterial chromosome by the prophage genome, with the result that the whole or part of the bacterial prophage locus would be deleted; the fact that lysogenic bacteria which lose their prophage, either spontaneously or after irradiation, can be re-lysogenized with normal efficiency by the same phage shows that the chromosomal location remains intact after lysogenization. The second argument against insertion runs as follows. When two bacteria carrying genetically marked prophages are mated, some progeny bacteria are found which carry new, recombinant prophages. If the prophage chromosome and the bacterial chromosome formed one continuous structure, genetic exchange between the prophage regions should often lead to the recombination of *bacterial* markers closely linked to the two extremities of the prophage region; but this does not seem to happen (Jacob and Wollman, 1957; 1961, p. 290).

On the other hand, the existence of transductional heterogenotes (Section VD2) is good evidence of adherence. Prophage is accordingly visualized as a phage chromosome having a short C region, which synapses with a homologous region of the bacterial chromosome, with two free arms on either side. Recombination can occur between related prophages, located at different sites in doubly lysogenized bacteria, without vegetative multiplication of the phages; such recombination may be thought to result from contact and pairing between the free arms of the prophages. Finally, it should be emphasized that prophage is much more than a viral gene; it is the whole phage chromosome, long enough to contain about 100 genes. Mutations in prophage genes may result in various defects in the capacity of the bacteria to produce phage, but unless such mutations occur in the C region the defective prophage continues to lysogenize the cell and its descendants, and to confer immunity upon them. Moreover, the normal lysogenic condition may be restored by reverse mutation. On the other hand, loss of lysogeny by bacteria is due to shedding of the whole prophage chromosome and can be restored only by re-infection. It is therefore quite different from the loss of a character as a result of mutational alteration of a gene to an allelic state.

E. PHAGE CONVERSIONS

We have seen that virulent phages employ the biochemical machinery of infected cells to express the functional activity of their genes, by making enzymes and other proteins exclusively directed to the synthesis of new phage particles. This is also the case with temperate phages whenever the onset of vegetative multiplication, resulting from infection or the induction of lysogenic strains, ushers in the lytic cycle. Cases are known, however, where phage genes in the prophage state express themselves by changing the bacteria phenotype. For example, the ability of *C. diphtheriae* to produce diphtheria toxin is determined by lysogenization with certain temperate pages. Toxigenic strains which lose their prophage also lose their toxigenicity; non-toxigenic strains do not harbour these prophages but, following lysogenization, every lysogenic clone becomes toxigenic (Groman, 1953). Moreover, genetic crosses between related *Corynebacterium diphtheriae* phages may result in loss, by some of the progeny phages, of the ability to confer toxigenicity as a result of recombination (Groman and Eaton, 1955). Again, *Salmonella* strains characterized by the somatic antigens 3, 15 are lysogenic for phage ϵ^{15}; other strains which possess antigens 3, 10, but not 15, are sensitive to phage ϵ^{15}, but when lysogenized by it are converted to the antigenic type 3, 15 (Iseki and Sakai, 1953). Conversions of this sort, however, are not solely dependent on the establishment of lysogeny, since the altered phenotype can be expressed very soon after infection by cells in which the lytic cycle has been initiated (Uetake, Luria and Burrows, 1958; Barksdale, 1959). Not only, then, may bacterial viruses incorporate host genes into their genetic structure, but bacteria may also express the activities of viral genes in ways indistinguishable from those of their own.

VI. Resistance and Immunity to Phage Infection

To avoid confusion, it should be clearly understood that the words "resistance" and "immunity" have come to have rather precise meanings, and denote quite distinct mechanisms whereby bacteria protect themselves against phage infection. A bacterium is said to be *resistant* when the structure of its cell wall prevents adsorption and attachment of the phage, irrespective of whether the phage is virulent or temperate. The term *immune*, on the other hand, is restricted to the protection conferred by lysogeny against lytic infection by the same phage, or mutants of it which share a common c_1 locus (Section V D 1). Operationally, however, the distinction is not always clearcut. For example, lysogenization of *Salmonella typhimurium* by phage P22 decreases the rate of adsorption of the same phage (Garen and Kozloff, 1959; see also Boyd, 1954), probably due to conversion of surface antigens by the prophage. Again, lysogenization by various temperate phages plays a major role in determining the specific immunity patterns of strains of *Salmonella typhi* against lytic infection by the virulent and quite unrelated series of Vi typing phages; the typing phages can still infect and kill the lysogenized cells but cannot multiply in them (Felix and Anderson, 1951; review: Anderson, 1962). A similar phenomenon is the immunity conferred against infection by phage T4 r_{II} mutants by lysogenization with λ prophage (Benzer, 1957; see C below).

A. RESISTANCE

The attachment of phages to bacteria is determined by the interaction of specific receptors on the phage tail fibres with complementary molecular groupings in the bacterial cell wall. The general nature of this interaction has already been discussed in Section IV, A 1 and A 3. Certain molecular groupings, recognized as antigens, may be widely shared by different bacterial species and genera, thus accounting for the apparent lack of specificity of attachment displayed by many phages. For example, the temperate phages P1 and P2 are broadly infective for strains of *Shigella* as well as of *E. coli*, while the transducing phage P22 infects all *Salmonella* species which possess the somatic antigen 12. On the contrary, possession of a common antigen to which a phage attaches by no means implies a common sensitivity to the phage, since susceptibility to infection depends on many factors besides adsorption. Another kind of apparent non-specificity is found in the simultaneous acquisition of resistance to several phages (i.e. T3, T4 and T7) as a result of a single mutational step in sensitive bacteria. That this is due to overlapping of molecular groupings within complex attachment sites, and not to lack of specificity, is revealed by chemical analysis of the cell walls of such mutants, as well as by the existence of mutants singly resistant to each phage (Section IV A 1). In fact, analysis of *host-range mutants* of phage shows that the specificity of attachment is exceedingly high. If sensitive *E. coli* B is plated with an excess of wild-type T2 phage (designated h^+) a few colonies of *E. coli* B arise, the cells of which have the inheritable property of resistance to T2; these resistant bacterial mutants are designated B/2. If, now, an excess of the wild-type phage is plated with the resistant B/2 bacteria, a few plaques will arise from mutants of the phage, called T2*h*, which have acquired the ability to plaque on both B/2 and B. Again, by plating B/2 bacteria with T2*h* mutant phages, new bacterial mutants (B/2/*h*), resistant to both wild-type and T2*h* phages can be isolated. Similarly, phage T2*h* can yield T2*h'* mutants which plaque on B, B/2 and B/2/*h*. This process, apparently, can be repeated indefinitely (Baylor *et al.*, 1957).

An extensive genetic analysis of host-range mutants of phage T2 by Streisinger and Franklin (1956; Streisinger, 1956), showed that host range is determined by a single functional locus (cistron) on the phage chromosome; mutation at any one of many sites within this locus can modify the tail protein and lead to a change in host specificity. This investigation raised the interesting question of what is meant by the term "wild-type", for it was found that while crosses between independently isolated wild-type (h^+) phages gave rise to *h* type recombinants which could plaque both on wild-type *E. coli* B and B/2, crosses between *h* mutants did not yield recombinants of h^+ type, which had formerly been regarded as the "wild-type"; thus it seems that it is the *h* mutants which are genetically homogeneous, while the h^+ mutants are genetically diverse, although, of course, all mutants of both types produce functional tail protein.

B. Immunity

In conjugal crosses between male and female strains of *E. coli* K–12, the male bacteria transfer their chromosomes to the females in a specifically oriented way, such that a particular extremity of the chromosome is always the first to be transferred and is thereafter followed by the various male genes in the order of their arrangement on the chromosome; under standard conditions, chromosome transfer proceeds at a constant rate, so that any particular gene always begins to enter the female cells at a specific time after the commencement of mating (Wollman *et al.*, 1956). When an inducible prophage such as λ, at its location on the chromosome of a lysogenic male bacterium, is transferred to a non-lysogenic, non-immune female during conjugation, as soon as it penetrates the female bacterium it comes off the chromosome and enters the vegetative state, so that the zygote lyses and liberates infective phage particles. Such zygotes constitute "infectious centres", which can be scored by the number of plaques they produce when plated on sensitive bacteria. This phenomenon is known as *zygotic induction* (Wollman and Jacob, 1957), and only occurs when the male is lysogenic and the female is sensitive; it is not found when the male is sensitive and the female is lysogenic, although the zygotes formed in the two crosses are genetically identical (ly^+/ly^-) with respect to lysogeny, nor when both parents are lysogenic. The only essential difference between the crosses lies in the *cytoplasm* of the female; zygotic induction occurs when the prophage is introduced into the cytoplasm of a sensitive cell, but not when it enters the cytoplasm of an immune cell. This gave rise to the idea that the cytoplasm of an immune cell contains a diffusible *repressor* substance which prevents the functional activity of the prophage genes; when the prophage encounters a cytoplasm which lacks repressor, its genes are released from inhibition and initiate vegetative growth.

The fact that treatment of cells, infected by temperate phage, with agents which specifically inhibit protein synthesis (as well as other metabolic and environmental factors—review: Jacob and Wollman, 1959) results in all, instead of only a fraction, of them becoming lysogenized (Bertani, 1957) suggested that the cytoplasmic repressor might not be a protein. Fisher (1963) has recently shown, by means of a special system of conjugation between lysogenic males and sensitive females, that immunity to infection by λ phage can be *passively* transferred in the absence of chromosomal or prophage transfer. As the result, the females are rendered insusceptible to subsequent challenge by free λ phage. After transfer to sensitive female bacteria this passive immunity decays rather rapidly, and is immediately destroyed by about one third of the normal inducing dose of u.v. light. This strongly suggests that induction of lysogenic bacteria by u.v. light is due to destruction of repressor. Furthermore, when cultures of lysogenic male cells are treated with specific inhibitors of

DNA, RNA or protein synthesis, only those cultures in which RNA synthesis has been prevented lose the capacity for passive transfer of repressor; the repressor therefore appears to be composed of RNA (Fisher, personal communication).

Repressor must not only be produced by a phage gene but must also have a genetic site on which to act. Two types of mutation to virulence may therefore be envisaged. A mutation in the repressor gene itself would yield a phage which could not produce repressor and would therefore be virulent for sensitive cells, but not for lysogenic cells whose cytoplasm already contained repressor. On the other hand, mutation in the site of action of the repressor would prevent repressor from any source from shutting off the activity of the phage genes; such a mutant phage would be virulent for both sensitive and lysogenic hosts. Mutant phages of these two types have been isolated (see Jacob et al., 1960). A similar regulatory system, involving a genetically determined cytoplasmic repressor which acts on a region of chromosome (operator) actuating a series of genes concerned in a biochemical sequence, is responsible for the control of lactose fermentation in E. coli (Jacob and Monod, 1961).

Non-inducible prophages do not show zygotic induction; in addition, there is some evidence that their form of attachment to the bacterial chromosome is different from that of inducible prophages—they may be inserted (Jacob and Wollman, 1957). Nothing is known about their immunity mechanism. In the case of the non-inducible phage P2, which has three alternative sites of attachment, it is clear that site blockage is not a factor in immunity, since this is fully attained by cells lysogenized at only one site (Bertani, 1958). For a review of other data and concepts about immunity, see Whitfield (1962).

C. Exclusion and Other Related Phenomena

When bacteria are mixedly infected with two related phages, each doubly infected bacterium usually liberates both infecting types as well as new recombinant types of phage. In the case of mixed infection with two unrelated phages, however, only one of the phages is usually propagated by each doubly infected bacterium. This phenomenon is called exclusion, and was investigated in some detail by Luria and Delbrück (1942; Delbrück, 1945b; review: Adams, 1959, pp. 319–330), using the T series of virulent phages. One method used was to plate about 100 of the mixedly infected bacteria on to a lawn comprising equal numbers of reciprocally resistant indicator cells. Bacteria which liberated only one phage type thus yielded plaques which were turbid, though otherwise characteristic of the type, since it could lyse only half of the indicator cells; but if both phages were liberated clear plaques were produced. In the case of the pairs of phages T1 + T2 and T2 + T7, all the bacteria yielded only phage T2; none liberated both phages in a single burst. When one of the phages was added at various times before the other it was found, in the case of T1 and T2, that infection by T1 must have a six-minute start in order to compete with T2 on an equal basis; under these conditions, the bacteria that yielded T1 liberated this phage alone. In the case of T1 and T7, T7 was dominant in synchronous infection, but could be completely excluded by giving T1 a four-minute start. The three phages could thus be arranged in an order of dominance T2 > T7 > T1. In some cases the excluded phage has the effect of depressing the burst size of its dominant partner. There are two lines of evidence that exclusion is not due to interference with adsorption or DNA injection. One is that the depression of burst size by the excluded phage is removed if its adsorption is prevented by antiserum; another is the fact that if *E. coli*, lysogenized by λ phage, is induced by u.v. light and then superinfected with phage T5, the development of phage λ is prevented, even when the induction precedes the super-infection by nearly 40 minutes. In this case, the excluded phage is already in the cell and in the vegetative state at the time of super-infection (Weigle and Delbrück, 1951). In contrast, the related phages T2, T4 and T6 do not exclude one another but yield mixed bursts which contain recombinants in addition to the parental phages.

The mechanism of exclusion is not known, but two factors may play a role in determining it. First, studies of the sensitivity to ultra-violet irradiation of phages and their hosts, with respect to the productivity of subsequent infection, have shown that while the integrity of the host nucleus is not required for vegetative reproduction of the T-even phages, it is essential for most other phages (see Section VII D 4). It is also known that infection by the T-even phages is followed by destruction and disappearance of the host nucleus (Luria and Human, 1950). This would clearly give the T-even phages an overwhelming advantage in mixed infection with other phages. Secondly, the T-even phages display a form of exclusion which has been found to operate even when an infected cell is superinfected *with the same phage strain* some minutes later. Thus, if bacteria are initially infected with un-labelled phage, and later superinfected with genetically marked phage whose DNA is labelled with ^{32}P, not only do the markers of the super-infecting particles fail to appear among recombinants, but the phage's DNA is broken down into a low molecular weight form. This *super-infection breakdown* appears to be related to the increased DNAase activity of bacteria infected with T-even phages (review: Stent, 1959).

One of the most intriguing examples of exclusion, which is not at all understood, is the specific inability of a group of mutants of phage T4 (designated r_{II}; see Section VII B 3) to replicate in *E. coli* K-12 lysogenized by λ phage; other mutants of phage T4 can infect this strain normally, while non-lysogenic K-12 strains are fully susceptible. The mechanism of this exclusion is important because the function which is lost in r_{II} mutants is the one whose genetic determinant has been subjected to the finest possible degree of genetic analysis (Benzer, 1957; see Section VII B 3).

VII. The Phage Chromosome

There is now such an incontrovertible weight of evidence that the genetic material of both phages and bacteria consists exclusively of DNA that we may assume this to be so. The question arises as to how the genetic material is organized into a functional structure, i.e. what is the nature of the phage chromosome. The chromosomes of both bacteria and phages are too small for their behaviour to be defined morphologically with any degree of precision, so that most of our knowledge of them has had to be inferred from less direct evidence. Since the discovery that infection by phage is fundamentally a genetic phenomenon initiated by the injection of its DNA into the host cell (Hershey and Chase, 1952), and the subsequent elucidation of the physico-chemical structure of DNA (Watson and Crick, 1953a), three main tools have been used to explore the way in which the DNA is organized in the phage particle and in infected bacteria. These are genetic analysis, the employment of physical-chemical techniques to investigate the organization and behaviour of DNA at the molecular level, and radiobiological procedures. In general, the results of these different approaches have tended to support and complement one another, so that a rather unified picture is now emerging. The focal point of this unity is the model for DNA structure proposed by Watson and Crick (1953a) and now generally accepted as correct, so that results coming from various fields of study tend increasingly to be interpreted in terms of it.

A. THE PHYSICO-CHEMICAL STRUCTURE OF DNA

Chemical analysis of DNA showed that it comprises a very long-chain polymer made up of alternating molecules of deoxyribose–sugar and phosphate coupled together by phosphate–diester bonds. To each sugar is attached a nitrogenous base, of which there are four kinds: the two purines, adenine (A) and guanine (G), and the two pyrimidines, thymine (T) and cytosine (C). Each unit of the polymer, consisting of base–sugar–phosphate, is called a *nucleotide*, so that the polymer is a polynucleotide (Fig. 2(a)). From the chemical point of view it is found that in DNA, from whatever source, the ratio of purine to pyrimidine bases is unity, i.e. that $A + G = T + C$.

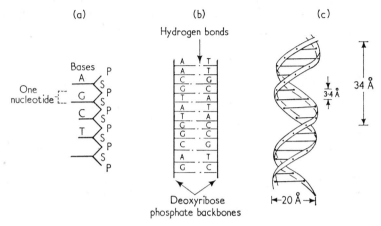

FIG. 2. The structure of DNA (Watson and Crick, 1953a).
    (a) Diagram illustrating the base–deoxyribose–phosphate arrangement of a single polynucleotide chain: P = phosphate; S = sugar (deoxyribose); A, G, T and C = adenine, guanine, thymine and cytosine, respectively.
    (b) Diagram showing specific base-pairing between the two polynucleotide chains of the double helix.
    (c) Diagrammatic representation of the double helix, giving dimensions.

X-Ray diffraction analysis of the way in which these molecules are arranged shows that the polymer has three essential structural features.

(*a*) The bases, which are flat structures, lie at right angles to the long axis of the fibre and are stacked one above the other like a pile of pennies;

(*b*) The fibre is arranged in the form of a helix.

(*c*) The fibre consists of more than one polynucleotide chain.

In the Watson–Crick model, which fits all the physico-chemical data as well as offering a plausible explanation for the biological attributes of genetic material, there are two polynucleotide chains (or strands) wound helically around one another so that the bases on each strand face inwards and are coupled together by hydrogen bonds (Fig. 2 (b), (c)). Since the purine bases (A and G) stick out further from the sugar–phosphate "backbones" than do the pyrimidine bases (T and C), the uniform diameter of the double helix can only be preserved if a purine on one strand always pairs with a pyrimidine on the other; thus, the requirement for equivalence between the purine and pyrimidine bases is satisfied. Moreover, uniformity of structure also depends on the orientation of the paired bases with respect to one another; this intro- duces the further restriction that, assuming the most stable distribution of hydrogen atoms on the bases, adenine (A) can only pair with thymine (T), and guanine (G) with cytosine (C) (Fig. 2 (b)). On the other hand, the model involves no restriction whatever on the *sequence* of bases along any one strand. The most important feature of the model is the necessity for *specific* base-pairing, since this means that each strand of the duplex is a mirror image of the other and so can serve as a template for its synthesis. Thus, replication of DNA is explained by separation and unwinding of the two strands so that newly synthesized nucleotides can bond specifically to the appropriate bases, now exposed, on each original strand. Subsequent polymerization of the backbones of these nucleotides then yields two pairs of strands (duplexes) each identical with the original one; since each new daughter duplex comprises one strand conserved from the original duplex and one newly synthesized strand, this method of replication is called *semi-conservative*. It has recently been shown to operate in *E. coli* (Meselson and Stahl, 1958; see Section VII C 4).

In addition to accounting for replication of DNA, the Watson–Crick model also explains how the genetic material may carry hereditary information in the form of a chemical code, since the only possible irregularity which could serve as a code is the sequence of the four bases, or pairs of bases, along the polynucleotide duplex. Thus, each base, or base pair, represents one letter of a four-letter alphabet from which is constructed the words that represent each of the twenty amino acids found in biological proteins (see Crick, Griffiths and Orgel, 1957). From this it follows that mutation probably results from substi- tution of a base pair (or sequence of pairs) by another (or others), so that the code is altered in such a way that one amino acid is replaced by another in the derivative protein; alternatively, if the base substitution makes "nonsense", no protein will be synthesized.

B. GENETIC ANALYSIS

Genetic analysis of phage has not only been of value in elucidating many aspects of the infective process, but has also provided a novel and refined means of attacking such problems in pure genetics as the mechanism of recombination; this latter aspect will be ignored here. The relevance of genetic analysis to the various stages of infection has already been discussed in previous sections; this section will therefore be mainly confined to a summary of the nature of the phage genetic system and how it has been used to investigate chromosome structure.

1. Mutagenesis in phage

Although phage DNA embodies all the potentialities of life, it can only express itself in the infected cell; the phage particle itself is metabolically inert. In conformity with this, it is found that treatment of a phage suspension with physical or chemical mutagens is not usually followed by any significant increase in the frequency of mutation above the spontaneous level, although the particles are inactivated exponentially by some of them (Section VIII D 1). An important exception is treatment with nitrous acid, which is able to induce mutations directly, not only in free phage particles (Tessman, 1959; von Vielmetter and Wieder, 1959) but also in tobacco mosaic virus (see Gierer, 1960) and transforming preparations of pneumococcal DNA (Litman and Ephrussi-Taylor, 1959). Nitrous acid has a direct deaminating action on the bases of DNA, changing adenine to hypoxanthine, guanine to xanthine, and cytosine to uracil. While transmutations to xanthine may be lethal since this base cannot be properly incorporated in DNA, the incorporation of uracil presents no difficulty. Uracil, however, is an analogue of thymine and would pair specifically with adenine, so that the nitrous acid transmutation of cytosine to uracil would lead, on replication of the DNA, to substitution of the original cytosine–guanine base pair by uracil–adenine; at the next replication the adenine would pair naturally with thymine, so that two replications would yield DNA molecules in which an original cytosine–guanine base pair had been changed to thymine–adenine. Among other chemical mutagens, which have a direct chemical action on DNA bases and are mutagenic for free phage particles, is the alkylating agent, ethylmethane sulphonate (EMS) (Loveless, 1958, 1959).

The fact that the only effective mutagens for free phage particles are those which can produce direct transmutation of DNA bases, implies that other mutagenic agents can only effect base substitutions in replicating DNA. Presumably, their killing action is therefore not due to induction of "lethal mutations" but to destruction of the integrity of the DNA molecule or to the production in it of "lesions" which prevent subsequent replication.

A group of chemical mutagens to which particular attention has recently been paid are the *base analogues* which are able to replace specific DNA bases in phage when infected cells are grown in media containing them; for example, replacement of thymine by its analogue 5-bromouracil is highly mutagenic (Litman and Pardee, 1956). By means of fine structure genetic analysis of phage T4, the sites and relative positions of large numbers of independent mutations have been located within a small region (called r_{II}) of the phage chromosome determining a single character (Benzer, 1957; see Section VII B 3). When the sites of spontaneous mutations were compared with those of mutations induced by 5-bromouracil, two important facts emerged. First, the mutational sites of neither class were distributed uniformly along the chromosome, but tended to be concentrated at a small number of particular sites, which Benzer (1957) called "hot spots"; secondly, the spontaneous and induced mutations showed quite different "hot spots", while the coincidence of individual mutational sites of the two classes was negligible (Benzer and Freese, 1958). Subsequent analysis of the spectrum of proflavine-induced mutations showed that, although these were more uniformly distributed, the sites were quite distinct from those induced by base analogues (Brenner, Benzer and Barnett, 1958). Moreover, base-analogue-induced mutations were not reversed by proflavine and *vice versa*. This work suggested that different mutagens may act selectively on different specific components of a single gene, which are probably the individual bases.

Very recent studies of the interaction of acridines with DNA have shown that acridine molecules can slide between adjacent pairs of bases, with some unwinding of the double helix (Lerman, 1961), and it has been suggested that their mutagenic action may be due to deletion or addition of a base pair, rather than to substitution. This may have an important bearing on our conception of the nature of mutagenesis and of how the genetic code is translated into functional terms, since it has also been observed that while mutant phages produced by base analogues can synthesize fully functional, though altered, proteins (e.g., host–range or lysozyme mutants), acridine mutants fail to do so and are restricted to those mutant types which involve a dispensible function (e.g. r_{II} mutants of phage T4) (Brenner *et al.*, 1961 b; see also Crick *et al.*, 1961).

2. Recombination analysis

The occurrence of genetic recombination between closely related phages can be demonstrated by mixedly infecting sensitive bacteria with mutant particles which differ in two or more observable characters. Among the progeny particles are found the two parental types together with two new recombinant types which display the characters of both parents in reciprocal combinations. For example, two mutants of phage T2 which differ in host range (h^+ or h) and in plaque type (r^+ or r), may be crossed; one is genetically labelled with a host-range mutation ($h.r^+$) and gives small, clear plaques when plated on a mixture of *E. coli* B and B/2 (see Section VI A); the other mutant is wild-type for host range but is marked by an r mutation ($h^+ r$) and yields large, turbid plaques on the mixed indicator (Section II B 2). When *E. coli* B is multiply infected with these two mutants ($h.r^+ \times h^+r$) and the progeny particles plated on the mixed indicator, in addition to the two parental types of plaque, large clear plaques ($h.r$) and small, turbid plaques (h^+r^+) are found (Hersey and Rotman, 1949; see Plate 4). Approximately equal numbers of the two reciprocal recombinant types appear among the progeny while, under standard conditions of infection, the proportion of recombinants to total progeny, i.e. the *frequency of recombination*, is constant. When different genetic markers are used, however, the frequency of recombination may vary widely. By applying orthodox genetical principles, according to which the distance between two markers is proportional to the frequency of recombination between them, the relative locations of various markers can thus be mapped on the phage chromosome. The study of a wide range of phage markers, especially in the T-even phages, has revealed that the phage genome is haploid and that all the markers are arranged linearly on a single linkage group or chromosome (reviews: Adams, 1959, pp. 331–364; Levinthal, 1959). By analysis of an extended range of mutations in phage T4, it has been found that as markers approach opposite extremities of the chromosome, the recombination frequency between them begins to fall, indicating linkage between the two ends of the chromosome. (Streisinger, G, Edgar, R. and Harrar, G, personal communication, 1961). Whether this surprising finding really means that the phage chromosome is a continuous structure or is due to an anomaly of the mechanism of recombination in phage, has not yet been resolved (see Section VII C 1).

So far we have considered phage recombination as if it took place in a normal mating system, directly amenable to classical genetic analysis. We have also seen, however, that phage reproduction is effected through the separate synthesis of its components in "pools" within the infected cell which are later randomly withdrawn and assembled into mature particles (see Section IV C). It seems improbable, and there is no evidence at all, that recombination can take place between mature phage particles, so that it must be assumed to occur between the replicating phage genomes in the DNA pool. This means that phage recombination must be interpreted, not in terms of static pairs of chromosomes isolated in individual zygotes, but as a dynamic system in which mating occurs randomly within a multiplying *population* of chromosomes, each member of which can indulge in a number of successive mating events, some of which may be incestuous. In such circumstances we cannot hope to discover the outcome of single mating events, and must rather regard recombination in phage as a problem in population genetics which requires mathematical treatment for its analysis (Visconti and Delbrück, 1953). This approach leads to the prediction that the frequency of recombination between two markers should be lowest among the first-formed particles, whose DNA was withdrawn early from the pool, and should then increase as a result of multiple rounds of mating; this has been confirmed experimentally by analysis of phage from prematurely lysed cells. Moreover, under conditions of lysis inhibition, the proportion of recombinants in the total yield increases linearly with time for about an hour, to reach a plateau when intracellular multiplication ceases (Levinthal and Visconti, 1953). A further complication of this system arises from the fact that about as many phage equivalents of DNA remain in the pool, and are lost at lysis, as are incorporated into particles (Fig. 1) so that the statistical assessment of rare recombination events becomes difficult, even in single-burst experiments. Nevertheless, these considerations in no way invalidate the inferences to be drawn from genetic mapping, since crosses performed under standard conditions yield reproducible results, while the effects of multiple rounds of mating can be compensated for mathematically. The only conclusion that cannot be drawn is that the frequency of recombination indicates the distance between two markers *as a proportion of the total length of the chromosome*, since the former varies with the experimental conditions while the latter remains constant; that is to say, genetic analysis permits the relative, but not the absolute, distances between markers to be measured.

There are two aspects of phage recombination which suggest that the mating event may be different from that operating in higher organisms.

(*a*) Absence of reciprocal recombinant types. There is rather convincing statistical evidence, from single-burst experiments in both T2 and T1 crosses, that reciprocal recombinant types do not issue from a single recombination event, even though both types may be found among the progeny particles (Hershey and Rotman, 1949; Bresch, 1955); this suggested that recombination was probably not mediated by a physical exchange between the mating chromosomes, and generated the idea that the recombinant chromosome might arise, during the replication of the paired parental chromosomes, from a replica which began by copying one chromosome and then switched to copy the other. This is known as the *copy-choice* model for recombination. However, recent experiments on λ phage, in which the inheritance of isotopic labels from the DNA of the parental phages has been correlated with that of genetic markers, points to an actual physical transfer of the parental DNA to recombinant chromosomes (Meselson and Weigle, 1961).

(b) Phage heterozygotes. About two per cent of the progeny emerging from "single factor" crosses (e.g. $r^+ \times r$, or $h^+ \times h$) consist of single, heterozygous particles which, on subsequent infection, yield equal numbers of both parental types together with 2% of newly formed heterozygotes; these particles contained both parental alleles of the marker which segregated again at the first replication of the chromosome. Heterozygous particles of this kind arise with the same frequency irrespective of the particular marker studied. The progeny of particles heterozygous for a particular marker are always found to be recombinant for other markers, closely linked on either side of it, in which the two original parents differed (Levinthal, 1954); this suggested that the formation of heterozygotes might be an integral part of the recombination process in phage. No comparable situation has been reported in any other organism. While nothing is known of the genetic structure or function of heterozygotes, their properties can formally be explained in terms of a single chromosome consisting of double-stranded DNA in which, at the site of the base-pair alteration which produced the mutational difference, one of the strands has inherited a base characterizing the wild-type, while the other strand has a mutant base. Suppose, for example, that the mutation from r^+ to r has been the consequence of a substitution of the base pair A–T by the base pair G–C at a particular site; the DNA duplex of the heterozygote would then have the anomalous base pair A–C (or T–G) at this site, and at the first replication would yield daughter duplexes of constitution A–T and G–C, i.e. the two parental base pairs would be reproduced and would thereafter breed true (See Section VII A).

3. The structure of the r_{11} region of phase T4

We have already referred to the plaque-type mutants known as r (rapid lysis) which produce larger and clearer plaques than do wild-type (r^+) particles (Section II B 2: Plate 1). When the mutational sites of r mutants of phage T4 are mapped by genetic analysis, they are found to fall into three clusters, r_I, r_{II} and r_{III}, which are well separated on the chromosome. Mutants of the r_{II} category differ from the others in being unable to multiply in *E. coli* K–12 lysogenized by λ prophage (which we will call "K" for short), although the bacteria are infected and killed (Benzer, 1957). When K cells are mixedly infected with wild-type and r_{II} mutant phages, the r_{II} particles multiply normally, so that they comprise about half the progeny particles. This shows that the r_{II} mutants are unable to promote the synthesis of some diffusible factor necessary for their growth, but which the wild-type phage can provide for them. Benzer found that when K cells were mixedly infected with certain pairs of r_{II} mutants normal lysis occurred, so that these mutants were defective in different functions associated with the r_{II} state and could therefore complement one another in producing normal growth and lysis. Other pairs of r_{II} mutants failed to complement one another and were therefore held to be defective in the same function. Analysis of several thousands of r_{II} mutants in this way revealed that each belonged to one or the other of two functional groups, A and B; no two mutants from the same group could complement one another, whereas complementation occurred between any Group A and any Group B mutant.

When the relative positions of a large number of r_{II} mutational sites were mapped by means of genetic crosses in *E. coli* B, in which r_{II} mutants grow normally, they were found to be arranged linearly within a very small segment of the T4 chromosome; moreover, all the Group A mutations were clustered in one region, while the Group B mutations were similarly located together in an adjacent region. These two regions of chromosome, each of which determines a different function, were termed *cistrons* (Benzer, 1957); a cistron is thus defined as a functional unit of the chromosome and is subdivisible into many mutational sites which are separable by recombination.

If any pair of non-identical r_{II} mutants of the same functional group are crossed by mixed infection of *E. coli* B, recombination between the sites of mutation results in the formation of wild-type (r^+) recombinant particles; these, unlike the parental particles, can plaque normally on K. On the other hand, *all* the progeny, which are predominantly parental r_{II} particles, yield plaques on B. Thus, the proportion of r^+ recombinants to total progeny, i.e. the recombination frequency, can be simply and accurately assessed by relating the number of plaques on K to the number on B. The method is sufficiently sensitive to detect one r^+ recombinant among 100,000 parental particles, so that the r_{II} system is ideally suited to fine-structure genetic analysis and has a resolving power in excess of that required to separate adjacent nucleotide pairs if mutations could be found that close together. The T2 chromosome is known, from chemical analysis, to contain about 2×10^5 base pairs. By translating his genetic data into these physical terms, Benzer (1957) calculated that, among his series of mutants, the nearest mutational sites separable by recombination were about 2·5 base pairs apart. Since the method of calculation involves an error which is probably less than a factor of five, it seems likely that the units of mutation and of recombination are, in fact, individual base pairs.

The picture of the phage chromosome presented by genetic analysis is therefore compatible with one double helix of DNA, of the order of 10^5 base pairs (equivalent to 34 μ) long, which possibly forms a continuous loop in infected cells. This DNA thread can be divided into small regions known as cistrons, which determine specific biochemical functions and which are of the order of 1000 base pairs long, so that the phage chromosome possesses about 100 cistrons. Each cistron, in turn, is made up of a sequence of mutational sites which can probably be equated with individual base pairs.

4. Host-controlled variation

This phenomenon, sometimes referred to as *phenotypic modification*, consists in an alteration of host range in *all* the progeny of a phage particle following a single growth cycle in a particular host; it thus differs strikingly from mutational modifications of host range, which involve only a minute fraction of progeny particles and arise independently of the host. The phenomenon may best be illustrated by an example. A phage plates with normal efficiency on host A (EOP$=1$) but with only a low efficiency on host B (EOP$=10^{-5}$); the particles isolated from one of the plaques which arise on B are now found to plate with equal efficiency on both A and B bacteria. So far there is nothing to distinguish this from host-range mutation. If, however, the particles with the extended host range are passed through a single cycle of growth on A, all the progeny particles plate with high efficiency on A bacteria only, i.e. they behave like the original phage in having a restricted host range.

Host-controlled variation of this kind is common and many virulent and temperate phages are subject to it (Luria and Human, 1952; Bertani, 1953; Anderson and Felix, 1953; Garen and Zinder, 1955; Lederberg, S., 1957). It appears to be frequently, if not exclusively, associated with lysogenization of one of the bacterial strains with a specific but unrelated prophage which immunizes the cell against the infecting phage. In many cases it has been shown that the infecting phage may attach and inject its DNA into the immune host cells, but cannot multiply in them. The ability of a small fraction of the infecting particles to overcome this immunity and yield normal infective progeny does not appear to be due to mutation in the phage, since the proportion of infectable host cells varies with their physiological condition and with the multiplicity of infection. Thus, the ability of the phage to plaque on the lysogenic host is dependent on the presence of exceptional bacteria rather than on exceptional particles; once particles have succeeded in establishing infection, their progeny become phenotypically modified so that the infection can spread through the surrounding, immune cells to produce a plaque (Lederberg, S., 1957). It has recently been shown that the immunity of the lysogenic host is due to its ability to break down the DNA of the infecting phage. Those occasional cells which do permit phage multiplication *alter the phage DNA* (but not, presumably, its bases) in some unknown way so that it can no longer be broken down. The DNA of all the progeny particles is modified in this manner. When the modified particles infect the primary host, all the newly synthesized phage genomes lose the modification, which is therefore not inheritable, so that the progeny which contain them can no longer infect the lysogenic host. On the other hand, the small proportion of progeny particles whose DNA contains even one modified polynucleotide strand conserved from the infecting particles, retains full ability to infect the lysogenic host (Arber and Dussoix, 1962; Dussoix and Arber, 1962).

In the *Salm. typhi* Vi-typing system, the specificity of some of the typing phages is due to host-range mutations, while that of others is a result of phenotypic modification (Anderson and Felix, 1953). The difference between these two types of variation has been clearly demonstrated by the fact that while the distribution of host-range mutants among wild-type populations of the typing phage is clonal, phenotypically modified adaptations of the phage show a Poisson distribution, i.e. each particle has an equal but small probability of infecting the immune host cells and becoming modified. (Anderson and Fraser, 1956).

C. PHYSICO-CHEMICAL ANALYSIS

1. Chromosomal structure of phage T2

Much effort has been devoted to attempts to characterize the organization of DNA within phage heads; in general, the DNA was released by osmotic shock, purified as gently as possible and then analysed with respect to its homogeneity and molecular weight, as well as by autoradiographic methods. The principal reason for failure to obtain consistent results in these experiments is the marked susceptibility of DNA to fragmentation by shearing forces, so that even the use of a syringe to transfer the extracted DNA can markedly reduce its mean molecular weight (Davison, 1959). Recent assessments of the organization of phage T2 DNA in the light of this finding, by two groups of workers (Davison *et al.*, 1961; Rubenstein, Thomas and Hershey, 1961), have agreed that all the DNA in each particle is present in a single structural entity of molecular weight about $1\cdot3 \times 10^8$. When intact DNA preparations are stirred at various speeds, the DNA breaks successively into half, and then into quarter, fragments at critical rates of shear; this behaviour appears to be incompatible with a continuous DNA loop and suggests that, whatever configuration the

DNA may adopt during recombination in the infected cell, it is not continuous in the phage head (Rubenstein *et al.*, 1961).

2. Chromosomal structure of phage ΦX 174

This phage, which is infective for *Shigella* and *E. coli* C, is among the smallest of the known viruses, with a mean diameter of about 20 mμ. It is polygonal in shape, being made up of 12 morphological sub-units located at the vertexes of an icosahedron, and does not possess a tail (Tromans and Horne, 1961). This phage is therefore closely similar in appearance to many small plant and animal viruses. How it transfers its genetic material to host cells is unknown. A unique feature of phage ΦX 174 is that although its genetic material consists of DNA, this DNA is in the form of a *single* polynucleotide chain. The evidence for this is twofold: first, unlike double-stranded DNA, every disintegration of incorporated ^{32}P is lethal; secondly, the ratio of purine to pyrimidine bases is not unity (Section VII A) (Sinsheimer, 1959a,b). The single-stranded DNA in each particle has a molecular weight of about $1 \cdot 6 \times 10^6$ and contains only a few thousand nucleotides. Since this is equivalent to only a few cistrons, the potentialities of the phage for protein synthesis must be severely limited. The single-stranded DNA, by itself, is infective for protoplasts of the host, but with much lower efficiency than the intact particles. There is good evidence that, on infection, strands of DNA are formed which are complementary to those of the infecting particles, and that DNA replication occurs in a normal, double-stranded DNA pool; however, when the DNA of the pool is isotopically labelled, very little of the label is ultimately transferred to the single-stranded progeny particles (Sinsheimer, personal communication, 1961). Genetic recombination has been observed to occur in this phage. There is also evidence to suggest that the phage carries its single-stranded DNA in the form of a closed loop and that only in this form is the DNA by itself infective for protoplasts (Sinsheimer, 1962).

3. RNA as genetic material of phages

Until very recently, one of the peculiar features of host–virus relationships in general was that while the great majority of plant and animal viruses have RNA as their genetic material, bacterial viruses contain only DNA, despite the fact that no striking differences are apparent between the metabolism of bacterial and animal cells. However, Loeb and Zinder (1961) have now reported the isolation of a phage which contains only RNA as its nucleic acid, and which specifically attacks only male strains of *E. coli* harbouring the sex factor.This RNA phage is very small, having approximately the same dimensions as the single-stranded DNA phage, ΦX 174 (see previous sub-section); like ΦX 174, it is polygonal in shape and appears to lack a tail. Otherwise the RNA phage behaves similarly to DNA phages but is characterized by an unusually large burst size, which may be as high as 20,000 plaque-forming units (Loeb and Zinder, 1961). DNA synthesis by the host is not necessary for phage reproduction (Cooper and Zinder, 1962). The molar ratios of the four bases of the phage RNA are: adenine $= 1 \cdot 0$, guanine $= 1 \cdot 17 \pm 0 \cdot 03$ cytidylic acid $= 1 \cdot 21 \pm 0 \cdot 06$ and uridylic acid $= 1 \cdot 13 \pm 0 \cdot 07$; presumably the RNA occurs as a single strand.

In addition, Loeb (1960) isolated in New York a number of other *E. coli* male-specific phages which fall into three serological groups, but the type of nucleic acid contained by these phages is not yet known. G. A. Maccacaro (personal communication, 1961) has independently obtained a series of *E. coli* male-specific phages from Milan sewage; the single representative of these which has been analysed is similar to the New York isolate in having RNA as its nucleic acid and in displaying a very high burst size. This suggests that RNA phages may be associated directly or indirectly with the sex factor which confers the male state on *E. coli*. One of the functions of the sex factor, which is itself composed of DNA, is to determine the synthesis of a surface entigen, which can temporarily be removed by treatment with periodate and which is necessary for the formation of conjugal unions with female bacteria (Sneath and Lederberg, 1961). Since treatment of male bacteria with periodate destroys, for a time, their capacity to adsorb the RNA phage *parri passu* with their ability to mate, although the treated cells retain their sex factor, the specificity of the phage is probably due to its adsorption affinity for the male antigen (Dettori *et al.*, 1961). Why such an affinity should be associated with RNA phages is quite unknown.

4. Chromosomal replication

The mode of replication of DNA in *E. coli* was studied by Meselson and Stahl (1958) by the method of density gradient centrifugation. All the nitrogen in the DNA bases of the bacteria was first replaced by "heavy" nitrogen (^{15}N) by growth in medium containing only ^{15}N as a nitrogen source, so that their DNA became denser than normal. The bacteria were then transferred to fresh, ^{14}N medium, so that DNA strands newly synthesized after transfer would contain only ^{14}N and therefore be of normal density. At intervals during multiplication in the ^{14}N medium, samples of the bacteria were removed and their DNA extracted, its density then being measured by centrifugation in a caesium chloride density gradient. Before the commencement of multiplication, the density of the bacterial DNA was exclusively that of ^{15}N–DNA; at the end of the first generation all the ^{15}N–DNA had disappeared and had been replaced by DNA having a density midway between that of ^{15}N– and ^{14}N–DNA, the so-called "hybrid" DNA (^{15}N–^{14}N); thereafter the amount of hybrid DNA remained constant while pure ^{14}N–DNA began to appear and increased in amount with each succeeding generation. Provided that the DNA molecules examined consisted of double helices (duplexes), as now seems certain, and not of aggregates of duplexes, these findings are only compatible with the semi-conservative mode of replication proposed by Watson and Crick (1953a), wherein the two strands of the double helix separate and each then acts as a template for the synthesis of a new strand; thus, each of the daughter duplexes is "hybrid", containing one old strand and one newly synthesized strand (see Section VII A; Meselson and Stahl, 1958).

Attempts to apply this method of investigation to the replication of phage DNA have yielded results which at first sight appear conflicting. In the case of phage T4, the phage DNA extracted from infected cells at intervals after infection, and having a molecular weight about 2×10^7, does not appear to contain hybrid molecules; if however, the molecular weight of the extracted DNA is first degraded to the order of 10^6 by sonication, then hybrid molecules are found (Kozinski, 1961). The existence of hybrid molecules can best be interpreted in terms of semi-conservative replication, but, in addition, some mechanism must exist whereby these molecules, instead of remaining together in the DNA of the chromosome to which they initially belonged, become distributed among larger molecules which are not hybrid, with the result that they are only revealed when these larger molecules are broken down. Since the genetic material of phage T4 undergoes approximately five rounds of mating in the DNA pool during the growth cycle, it seems likely that this redistribution of hybrid DNA molecules can be accounted for by genetic recombination (Section VII B 2). The temperate phage, λ, on the other hand, undergoes only about 0.5 rounds of mating during the growth cycle, and here the development of hybrid DNA molecules during replication can be demonstrated directly and without sonication (Meselson and Weigle, 1961).

D. The Radiobiology of Phage Infection

The effects of subjecting phage particles to various forms of radiation have been studied in order to reveal new facts about phage behaviour as well as to elucidate the mechanisms of radiation damage. While the former aim has undoubtedly been the more rewarding, many of the facts which have emerged have proved complex and conflicting in their nature and have generated new problems rather than solved old ones. Nevertheless, much of the information obtained from radiation studies, which previously seemed ambiguous, can now be seen to make sense, while various discrepancies in the behaviour of different phages and bacterial hosts have stimulated some productive interpretations. In this section, only those experimental findings which have led to meaningful conclusions about the nature of phage infection will be summarized (reviews: Stent, 1958; Adams, 1959; Stahl, 1959).

In general, the most profitable results have come from two kinds of investigation. The first involves the effects of u.v. light or X-rays on phage particles or on phage–bacterium complexes. In the second, the phosphorus atoms linking the nucleotides of the phage DNA are replaced by radioactive phosphorus (^{32}P), by propagating the phage in bacteria growing in a medium containing a known high specific activity of the isotope; since the half-life of the radioactivity of ^{32}P is about 14 days, the effects on the behaviour of the phage particles (or of the phage–bacterium complexes) of the decay of ^{32}P atoms to sulphur are observed by assaying them from day to day for the number of plaques (or infectious centres) (Hershey *et al.*, 1951). In practice, therefore, the effect of radiation or of ^{32}P decay is assessed in terms of the proportion of surviving particles as a function of dosage, surviving particles being defined as those that retain the ability to form plaques on sensitive bacteria.

1. The theory of inactivation by radiation

When a suspension of phage particles is treated with X-rays, or subjected to the decay of incorporated ^{32}P atoms, the number of surviving particles is found to decrease exponentially with dosage (or with the proportion of ^{32}P atoms which have decayed) over the entire dose range, i.e. if the logarithm of the number of survivors is plotted against dosage, a straight line is obtained. This is termed a "one hit" type of response and signifies that a quantum of radiation energy (or the decay of a ^{32}P atom) has a constant probability of inactivating a phage particle which behaves as a single susceptible target. A decrease in this probability indicates increased resistance of the phage and is revealed by a decrease in the rate of decline of the survival curve, i.e. its slope becomes less. In the case of u.v. irradiation of the T-even phages, the survival curve may depart slightly from the exponential and show a small shoulder, but this is usually insignificant enough to be ignored for practical purposes.

Let us now suppose that a phage particle contains two targets instead of one, the survival of only one of which is requisite for viability; at low doses of irradiation, the probability that both targets will be simultaneously inactivated by "hits" is negligible, so that nearly all the particles will survive and the survival curve will remain flat. With greater dosage, however, an increasing proportion of particles will be left with only one active target and will therefore subsequently decline as an exponential function of the dose. An increase beyond unity in the number of targets, which may be construed as phage genomes in an infected cell, is therefore accompanied by a deviation of the survival curve from the "one hit" type. At low dosage the curve is no longer exponential but shows a shoulder; as the dosage increases, the curve becomes steeper and finally falls exponentially with the same slope as

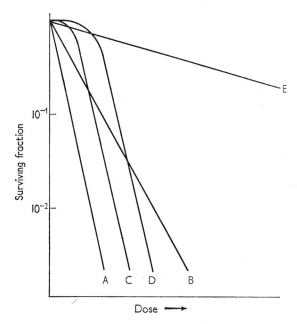

FIG. 3. Diagram illustrating the types of survival curves which may be obtained when suspensions of phage or of phage–bacterium complexes are treated with increasing doses of radiation. Curves A, B and E are "single hit" curves, showing progressively decreasing sensitivity of a single target.
Curves C and D are "multi–hit" curves, showing progressive increase in the number of targets, each of which has the same sensitivity as the single target exemplified by curve A.

that of a single target. This type of curve is called "multi-hit". The greater the multiplicity of targets, the bigger is the shoulder of the curve and the higher the dosage at which the exponential part of the curve commences.

These principles may be summarized by a comparison of the curves of Fig. 3. Curves A and B are exponential throughout the dosage range and indicate that in each case a single target is involved. Curve B, however, is less steep than curve A; this means that target B is less likely than target A to be inactivated per quantum of radiation to which it is exposed, i.e. is more resistant. This resistance could be due to target B being smaller than target A, or to the possession by target B of fewer vulnerable regions than target A so that the probability of a "hit" involving such a region is less. Curve C, on the other hand, has a shoulder at low dosage but ultimately becomes exponential with the same slope as curve A, indicating that C is composed of more than one target unit, each of which is sufficient for survival and has the same sensitivity as A; similarly, curve D represents a greater multiplicity of target units than C.

2. Multiplicity reactivation

If a suspension of phage T2 or T4 is irradiated at high u.v. dosage, it is found that virtually none of the complexes liberate phage when *E. coli* B is infected at low multiplicity. As soon as the multiplicity is increased, however, so that the bacteria become infected by more than one inactivated particle, phage is liberated with a high probability. Thus, the DNA of two or more inactivated particles can cooperate in producing normal progeny (Luria, 1947). This phenomenon is called "multiplicity reactivation". Luria (1947) proposed that each particle possessed a number of different, but equally sensitive, sub-units, all of which were required for reproduction but only a proportion of which might be inactivated by the irradiation; if a cell were infected by two phages which between them possessed one complete set of undamaged sub-units, then a reassembly of these sub-units could yield active phage. With our present knowledge of phage reproduction we may interpret these sub-units as genes and assume that recombination is the mechanism whereby a fully functional genome can be reconstituted from the damaged ones. Luria's hypothesis, as it stands, would predict that, if the mean multiplicity of infection was 2, a stage would be reached, as the irradiation dosage increased, where the damage to the two genomes would overlap with high probability, so that the formation of an intact genome by recombination would no longer be possible; beyond this point, therefore, the survival curve should fall exponentially with the same slope as for single infection. Thus, increasing multiplicity of infection should yield a family of curves comparable to C and D in Fig. 3, where A represents the curve obtained for single infection. Such curves have, in fact, been found for some phages such as *Salm. typhi* Vi (Bernstein, 1957). However, in the case of the T-even phages, as well as of phage T5, the slopes of the multiplicity reactivation curves at high dosage proved to be much less steep than those for single infection. To explain these results, the original Luria hypothesis was modified by assuming that the phage genome contains two different kinds of sub-unit with respect to radiosensitivity, one of which is reactivable with high efficiency in multiple infection, while the other, called "vulnerable centres" (Barricelli, 1956), is not. According to this idea, in single infections, where multiplicity reactivation cannot occur, the phage is rendered inactive if either a reactivable sub-unit or a vulnerable centre sustains an effective "hit"; in multiple infection, on the other hand, the effect of "hits" on the reactivable sub-units tends to be fully compensated by the efficiency of reactivation, so that the slope of the survival curves will be less steep. In practice, the curves for phage T4 were found to fit the data on the assumption that the "target" comprised about 40% vulnerable region and 60% reactivable region.

If this hypothesis is true, the question of the nature of the vulnerable centres arises. In the case of the T-even phages they can be interpreted plausibly in terms of our knowledge of the metabolic prerequisites for multiplication (Section IV C 4) and of the fine structure of the phage chromosome as revealed by Benzer's (1957) analysis of the r_{II} region of phage T4 (Section VII B 3). We have seen that the presence of 5-hydroxymethyl cytosine (HMC) in place of cytosine in the T-even phages demands the early synthesis of a number of new enzymes (non-precursor protein) before replication of the phage DNA can commence. The phage genes determining the synthesis of these enzymes might be expected to behave as vulnerable centres, since the initiation of DNA synthesis, and therefore of phage recombination in the DNA pool, depends on them. Thus, in doubly infected cells, inactivation of the function of the same gene (cistron) in both phage genomes by a "hit", involving any site (i.e. base pair of the DNA) on each of them, would prevent the commencement of DNA synthesis and therefore the possibility of recombination and multiplicity reactivation for any gene. In the case of cistrons determining other functions, however, damage sustained at different sites within an homologous pair of cistrons can be made good by recombination, so long as DNA replication can occur, although in single infection such damage would be lethal in the same way that single mutations are lethal. From this it follows that, in multiplicity reactivation, the "target size" of a gene determining precursor protein could be regarded as being the whole cistron, while that of other genes comprises only sites within the cistron and is therefore of the order of 1000 times smaller (Section VII B 3). From the point of view of target theory, therefore, a small number of vulnerable centres could appear to occupy a relatively large region of the chromosome.

Evidence favouring this interpretation comes from studies of the effects of irradiation on phage T4 when *E. coli* K-12 lysogenized by λ phage, instead of *E. coli* B, is employed as host. In this system, effective multiplication of the phage depends upon the functional activity of the A and B cistrons of the r_{II} region (Section VII B 3), so that the A and B cistrons should behave as additional vulnerable centres; this was found to be the case experimentally (review: Stahl, 1959). Multiplicity reactivation of the type shown by the T-even phages is also given by phage T5, whose DNA contains ordinary cytosine and not HMC. This does not invalidate the theory, however, since all these phages share the ability rapidly to destroy the host nucleus on infection, an ability not possessed by phages T1, T3 and T7, which show little or no multiplicity reactivation. Although phage T5 does not have to synthesize HMC, it may still be dependent on the activity of its own genome for the initiation of multiplication.

Before leaving the subject of multiplicity reactivation, some mention should be made of *cross-reactivation* or, more precisely, *marker rescue*. The experimental approach to this phenomenon is to mixedly infect bacteria with irradiated, genetically marked phage of one type, together with unirradiated phage of complementary genotype; the progeny particles, predominantly derived from the unirradiated parent, are then examined for the inheritance of genetic markers from the irradiated parent. Studies of this sort have provided evidence of the recombinational nature of multiplicity reactivation as well as quantitative information about the nature of u.v. damage. For example, a comparative assessment of the rescue of markers from the irradiated parent, whose positions on the chromosome are known from genetic mapping, has revealed that unlinked markers are independently knocked out by the irradiation with about equal probability, while closely linked markers tend to be knocked out together, indicating that the majority of u.v. "hits" result in discrete lesions whose effects on the phage chromosome are strictly localized (Doermann, Chase and Stahl, 1955).

3. The Luria–Latarjet experiment

In this type of experiment, first performed by Luria and Latarjet (1947), instead of irradiating the free phage particles, singly infected phage–bacterium complexes are irradiated at intervals after infection and the proportion of surviving infectious centres is then plotted as a function of dosage. This experimental approach was introduced as a method of studying the kinetics of the intracellular development of phage; it was thought that phage multiplication would be reflected in a series of multi-hit curves (e.g. Fig. 3, curves C and D), from whose characteristics the number of intracellular particles could be calculated. Using an improved technique, Benzer (1952) found that with phage T7 the exponential curves were much as expected in that they were roughly parallel and differed mostly in the size of their shoulders. Similar results have since been obtained with phages T1, T3 and λ. With phage T2, however, the curves obtained were quite different; up to six minutes after infection only a slight increase in u.v. resistance was found, but thereafter resistance rose rapidly until, at nine minutes, it had increased about twentyfold (Fig. 3, curves A, B and E; Benzer, 1952). Phages T4, T6 and T5 conform to the T2 pattern in this type of experiment as in multiplicity reactivation experiments.

The difference in behaviour of the two groups of phages in the Luria–Laterjet experiment can be interpreted along the same lines as before. The T-even phages are characterized by the need to synthesize a number of enzymes before DNA replication can begin, and we have seen (Section IV C 2) that these functions are performed prior to six minutes after infection, when DNA synthesis starts; before six minutes, then, no marked change in the resistance of the complex over that of free phage would be expected. From the sixth minute onwards replication of DNA is taking place and the opportunity for recombination is inceasing, so that the rapid development of resistance is ascribable to multiplicity reactivation; by this time, however, the vulnerable centres have already fulfilled their function, so that the high efficiency of multiplicity reactivation can achieve the maximum scope provided by the large number of rounds of mating which characterizes these phages. Phages T1, T3, T7 and λ, on the other hand, not only probably lack vulnerable centres as we have interpreted them, but also show only a small number of rounds of mating, so that their inherent capacity for multiplicity reactivation is insignificant.

When X-rays are employed in Luria–Latarjet experiments with the T-even phages, the same trends are observed but the results are less marked than when u.v. light is used. On the other hand, the effects of ^{32}P decay on the output of phage from cells singly infected with radioactive T2 are very clearcut; for the first five to six minutes the complexes show little or no change in resistance, while at nine minutes virtually complete resistance to ^{32}P decay has been attained (Stent, 1955; Symonds and McCloy, 1958). The simple explanation of this stabilization seemed to be that at nine minutes nearly every infected bacterium contains at least one ^{32}P-free replica of the phage chromosome. This interpretation, however, was contradicted by the finding that when not only the phage but also the bacteria and the medium contained a high specific activity of ^{32}P, the same stabilization of the complexes occurred (Stent, 1955). Multiplicity reactivation could account for this second finding; this also was excluded, however, since in other experiments no multiplicity reactivation was observed to follow the ^{32}P inactivation of phage, even when the decay was allowed to occur after infection (Stent and Fuerst, 1955). Stent therefore proposed the unorthodox hypothesis that, during replication, the information contained in the DNA of the infecting particle might be transferred to an intermediate substance, such as protein, which is not destroyed by ^{32}P decay. Recently, however, it has been shown that multiplicity reactivation of ^{32}P inactivated phage particles *does* occur, provided the host bacteria are also made radioactive (Symonds and Ritchie, 1961); the postulation of an insensitive intermediate in DNA synthesis is, therefore, no longer necessary.

4. Effect of radiation of the ''capacity'' of host bacteria (review: Stent, 1958)

Bacteria which have been sterilized, i.e. have lost the ability to multiply and form colonies, by treatment with u.v. light or X-rays, or by the decay of incorporated ^{32}P, vary widely in their "capacity" to support the growth of various types of unirradiated phage. This difference is most clearly seen in the case of the T series of phages and *E. coli* B, on which they all plaque with comparable efficiency. Thus, the capacity of *E. coli* B bacteria to yield progeny particles following infection with phages T2, T4 and T6 is highly resistant to u.v. irradiation; for example, when only an estimated 1 in 10^{13} of the bacteria survive as colony formers, one third can still act as infectious centres. On the contrary, a dose of u.v. which scarcely affects the capacity for reproduction of the T-even phages may reduce that for phages T3 and T1 by a factor 10–100. Owing to this, the meaningful analysis of Luria–Latarjet curves with these phages becomes very difficult. The capacity of host bacteria for other phages such as λ and P22 is similarly sensitive to u.v. irradiation. This supports the conclusion previously reached that while the reproduction of the T-even phages is self-supporting, that of most other phages is, to some extent, host-dependent. The effect of ^{32}P decay in reducing the capacity of bacteria to support the growth of this latter group of phages suggests that their dependence is on the integrity of the host's genome.

It further transpires that there is an inverse relationship between the radiosensitivity of the phages themselves and that of the capacity of the host bacteria to reproduce them; thus, the T-even phages are highly sensitive to radiation and to ^{32}P decay, while those phages which are host-dependent are relatively resistant. Stent (1958) therefore suggested that the relative radio-resistance of the host-dependent phages might be due to the repair of damage to their chromosomes by interaction (possibly recombination) with the nucleus of the host. The small number of rounds of inter-phage matings associated with these phages might also be due to replacement of these matings, which Stent visualized as playing a necessary role in the reproductive process, by phage–host matings; in this way, the effect of radiation in reducing the capacity of the host could also be explained. There are some additional facts to support this concept, which fits well into the general picture of multiplicity reactivation and Luria–Latajet experiments. For example, it is known that genetic homology exists between the chromosome of λ prophage and that of its host and that some form of recombination can occur between the two (Section V D 2). Again, Weigle (1953) found that if host bacteria were lightly irradiated with u.v. light prior to infection with u.v.–inactivated λ phage, the proportion of phage survivors increased by as much as a hundredfold; this "u.v.–reactivation" could be due to the stimulating effect which small doses of u.v. are known to exert on genetic recombination (Jacob and Wollman, 1955). Moreover, Weigle discovered that among the u.v.–reactivated particles there existed a very high proportion of new phage genotypes which revealed themselves as different plaque-type "mutants". Results of a similar kind have since been reported for phages T1 and T3 (review: Stent, 1958).

Acknowledgement

I wish to thank Dr N. D. Symonds for the benefit of many illuminating discussions, and for his invaluable criticisms during the preparation of this review.

CHAPTER 3

Pathways of Virus Infection

A. W. DOWNIE

*Department of Bacteriology, The University,
Liverpool, England*

I. Introduction

In recent years the emphasis in virus research has tended to be on the mechanisms of infection at the cellular level. But in order to parasitize sysceptible cells in a metazoan host, virus has to gain entry into the body of the host; in some instances it must then spread through the host tissues in order to reach cells particularly suitable for its growth; and, finally, it must eventually leave that host to infect the next. Knowledge of the mechanisms involved in this sequence may provide the means of practical control of diseases resulting from virus infection of animals or plants. This chapter is concerned then with the entry of virus, its mode of spread within the host and its eventual release from the host body.

Ideas in this field were at first based on clinical and epidemiological observations of those virus infections which led to overt disease. Thus, the clinical course of illness, the signs of involvement of various organs and the pathological changes noted in severe and fatal infections provided information from which the spread of the virus in the body could be surmised. The duration of the incubation period and epidemiological study of case to case spread served to indicate the probable mode of entry and excretion of the infecting virus. With the development of methods of identification and of quantitative estimation of viruses in body fluids or exudates, existing views were confirmed or modified. Finally, studies of experimental infections, which attempted to reproduce the diseases as naturally acquired, have served to bring our knowledge to its present state.

It may be noted, however, that while the conditions of natural infection can be closely simulated in the study of some animal and plant diseases, this is not possible in certain viral infections of man. Although experimental human infections have been profitably studied in diseases such as measles, mumps, rubella and influenza, experimental infections in human volunteers are not justifiable in diseases which may be attended by more serious consequences such as smallpox and poliomyelitis. In these, experimental studies with the causal viruses in susceptible animals may provide information on possible pathways of infection, but the results have always to be interpreted with caution. The experimental animal is often either much more or much less susceptible than the human host, and the route of infection and required dose may be quite different from those which are effective in natural disease in man. For example, the intravenous or intracerebral injection of large doses of poliomyelitis virus into rhesus monkeys helps little in our understanding of how this virus may travel from the mucosa of the alimentary tract to the anterior horn cells in human paralytic disease. Even the intracerebral injection of virus suspension in mice may tell us little of the natural mode of spread of virus within the central nervous system because of the disruptive trauma produced by the injection pressure in these small animals (Mims, 1960).

Most of the following discussion will of necessity be concerned with virus infections which are clinically manifest. Our appreciation of the prevalence and importance of latent or inapparent infection has been greatly increased in recent years by the discovery of many new viruses; but for the most part knowledge of their mode of spread is far from complete, and the question of latency will be discussed in later chapters.

II. Routes of Entry of Virus into the Host Body

Virus may gain entry to a new host by various routes. The route taken may be determined by the localization of susceptible cells, by the mode of excretion of virus from a previous host and by the ability of the virus to survive outside the animal body. While some viruses are relatively specific in their cell requirements—for example the viruses of the common cold and influenza multiply only in cells of the respiratory mucosa and the virus of molluscum only in the cells of the skin—other viruses may be able to multiply in a variety of cell types. In suitable experimental animals, viruses such as herpes simplex and vaccinia may produce disease when inoculated by the intradermal, intravenous, intranasal, intratesticular or intracerebral routes. In natural infection, however, the mode of entry is usually limited to one route. Herpes simplex virus, for example, infects through the skin and mucous membranes where growth in susceptible cells produces typical local lesions.

In virus diseases, as in infections caused by bacteria and protozoa, the routes of entry to be considered are:

Mucous membranes—respiratory route, alimentary route, other mucous surfaces such as those of the genital tract;
Conjunctiva and skin;
Subcutaneous tissues following wounds, insect bites or inoculation;
Placenta—in intrauterine infections.

A. RESPIRATORY ROUTE

The diseases spread by the respiratory route may be broadly sub-divided into two categories: those in which the incubation period is short and the infection remains confined to the respiratory mucosa, such as the common cold and influenza, and those in which, although the site of entry is believed to be the respiratory mucosa, the symptoms are referable to generalized infection with involvement of tissues elsewhere in the body. The exanthemata and mumps in man and dog distemper and some pox diseases of animals are of this latter kind, and in these the incubation period is usually at least 10 days and may be much longer.

1. Mechanism of transfer

In most instances the exact mechanism of transfer of virus to the respiratory mucosa is not precisely known. The virus is usually inhaled, either in infected dust or more directly in droplet nuclei from the mouth or respiratory tract of another infected person. Direct spread through relatively large droplets of respiratory mucus or saliva requires fairly close contact, as such droplets rapidly fall to the ground.

Dust may be infected by larger droplets expelled through the mouth or nose, or by infective material from the skin or by dried faeces—for example from the soiled plumage of sick birds in psittacosis. Clinical and pathological evidence indicates involvement of lung parenchyma in human psittacosis, suggestive of inhalation of virus in small particles deep into the respiratory tract. Epidemiological evidence of airborne spread of this virus to man has been obtained from the distribution of cases in the vicinity of premises where infected turkey carcases were being processed (Langmuir, 1961).

The importance of infection by inhalation of infected dust will depend on the ability of virus to survive outside the host organism. Like bacteria, viruses vary in their resistance to environmental conditions, although, because of the lack of sensitive methods for their detection, exact information is often lacking. The virus of smallpox seems to be particularly resistant. Advantage was taken of this many centuries ago by the Chinese, who used dried scabs inserted into the nose as a means of variolating susceptible children. In the early days of immunization with cowpox, the virus from vesicle fluid was preserved dried on cotton threads or on ivory points. Smallpox virus survives in crusts and dried pustule fluid for months at room temperature (Downie and Dumbell, 1947) and up to six months in raw cotton at suitable temperatures and humidity (MacCallum and McDonald, 1957). The resistance of this virus in bedclothes has been demonstrated by the occurrence of smallpox in laundry workers (Parker, 1952); but whether in such cases infection is conveyed by the hands to nose or mouth or through the air as contaminated dust has not been determined. Herpes simplex virus has similarly been recovered from dried crusts, but the virus of chickenpox cannot usually be isolated from such material by present methods of tissue culture (Weller, Witton and Bell, 1958; Taylor-Robinson, 1959).

The viruses of measles, influenza and the common cold appear to be less resistant to environmental conditions than the virus of smallpox. In such diseases droplet nuclei may well be important in the spread of infection for transmission was not entirely prevented by the nursing of patients in separate rooms in infectious diseases hospitals (Harries, 1935). Moreover the spread of measles was greatly reduced in schools by u.v. light irradiation of classrooms (Wells, Wells and Wilder, 1942), a result which suggested that infection in such a community was normally spread by droplet nuclei.

A good deal of study has been devoted to the importance of particle size, in relation to penetration into the lower part of the respiratory tract of man (Davies, 1949) and of animals (Druett et al., 1953, 1956, Hatch, 1961). Particles greater than 6 μ in diameter are retained in the nose and even with mouth breathing they would hardly penetrate deeper than secondary bronchi (Davies, 1949). At 2 μ, passage through the nose is considerable and a small proportion of the inhaled particles reach the alveoli. Retention is enhanced by slow and deep breathing. These observations on the inhalation of inert particles in man have been confirmed by observations on the infectivity for animals of bacterial aerosols. In guinea-pigs exposed to *Past. pestis* in aerosols of particle size 1 μ to 6 μ the infection was primarily pneumonic (Druett *et al.*, 1956 a). Similar results have been obtained in guinea-pigs and monkeys exposed to aerosols of *Past. pestis* by Goodlow and Leonard (1961). With *Brucella suis* in guinea-pigs much smaller doses were required to infect with aerosols of single organisms than with 12 μ particle aerosols. It was suggested that this was because *Br. suis* multiplied more rapidly on the surface of the lower reaches of the respiratory tract (Druett *et al.*, 1956b). Duguid (1946) concluded from his observations on the sizes of droplets and droplet nuclei resulting from sneezing, coughing and talking, that droplet spray was unlikely to give rise to true airborne infections unless very large numbers of pathogens were present in the secretions in the anterior part of the mouth. But this does occur in the acute stage of smallpox, chickenpox and measles, because of the release of virus from lesions in the buccal mucosa; and, in mumps, saliva from affected glands may have a high concentration of virus. Spread of these infections by droplet spray may, therefore, occur.

In some diseases infection may be transmitted by indirect contact; for example, by means of the hands contaminated from articles such as towels soiled by the respiratory mucus or saliva of an infected person. It may well be that the relative importance of droplet nuclei, dust, or other indirect contact varies in different diseases depending on the resistance of the virus to drying. The studies of Lovelock *et al.*, (1952) on transmission of the common cold showed that infection could be transmitted by droplet nuclei from persons suffering from natural colds or in mists produced by a Collinson-type spray from nasal secretions of such persons. However, little success was obtained in transmission experiments when secretions were painted on the outside of the nose, or when infective secretions were dried on strips of gauze which were then inserted within the nostrils for two hours. Experiments of this kind suggested that the viruses used were readily inactivated by drying and that indirect spread was relatively unimportant in transmission of the common cold. However, the low rate of transmission in many of these experiments may have been due in part to the variable susceptibility of adults to infection with common cold virus. As Williams (1960) has pointed out, in spite of many bacteriological studies on the potential importance of the mechanisms of spread, "What has not been attained is convincing evidence as to which of the various ways is most commonly employed by the pathogens causing natural human disease". This statement is applicable to virus and bacterial pathogens alike.

2. Infections confined to the respiratory tract

The commonest infections in this group are the common cold and influenza. Although infection by these viruses is followed by the appearance of antibody in convalescence, suggesting that virus antigen reaches antibody forming cells in mesodermal tissues, the cells damaged by virus appear to be limited to the respiratory mucosa.

In the common cold it seems to be chiefly the respiratory epithelium of the nose and nasopharynx that are involved, and infection is most readily induced by instillation of virus into the noses of volunteers who have little or no serum antibody to the strains used (Bynoe et al., 1961). The successful cultivation of common cold viruses was achieved by Tyrrell et al. (1960) and Tyrrell and Bynoe (1961) in cultures of human embryonic tissue or, in some instances, of monkey kidney cells; the pH of the medium was on the acid side of neutrality and cultures were incubated at a temperature a few degrees below normal body temperature. These conditions of temperature and pH are those found at the surface of the mucosa of the nasopharynx, so it would appear that common cold viruses have, in the course of their evolution, become adapted to grow and produce cell damage in such an environment. As yet there is no evidence that they produce lesions elsewhere in the body. It may be that, in adapting to environmental conditions as found in the nasopharynx, they have lost the ability to multiply in other situations.

In influenza, clinical and pathological observations suggest that the mucosa of the respiratory tract is primarily involved. Virus has occasionally been recovered from internal organs after death (Kaji et al., 1959, Flewett and Hoult, 1958) but this is exceptional. The observations of Hers and Mulder (1951 and 1961) indicate that the surface epithelial cells are chiefly affected and the changes in the human respiratory mucosa resemble those observed in the nasal mucosa of ferrets infected experimentally (Francis and Stuart-Harris, 1938). The examination by fluorescent-antibody techniques of cells from nasal washings of patients in the acute phase of influenza showed that the epithelial lining of the nasal passages contained virus antigen (Liu, 1956). However, examination of cells in bronchial mucus (Liu, 1961) and biopsy specimens from cases of uncomplicated influenza (Walsh et al., 1961) confirm the clinical evidence that the bronchial epithelium is frequently invaded. Extension of infection to the respiratory bronchioles and alveoli rarely occurs in uncomplicated cases. There is, however, evidence from the studies of Hers, Masurel and Mulder (1958) and Hers and

Mulder (1961) that influenza virus may occasionally produce an infection extending down to the alveoli with patchy pneumonic consolidation. This is most likely to occur in persons with chronic lung or heart disease, in whom presumably the mucociliary mechanism, being relatively inefficient, is less likely to prevent the spread of infection to the lower parts of the respiratory passages. In the series of fatal influenza infections studied by Hers and Mulder (1961) spread of virus to lung tissue was most commonly associated with bacterial infection, particularly by staphylococci. While the virus infection, by destroying mucociliary function, favoured the spread of *Staphylococcus* down the respiratory tract, it seems that the subsequent destructive effect of staphylococcal toxins permitted an extension of virus to the respiratory bronchioles and alveoli. The histological and cytological observations in influenza and the clinical course of the disease would seem to suggest, therefore, that the primary site of virus multiplication may be either in the nasopharynx or lower down in the trachea or bronchi.

3. Infections of respiratory tract by viruses also producing lesions elsewhere

Several viruses which sometimes cause respiratory tract infections are much less strictly limited to this tissue than are common cold and influenza viruses. Of these, the adenoviruses constitute an interesting group. They were first isolated from tissue cultures of tonsillar and adenoidal tissue removed from children without any obvious signs of virus infection—hence their name—but have since been shown to be capable of causing respiratory disease, especially in children. Such infections may take the form of atypical pneumonia, pharyngo-conjunctival fever or epidemic kerato-conjunctivitis. Enlargement of local lymph glands often accompanies these conditions. Moreover, adenoviruses have been found as a cause of mesenteric adenitis in children (Kjellén, 1955; Steyn and Bell, 1961) and one type, type 3, has been reported as a possible cause of gastroenteritis (Duncan and Hutchison, 1961). There is thus clear evidence that at least some of the adenoviruses possess a greater potentiality of tissue invasion than do the common cold and influenza viruses.

The adenoviruses also exhibit a tendency to persist in the tissues after primary infection, in a manner reminiscent of herpes simplex virus. In a two-year survey of the faeces of normal children they were found more often than were Echo viruses (Spicer, 1961). Apparently they can continue to survive in lymphatic tissue even after the development of specific antibodies. This prolonged latency in children suggests a well-adjusted host–virus relationship, and this theory is further supported by their behaviour in cultures of human epithelial cells as reported by Fisher and Ginsberg (1957). These workers found that in such cultures cytopathic changes appeared slowly and that the infected cells continued to metabolize.

Enteroviruses are occasionally associated with respiratory tract infection—Coxsackie A strains with herpangina and Echo viruses with pharyngitis, bronchitis, etc.—although these viruses are more often associated with disease in other parts of the body. In human volunteer experiments with Echo viruses (Tyrrell and Buckland, 1960; Buckland et al., 1961), respiratory symptoms sometimes followed intranasal infection, but abdominal distension and diarrhoea were also noted.

The Echo viruses and adenoviruses obviously differ from those of the common cold and influenza viruses in the variety of their pathogenic potentialities. The common cold and influenza viruses must be swallowed in large amounts by patients suffering clinical infection, but they produce no symptoms of intestinal or generalized infection. Perhaps they are less resistant to gastric acidity than enteric viruses, or they may be inactivated by bile or intestinal secretions, for they have not apparently been isolated from normal faeces in enterovirus surveys. The tissue culture methods used in such surveys probably were not suitable for the detection of common cold viruses, but there is little evidence that influenza virus persists even in the respiratory tract of patients or contacts for more than a few days. Perhaps virus might be demonstrated in the faeces of acute cases of influenza by suitable techniques, but the epidemiology of outbreaks does not suggest that faecal contamination is of any importance in the spread of the disease. The inability of common cold and influenza viruses to infect through the intestinal mucosa is paralleled by a similar inability of, for example, Bordetella pertussis or the pneumococcus to infect by this route; but there is no evidence to indicate that similar factors may be involved.

4. Viruses entering by the respiratory tract but producing generalized disease

In the exanthemata and mumps, the virus is believed to enter the tissue through the mucosa of the upper or lower respiratory tract. Evidence of the spread of measles by droplet nuclei has been mentioned previously; because of the small size of such infective particles, which may escape the filtering action of the nose and nasopharynx, the lower respiratory passages are subject to direct invasion, though this does not of course exclude the possibility of virus entry through the mucosa of the nose or nasopharynx. It has been shown that typical infection with the normal incubation period could be produced in human volunteers by spraying mumps virus (Henle et al., 1948) or rubella virus (Anderson, 1949) into the back of the throat. These experiments did not indicate the point in the respiratory tract at which virus gained entry to the tissues. However, in the most successful of Anderson's four experiments the infective material was atomized to give droplets of approximately 0.4 mμ diameter; droplets small enough to reach the smaller bronchioles and alveoli.

In the diseases under discussion 10 or more days elapse from the time of infection until the onset of illness, and during most of this period patients are not infectious. This is indicated by the occurrence of fresh cases at regular intervals of 10–16 days, depending on the incubation period of the disease under consideration. (For chickenpox, measles and mumps, see Pickles, 1939; for smallpox, see Dixon, 1948.) The control of smallpox by isolation of patients is based on the belief that patients are not infectious in the incubation period. Henle *et al.* (1948), in virological studies of children infected by mumps virus sprayed into the throat, provided more direct evidence by their failure to recover virus from the saliva until 11 days after exposure.

The spread of viruses throughout the tissues during the incubation period will be considered later. Here we are concerned with means by which virus gains entry. The lack of infectivity of patients in the incubation period must mean that infective virus is not discharged from the respiratory tract in significant amounts at this time. This raises several questions. Does the infecting particle multiply in superficial epithelial cells at the point of entry and, if so, why is the patient not infective for his contacts? If primary multiplication does not occur in superficial epithelial cells, how does virus reach the deeper tissues where multiplication is to take place? Definite answers to these questions are not possible from the evidence available. There is no clinical or pathological evidence of a primary lesion in respiratory mucosa in the early days of the incubation period. If virus does multiply in respiratory epithelial cells at the point of entry, virus released may be taken up by phagocytic cells and transferred within these to underlying lymphoid tissue. The small amount of virus liberated on the surface of the mucosa may be swallowed or, if discharged, be insufficient in amount to infect susceptible contacts. The observations of Duguid (1946) suggest that dissemination, to the environment, of bacteria in the trachea or bronchi does not readily take place unless inflammatory changes and excess secretion induce bouts of coughing. It is, however, apparent that the viruses of chickenpox, smallpox, measles, etc., do not, as does the virus of influenza, spread rapidly along the respiratory mucosa in the early days of the incubation period. Yet when clinical illness becomes manifest, numerous lesions appear in the throat and mucosa of the mouth, and the patient is then highly infectious. These mucosal lesions, however, result from infection of the lower epithelial layers by virus from the underlying capillaries. It is uncertain whether the virus at this stage is in some way different from the original infecting virus, whether it is a question of the number of particles reaching the epithelium or whether there is a difference in susceptibility of superficial and deeper epithelial cells of the mucosa.

Another possibility which might account for the lack of infectiousness in the incubation period is that there is no multiplication of virus in epithelium at the site of entry, but that the infecting particle is taken up by phagocytic cells and transported to deeper tissue. This seems to happen in infections with the tubercle bacillus, as primary tuberculosis of lymph glands in the neck may occur without evidence of a lesion in the mucosa of the upper respiratory tract. There is evidence of such an occurrence in infections of ferrets and dogs with the virus of dog distemper. This virus has some serological affinities with that of measles and resembles it in certain physical and chemical properties (Palm and Black, 1961). The illness induced by intranasal infection in the ferret is similar to that of the natural disease in dogs. Liu and Coffin (1957) followed the early stages of infection in the ferret by examining the tissues of animals for virus antigen by fluorescent antibody. The antigen was first detected in phagocytic cells in the respiratory mucosa and then it appeared in increasing amounts in the local lymph nodes from the second day onwards. Thereafter antigen was detected in other internal organs but was not found in the nasal or bronchial epithelium until after the seventh day, when the animals had become febrile. In similar studies on mice infected by the respiratory route with aerosols of ectromelia virus, this virus appeared to be taken up by phagocytic cells in the bronchioles and transported in these to underlying tissues (Roberts, 1963). These experimental observations suggest that a similar sequence of events in the exanthemata in man might explain the absence of spread of infection from persons incubating these diseases.

It has been suggested by Papp (1956) that the conjunctiva is the important route of entry in measles infection. The presence of conjunctivitis in many patients in the first few days of illness can scarcely be regarded as evidence of this site of entry, for at this time virus is already present in the blood and lesions appear in the mouth. She has claimed that the wearing of goggles by child contacts or the dropping of measles antibody on the conjunctiva will protect them from infection, but these observations have not so far been confirmed. Bynoe et al. (1961) succeeded in inducing colds in human volunteers by the conjunctival route. As they point out, however, fluid dropped into the conjunctival sac quickly reaches the nasal mucosa through the lachrymal duct. The conjunctival route produced the same number of colds as did the nasal. In their experiments with Newcastle disease virus in young chicks, Andrewes and Allison (1961) did not succeed in protecting contact chicks from infection by providing them with "spectacles".

The recent observations on "spontaneous" measles infection in monkeys raises interesting questions relating to latent infection in man. The disease may be produced experimentally in the monkey by spraying virus into the throat of susceptible animals (Blake and Trask, 1921). However, monkeys readily acquire inapparent measles infection through contact with man, and in consequence they become immune to experimental infections (Peebles *et al.*, 1957). The observations of Ruckle (1958), who isolated measles virus in tissue culture from 17 of 99 batches of monkey kidney cells, suggest that the inapparent infection in these animals may be generalized. There is, however, no evidence of the route by which virus enters the body of the monkey. Moreover, the source of infection is often not apparent. Recently trapped monkeys have no antibody in their blood and are susceptible to experimental infection with measles virus. Monkeys found to be immune may have had no known contact with humans clinically infected with measles. These observations suggest that subclinical measles infection may also occur in man and that the monkey may be a more sensitive indicator of such occurrence than susceptible human contacts. The epidemiology of the disease in man does not, however, support the view that such hypothetical subclinical infections play any part in the spread of the disease.

B. Alimentary Tract

Virus entering the mouth through direct or indirect contact may gain entry to the tissues through the buccal or pharyngeal mucosa. There may be a primary lesion in the mouth as in foot-and-mouth disease, in primary herpetic infection and in herpangina. In the first of these examples, primary lesions are rapidly followed by generalization with lesions in the skin, the skeletal muscles and elsewhere. In herpes simplex the primary infection in young children is often manifest as a general stomatitis, but even in young children the primary infection may not produce clinically apparent disease. In a group of children under three years of age kept under close supervision in an institute in Melbourne, 29 developed antibody to herpes virus during the 11-month period of observation; of these, 20 suffered from clinical stomatitis (Anderson and Hamilton, 1949). This gives a much lower rate of subclinical primary infection than that estimated by Scott—90% (Scott 1957). The carrier rate detectable by isolation of virus from saliva (or faeces) appears to vary with age. Buddingh and his colleagues (1953) found in healthy children in New Orleans that the salivary carrier rate decreased from 20% in children aged seven months to two years to 2·5% among adults. It is not certain whether the lower carrier rate with increasing age is due to increasing titre of antibody as a result of repeated antigenic stimulation, to increased thickness of the mouth epithelium or to other factors. The frequent finding of virus in the saliva of carriers supports the commonly held view that in latent herpes infections the virus survives in epithelial cells of the oral mucosa.

There is still uncertainty as to the site of initial penetration of poliomyelitis virus in the alimentary tract. Evidence has been brought forward from human studies, as well as from experimental infection in cynomolgus monkeys and chimpanzees, in support of both the oropharynx and bowel as sites of entry, so it may well be that either site may serve in different individuals. Virus has been found both in the wall of the pharynx and tonsils and wall of the bowel in fatal cases of poliomyelitis (Sabin and Ward, 1941a). However, observations of this kind are of little value in determining the tissue first infected, for in such cases virus will have been distributed by the bloodstream at an early stage of illness. Faber and Silverberg (1946) concluded from detailed histological study of the nervous system of fatal cases that the distribution of lesions in peripheral nerve ganglia and the CNS indicated the oropharynx rather than the bowel as the site of virus entry. On the other hand, Howe and Bodian (1941) concluded from similar studies that virus spreads to the CNS from the bowel more often than from the pharynx. Conclusions drawn from such histological observations were mostly based on the belief that virus reaches the nerve ganglia and CNS from the periphery along nerve pathways—a belief not now universally held (Bodian, 1956). The occurrence of bulbar paralysis following tonsillectomy has been regarded as evidence of the presence of virus in the tonsillar area; and bulbar poliomyelitis has been produced in cynomolgus monkeys by the operation of tonsillectomy following the application of virus to the pharynx (Faber et al., 1951). The more frequent occurrence of paralytic poliomyelitis in cynomolgus monkeys after simple feeding of virus than after feeding virus in capsules suggested to Faber, Silverberg and Dong, (1948) that in this animal the virus infected more readily through the oropharyngeal than through the intestinal mucosa. In clinical cases of poliomyelitis in humans, virus is usually present in the throat in the acute phase of the disease but cannot usually be recovered from this site at later stages when virus is still being excreted in the faeces. Many years ago, Aycock and Kessel (1943) observed that in families where case-to-case spread seemed to occur, infection was transferred from the initial case during the acute phase of the disease—that is, at a time when virus is most readily found in the throat. The value of such evidence is, however, doubtful because of the high carrier rate amongst family contacts and the possibility of transfer of virus from a carrier within the family. Much of the epidemiological evidence favours faecal contamination as a mode of spread of virus within human communities; but even so, from such a source the oropharynx might be as readily infected as the lower alimentary tract.

Little is known of the location of cells in which primary multiplication of poliomyelitis virus occurs. The finding of virus in throat swabs or faeces in cases of poliomyelitis, in contacts or in healthy carriers, might suggest that virus multiplies in the superficial epithelial cells of the mucosa. However, neither in experimentally infected monkeys nor in the tissues of fatal human cases is there any cytological evidence of viral damage in mucosal epithelium or underlying mesodermal tissue of the alimentary tract. It is evident that the necrotizing effect of poliomyelitis virus on epithelial and fibroblast cells, which is so strikingly apparent in tissue culture, does not occur in the intact animal. It seems that in the animal body cells other than those of the central nervous system are under hormonal, or other unknown physiological, control mechanisms which protect them against the cytopathic action of the virus. The low titre of virus found in lymph nodes of monkeys which have been fed virus might be due to collection of virus which had multiplied elsewhere (Wenner and Kamitsuka, 1957; Wenner et al., 1959). Thus in spite of the large amount of work done on this subject we are still ignorant of the exact site of implantation and multiplication of the virus in natural human infections. The difficulty in arriving at a definite decision is due in part to the failure of poliomyelitis virus to produce an obvious lesion, or even microscopically visible damage to the cells, at the site of initial multiplication, and partly to the fact that virus taken into the body by mouth, or by inhalation, may have ready access to both the oropharyngeal and the intestinal mucosa, for it has been shown by Barski, Macdonald and Slizewicz (1954) that this virus is resistant to gastric juice. The finding of virus in faeces is not of itself very helpful, as such virus might come from any part of the mucosa of the upper or lower alimentary tract—or from the secretions of liver or pancreas.

In infections with other enteroviruses—Echo and Coxsackie—we have no more exact knowledge of the site of penetration or multiplication than we have for poliomyelitis. Outbreaks of gastroenteritis due to different types of Echo viruses have frequently been reported in recent years. In these outbreaks symptoms might be due to extensive multiplication of virus in the mucosa of the alimentary tract; while such multiplication almost certainly occurs, virus is not necessarily confined to the bowel. Klein, Lerner and Finland (1960) reported two patients who suffered from vomiting, chills, abdominal cramp and diarrhoea and from whom Echo virus was found in blood serum as well as in rectal swabs.

The great majority of infections with enteroviruses remain sub-clinical, as indicated by the frequent finding of these viruses in the stools of healthy children. In these asymptomatic infections the type of cell in which virus multiplies is not known. However, antibody forma-tion frequently results, and it is probable that in such individuals virus spreads beyond the intestinal mucosa to antibody-forming cells in the submucosa or mesenteric lymph nodes. The presence of virus in stools could conceivably result from virus multiplication in the liver and excretion in the bile. The occurrence of sporadic cases, or occasionally outbreaks, of severe clinical illness in the form of aseptic meningitis, epidemic pleurodynia, etc. is evidence of the ability of at least certain strains of enteroviruses to spread throughout the body and multiply in various organs and tissues.

The alimentary tract is generally regarded as the route of infection in infectious hepatitis. This view is supported by the results of feeding infective material in capsules, and by the occurrence of waterborne outbreaks, such as that recently described by Anderson (1957). The site of initial multiplication of this virus is uncertain, nor are we better informed of the tissue in which virus multiplication takes place during the prolonged incubation period. This is considered later in the dis-cussion on serum hepatitis.

The infection of dogs known as salmon poisoning confined to a certain area of the North-west of the U.S.A., has an unusual mode of infection (Cordy and Gorham, 1950; Shope, 1954). Affected animals suffer from an acute, frequently fatal, infection after eating salmon or trout infected with meta-cercariae of the fluke *Troglotrema salmincola*. With the development of the fluke in the dog, acute symptoms appear, due to a virus or rickettsial-like agent (Philip, Hadlow and Hughes, 1954) acquired with the metacercariae; the disease can be artificially transmitted to other dogs with the blood of sick animals. In this instance, as possibly also in swine influenza, the virus, acquired by ingestion, is apparently derived from a parasitic worm, which had presumably become infected with virus from a mammalian host at an earlier stage in its life history.

C. OTHER MUCOUS SURFACES, CONJUNCTIVA AND SKIN

Virus infections of the genital tract in man occur by direct venereal contact; at least two viruses may be transmitted in this way, those of lymphogranuloma venereum and of inclusion conjunctivitis. While the former may spread to deeper tissues, the latter remains in the superficial epithelium, giving rise to a mild or asymptomatic infection in the female and a form of nonspecific urethritis in the male. The conjunctiva of the child at parturition is highly susceptible to contact infection during birth. Neither the virus of inclusion conjunctivitis nor that of lymphogranuloma survives long outside the body, but the mechanism of infection by direct contact of susceptible epithelial surfaces ensures transmission to fresh hosts. Indirect contact infection may also occur through fomites, and in swimming-bath conjunctivitis, caused by the virus of inclusion blenorrhoea, infection occurs through water infected by discharges from the genital tracts of infected bathers. Because of the susceptibility of the virus to mild chemical disinfectants, it is believed that chlorination eliminates this risk (Thygeson and Stone, 1942). The virus of trachoma, also transmitted by direct implantation on the conjunctiva, produces lesions only on the conjunctiva and immediately subjacent tissue.

The two outstanding virus infections confined to the skin of man, warts and molluscum contagiosum, like certain virus papillomas of animals, result from direct inoculation or contact, possibly through abrasions in the skin. The incubation period may be prolonged. Virus from plantar warts after being grown in cultures of monkey kidney monolayers through six passages, produced common warts on intradermal injection in 12 of 20 volunteers after periods of 3–12 months. An ultrafiltrate of material from two of these volunteers produced, within 8 months after inoculation, typical warts in 9 of 17 volunteers (Mendelson and Kligman, 1961). Like the virus of trachoma, the causal agents show a high degree of tissue and host specificity; after implantation they give rise to localized hypertrophy of skin epithelium, and show little tendency to invade deeper tissues. This contrasts with the behaviour of fowl-pox and cowpox viruses. Abrasions or minor wounds of skin are frequently the portals of entry in naturally acquired disease due to these viruses; but although hypertrophy and specific changes occur in the epithelial layers primarily invaded, the viruses invariably spread to the underlying mesodermal tissues.

In some virus diseases of plants, spread may occur through contact of the leaves of affected plants with those of a healthy plant. In this case, however, it is believed that injury to the plant cuticle through friction of contiguous leaves is necessary to allow transfer of virus to the susceptible cells of the healthy plant (Bawden, 1950).

D. Direct Implantation to Tissue Underlying Skin

Virus may reach subcutaneous tissues by direct implantation in one of three ways: through breaks in the skin resulting from injury, through inoculation by insects and by artificial inoculation. The first two categories, in contrast to the third, may be regarded as mechanisms operating in natural infections. Infection by artificial inoculation is usually incidental to prophylactic or therapeutic injections or to the taking of blood samples.

1. Implantation resulting from injury

This is a relatively infrequent mode of virus transmission, and the three instances selected for discussion, rabies, pseudorabies and B virus, all involve transmission of virus between unrelated animal species. Rabies is an example of a virus infection which depends for its overt manifestations in carnivores and man on severe trauma inflicted by the bite of an animal whose saliva contains virus. This dependence is probably due to the mechanism of spread of virus from the periphery to the CNS, as discussed in a later section. The likelihood of the disease developing appears to depend not only on the amount of virus in the saliva of the animal inflicting the wound but also on the location and severity of tissue damage caused by the biting. In man, bites on the hands and face are more likely to be followed by symptoms of rabies than bites elsewhere, because of the increased probability of damage to nerves (see Johnson, 1959). In cattle and in man, rabies is usually of a paralytic type, and infection of these hosts is of no value for the survival of virus in nature, whereas the long incubation period of the disease and the "furious" form which is encountered in carnivores such as dogs, foxes, wolves, etc., ensures it continuous transmission to fresh hosts. But the survival of virus in nature may depend more on the asymptomatic carrier state of vampire bats, skunks or other small carnivores (Johnson, 1958).

Pseudorabies in cattle is a fatal infection also involving the CNS. The virus is believed to gain entry through minor abrasions of the skin of cattle from contact with the infected snouts of pigs kept on the same premises (Shope, 1954). In pigs, which are the natural hosts, the virus produces only a mild, often inapparent respiratory infection, and virus may be present on their noses. Human infections with B virus (*Herpes virus simiae*) are occasionally acquired from the bite of a monkey carrying virus in its saliva. In the natural simian host, infection produces relatively trivial disease comparable to that caused by herpes simplex in man (Keeble, Christofinis and Wood, 1958).

It may be noted that in all these three diseases the outcome of infection in the "unnatural" host is usually fatal, while in the natural host, at least with pseudorabies and B virus, the infection is mild or even inapparent. This is possibly because implantation through injury is a purely accidental mode of virus entry and its rarity of occurrence has allowed no opportunity for the evolution of a host–virus relationship resulting in mild disease or inapparent infection.

2. Transmission by insects

This section is not concerned with the viruses which are responsible for diseases in insects, of which several hundred have been described, mostly affecting larvae of lepidoptera, hymenoptera and diptera (see Bergold, 1958); these viruses do not appear to parasitize other animals. We are concerned rather with diseases of animals for which arthropods serve as vehicles of transmission, although in some instances multiplication of virus within the insect may occur without producing obvious pathological effects. Insect transmission of virus infections to animals is usually effected by blood-sucking mosquitoes, sandflies or ticks. Transmission may be mechanical or may not occur until after the virus has multiplied in the insect vector—biological transmission.

Mechanical transmission by insects seems to be surprisingly rare in view of the wide opportunities which exist for its adoption in nature. One might expect that the enteric viruses which are excreted in faeces would be widely distributed by flies on both their feet and their mouth parts, but there is no convincing evidence that any virus infections are transmitted in this way. It is true that both blow-flies and house-flies have been shown experimentally to excrete poliomyelitis virus in the faeces after laboratory feeding on virus-infected human stools but there is no evidence either that the virus multiplies in such insects or that they constitute a source of infection in nature (Melnick and Penner, 1952). Theoretically, of course, it is possible that not only enteric diseases but also diseases such as trachoma and even smallpox, in which superficial lesions are both accessible and very heavily contaminated with virus, may be transmitted by such means, but it seems most unlikely that contaminated flies are of any real importance in this connection.

In certain infections of lower animals, however, mechanical, as opposed to biological, transmission by biting insects is an important, or even essential, mechanism. This has been shown for fowl-pox (Kligler and Ashner, 1929), rabbit fibroma (Kilham and Dalmat, 1955) and rabbit papilloma (Dalmat, 1958). In pig pox the work of Shope (1940) suggests that the louse may be important in transmission. It has been suggested by Fenner (1959) that mechanical transmission by arthropods will be implicated in the majority of animal diseases characterized by lesions of the skin, such as contagious pustular dermatitis of sheep, sheep-pox, lumpy skin disease and cowpox. This method of transmission has most intensively studied in myxomatosis by Fenner and his colleagues (Fenner and Woodroofe, 1953; Day et al., 1956). In

Australia this disease is spread amongst wild rabbits by various species of mosquito. The maxillary stylets become contaminated when the insect probes through virus infected skin but the virus does not apparently multiply in the mosquito. The mosquito may then transmit infection to healthy rabbits up to 20 days. In Britain the rabbit flea is believed to be the usual insect vector of myxomatosis, although in rabbitries in the South of England *Anopheles atroparvus* may be important in transmission (Andrewes, Muirhead-Thomson and Stevenson, 1956). This mosquito may retain infectivity for as long as 220 days over the winter, although survival of virus on the mouth parts of mosquitoes that have been killed lasts only a few days, which rather suggests that in this case natural transmission may not be purely mechanical.

In the typical mosquito-borne virus infections, transmission involves multiplication of virus in the insect vector. Infection of the vector is established by the ingestion of virus-containing blood. This is followed by a latent period of some days during which the mosquito does not transmit. At the end of this extrinsic incubation period, the virus has reached the salivary glands and the mosquito becomes infective and remains so for the rest of its life. The non-infective period, seen also in the mosquito infected with malarial parasites, is analogous to the incubation period of human diseases such as measles and smallpox during which the patient is not infectious because no virus is being discharged from the body.

The incubation period in the mosquito varies with the external temperature, as was shown by Davis (1932) for the yellow fever virus in *Aedes aegypti*. The vector relationships have been investigated extensively in relation to the transmission of St. Louis, Japanese B, Eastern and Western equine encephalitis (Chamberlain, 1958; Kissling, 1960). A certain specificity of vector is exhibited. In experiments with chickens infected with St. Louis encephalitis virus, *Culex pipiens* and *C. quinquifasciatus* were shown to be readily infected, and transmitted infection after 12 or 20 days, whereas representatives of other mosquito genera were much less readily infected and less efficient transmitters (Chamberlain, Sudia and Gillett, 1959). The titre of virus as determined by titration of ground-up insects had often reached a high value several days before the mosquitoes were capable of transmitting infection to the chicken by biting, indicating that transmission occurs only when virus has multiplied in the salivary glands. LaMotte has shown that the infection rate and transmission rate of mosquitoes infected with Japanese B virus increases with increase of virus concentration in blood meals (LaMotte, 1960). In *Culex pipiens*, virus was usually found only in the abdomen in the first week after feeding, but by the second or third weeks all parts of the mosquito were infected; after 48 days high virus titres were found in the head, proboscis and salivary glands, but little or no virus was present in the abdomen.

The observations of McLean (1955) on the multiplication of Murray Valley encephalitis virus in mosquitoes suggests that certain species fail to transmit virus because virus does not pass from the gut to the rest of the body. In *Anopheles annulipes* there was practically no multiplication of virus after feeding; but after injection of virus into the thorax, virus multiplied, and the insects became infective for chickens a few days later. There is no evidence of transovarial passage of virus in mosquitoes but, as in certain rickettsial infections, virus may pass to the eggs in the tick vectors of Russian spring-summer encephalitis and louping ill of sheep.

Man is only an occasional host to some of the viruses of the Arbor group, and the survival of these viruses appears to depend on a cycle of transmission between insect and birds or mammalian hosts. Viraemic infection of these normal hosts is necessary for the infection of the vector, but in most cases neither the animal host nor vector appears to suffer pathological effects. Serological surveys have shown that sub-clinical infections of man with Arbor viruses are common in endemic areas. Some of the viruses of this group, recently discovered in tropical regions of Africa and South America, have not yet been shown to produce clinical illness in man, although serological evidence of sub-clinical infection has been obtained. Perhaps in these instances the virus–man association has been of long duration.

While subclinical infection with Arbor viruses in man and other animal hosts may be of frequent occurrence, this is not peculiar to this virus group. Latent infections with adenoviruses and enteroviruses are of common occurrence and sufficiently extensive to elicit antibody formation. The lack of overt disease in many of the human beings infected with Arbor viruses might be attributable to the lack of ability of the virus to multiply sufficiently in a new species of host to induce pathological effects. But, then, in the natural animal host there is frequently sufficient multiplication to produce a viraemia of high titre, and yet illness does not result. Moreover, viruses on transfer to a new host species tend to produce severe and fatal disease, as with pseudo-rabies in cattle or B virus in man. It seems more likely that the occurrence of overt illness will depend on whether the extent and manner of multiplication of virus within host tissues is such as to produce marked cell damage. This subject is considered in Chapter 7.

The Arbor viruses have shown an extraordinary adaptability to multiply in such diverse hosts as insects and warm-blooded animals. The absence of pathological effects from their multiplication in these

V.I.—E.

hosts suggests the kind of relationship between virus and host usually attributed to long-continued association and mutual adaptation. The transmission of certain viruses of the group to successive generations of ticks through the egg might suggest that ticks were the original hosts of the virus which later became adapted to growth in warm-blooded animals. In other cases transovarial transmission would appear not to have been adopted because unnecessary. For example, in tropical and subtropical countries the presence of susceptible animal hosts and the prevalence of active mosquitoes throughout the year provide the conditions needed for continued survival of these viruses.

The insect transmission of virus infection in animals shows interesting parallels with the insect transmission of virus infection of plants. It should, however, be noted that in virus diseases of plants, transmission by insects is the common mode of infection, whereas in animal diseases it is *relatively* uncommon. Damage to, or puncture of, the rigid cell wall of plants is necessary for entry of virus, whereas animal cells, and particularly mucosal cells liable to surface contamination have a soft plastic membrane suitable for other mechanisms of virus penetration. Moreover, because of the static nature of plants, spread of virus amongst them requires transfer of virus sometimes over considerable distances, and this is effectively achieved through the agency of flying insects. On the other hand, the mobility of animal hosts ensures dissemination of many virus infections without the necessity of insect vectors.

In virus infections of plants, insect transmission may also be purely mechanical, usually by aphids, or biological by leafhoppers. In biological transmission, the leafhoppers have a non-infective incubation period until virus has multiplied in the insect and reached the salivary glands. The insects usually do not suffer from this virus infection and a certain specificity of insect vector is apparent. In leafhoppers, virus may be transmitted transovarially through many generations (Black, 1950) just as transovarian transmission of animal viruses may occur in ticks. It has been suggested that the biologically transmitted plant viruses were originally insect viruses which later became adapted to growth in plants (Maramorosch, 1955).

3. Artificial inoculation

Generalized virus infections normally acquired through the respiratory route may be transmitted by inoculation into subcutaneous tissues. For example, smallpox has occasionally been contracted through cuts in the skin by those making autopsies in undiagnosed cases, and in the eighteenth and nineteenth centuries variolation frequently produced a local lesion followed by a generalized smallpox eruption. In these instances, as in measles produced by injection of blood subcutaneously (Papp, 1959), the incubation period was generally a few days shorter than in the naturally acquired disease. This may have been the result of the larger infecting dose in the artificial infections, or the more rapid spread of virus to tissues (? lymphatic) suitable for multiplication. However, in chickenpox produced by inoculation of vesicle fluid into the scarified skin of young children, the incubation period was within normal limits (Bruusgaard, 1932).

The outstanding example of disease conveyed accidentally by inoculation is viral hepatitis. The disease has become more common in recent years because of the greater use of blood or plasma for transfusion, and the increased frequency of prophylactic or therapeutic injections and of withdrawal of blood for diagnostic tests. The person from whom infection is derived may be in the incubation period of an overt attack of the disease or be suffering from a subclinical infection. This inoculation infection, often called serum hepatitis, was regarded as being aetiologically distinct from naturally acquired infectious hepatitis because of: (a) the different routes of infection, (b) the absence of cross-immunity between the two forms of hepatitis, (c) the long incubation period in serum hepatitis as opposed to infectious hepatitis, and (d) the lack of infectivity of the stools in serum hepatitis. It is doubtful if, in the light of more recent knowledge, this differentiation is justifiable. Successful cultivation of the virus of infectious hepatitis has been reported in tissue cultures of Detroit 6 cells (Rightsel et al. 1956, 1961) and human embryo lung cells (Davis, 1961). It would appear that there are several different immunological types of infectious hepatitis virus (Rightsel et al., 1961), so that the lack of immunity between infectious hepatitis and serum hepatitis observed in human experiments is of doubtful significance. Moreover, it has been shown that infectious hepatitis virus may be transmitted by blood transfusion (Francis, Frisch and Quilligan, 1946; Harden, Barondess and Parker, 1955); virus may be present in the blood before the appearance of clinical illness and for some time afterwards. Clinically there would appear to be no difference between viral hepatitis contracted by contact and that transmitted by inoculation. It is generally agreed that the incubation period of infectious hepatitis as usually acquired is 20–40 days, and the cases of this infection conveyed by inoculation have generally had an incubation period of less than 40 days (Capps, Sborov and Scheiffley, 1948). But the incubation period of cases labelled serum hepatitis has varied from less than 40 days up to 100 days or more. It is obvious that the shorter incubation period is within the range met with in infectious hepatitis. The longer incubation periods in some cases of serum hepatitis might conceivably be due to

the duration of the carrier state of the donor. It seems possible that in
the donor whose infection has lasted for months, the amount of virus
in the blood might be less than in the earlier phase, the virus might
have become attenuated or the blood in which virus was transferred
might contain low-grade antibody which might delay multiplication
of virus in the recipient. This last possibility receives some support
from the observation of Boggs *et al.* (1961). In volunteers inoculated
with culture virus neutralizing antibody and virus were occasionally
present in blood at the same time. Stokes *et al.* (1954) record the case
of a blood-donor whose blood was apparently infective over a period of
five years. In 1945, when the condition was first detected, the incubation period in three recipients of his blood was 41, 41 and 43 days;
in 1950 the incubation period in a recipient was 68 days. The stools of
this last patient were not infective when given orally to eight volunteers,
but, it is difficult to attach much importance to this negative feeding
experiment, for the stools of typical infectious hepatitis patients may
cease to be infective after a few weeks or months.

That the incubation period of viral hepatitis is not wholly dependent
on the route of inoculation is suggested by the observations of Francis
et al. (1946) and Harden *et al.* (1955) on cases of transfusion hepatitis
in which the incubation periods in the recipients were unusually short—
11 and 14 days to onset of illness and 21 and 30 days to onset of jaundice. In each case the donor developed clinical hepatitis a few days
after donating blood, so that virus titre in the transfused blood may
have been high and antibody was unlikely to have been present.

Prolonged viraemia in the absence of clinical illness or signs of
hepatic insufficiency is illustrated in one of the cases quoted by Stokes
et al. (1954). This patient may have transmitted hepatitis to her infant
in utero, as the child became jaundiced at the age of two months. The
blood of this child was icterogenic at the age of nine months and the
mother's serum was likewise infective two years and eleven months
after the birth of the child; she had shown no clinical illness and
laboratory tests showed no evidence of hepatic insufficiency.

It would seem to the writer that for the time being the virus of serum
hepatitis is best regarded as one of several serological types of hepatitis
virus which normally infect by the alimentary tract but may be
transferred by inoculation of blood of apparently healthy individuals.
If the observations of Rightsel *et al.* (1961) and Davis (1961) can be
confirmed, detailed study of virus strains isolated from hepatitis
infections, contracted naturally or conferred by inoculation, may serve
to elucidate the outstanding problems in the pathogenesis of viral
hepatitis in man. That infections with these viruses are widespread is
evident from the protective effect of γ-globulin (Krugman *et al.*,

1960), but there is at present no obvious explanation for the continued viraemia and apparent lack of antibody response in some of those infected. It has been suggested that such individuals may have been infected with the virus in early foetal life and that a state of immune tolerance has developed between host and virus. Definite evidence of such an association is, as yet, lacking.

The primary site of virus multiplication following ingestion or inoculation of hepatitis virus is unknown. Virus has frequently been found in the blood in the absence of hepatitis or before symptoms suggestive of liver involvement have appeared. The clinical picture and histological evidence from biopsy material indicate that liver damage may be severe in clinical cases. Electron-microscopical studies of biopsy material reveal masses of virus-like particles not only in liver cells but also in endothelial cells of the liver sinusoids (Bearcroft, 1962).

E. Entry of Virus through Placenta

Infection of the human foetus *in utero* with the virus of rubella has attracted much attention in recent years. An attack of rubella occurring during the first three months of pregnancy is followed in 10–30% of patients by the birth of a baby showing congenital abnormalities. Whether transfer of virus to the foetus is preceded by growth of virus in the placenta is unknown. It seems likely, as suggested by Burnet (1960), that in other generalized virus infections of the mother at this stage of pregnancy, infection of the foetus is more likely to be followed by its death and consequent abortion; survival of the foetus with congenital abnormalities is therefore probably a consequence of the relatively low virulence of this virus for the human host.

In animals, the most striking example of intra-uterine virus infection is that of lymphocytic choriomeningitis in mice. This was first detected in a colony of mice in 1934, when it was estimated that 40–50% of the colony of 2000 animals were infected (Traub, 1936). From the uninfected animals a virus-free stock was built up. The progeny of infected females were kept segregated and the progress of the endemic infection in this sub-colony followed over several years (Traub, 1938, 1939). The presence of virus in infected animals showing no symptoms could be detected by injection of blood or tissue suspensions intracerebrally into mice of virus-free stock. In the infected stock, symptoms were observed only in animals up to six weeks of age; the morbidity was 20% and the mortality 4·4%. At this time (1935) only some of the mice infected *in utero* showed symptoms, and young mice infected after birth through contact with infected adults often developed latent infections. The urine and nasal secretions of infected animals contained virus, and it was believed that infection by contact occurred by the nasal route. By 1937, among the infected stock all animals became infected *in utero* and the disease was now entirely subclinical. Virus was present in blood and tissues of these animals (especially spleen, lymph glands, liver and uterus—Traub, 1960), and they were completely immune to inoculation with virus. On the other hand, animals from the virus-free stock which recovered from experimental infection failed to carry virus and had an incomplete immunity to intracerebral challenge infection (Traub, 1938); the serum of such animals contained antibody (Traub, 1960). The persistent, often lifelong, presence of virus in the tissue of mice infected *in utero*, associated with a high degree of immunity in the absence of antibody, is perhaps the most striking example of immune tolerance in the virus field (Burnet and Fenner, 1949). Because of the lack of methods for detecting or titrating the virus of rubella, no information is available as to the presence of rubella virus, or antibody to it, in the tissues of babies showing congenital malformations due to infection with this virus in foetal life. The cultivation of rubella virus, recently reported by Parkman *et al.* (1962), if confirmed, may provide a means whereby this information may be obtained.

Another virus infection which may pass to the foetus is that due to salivary gland virus. Its presence has been demonstrated by the finding of typical cytomegalic inclusions in the tissues of babies dying from various diseases (Farber and Wolbach, 1932). Such infections are for the most part inapparent, although there may occasionally be evidence of generalized disease in the new-born as shown by the presence of erythroblastosis, thrombocytopenia, purpura, jaundice and splenomegaly in the absence of blood group incompatibility (Cappell and McFarlane, 1947; Smith and Vellios, 1950). Microcephaly, cerebral calcification and chorioretinitis have also been noted and suggest a diagnosis of congenital toxoplasmosis (Guyton *et al.*, 1957). Asymptomatic infection with this virus frequently occurs in the early years of life (Rowe *et al.*, 1958a) and the survival of the baby infected *in utero* is consistent with the low virulence of the virus.

Transplacental infection with viruses producing generalized infection in the mother, such as those of variola, chickenpox and poliomyelitis, may be deduced from the fact that when these diseases occur in the mother in the last few days of pregnancy, symptoms in the baby develop within a few days of birth (smallpox: Marsden and Greenfield, 1934; chickenpox, Ehrlich, Turner and Clarke, 1958; poliomyelitis: Swarts and Kercher, 1954). It seems likely that when infection of the foetus with these more virulent viruses occurs earlier in pregnancy, it may be overlooked because of death of the foetus and consequent abortion or premature labour. Some of the babies showing symptoms of generalized cytomegalic inclusion disease (due to salivary gland virus) have been premature.

III. Spread of Virus within the Host

From the site of entry the spread of virus is determined by the nature of the virus and the susceptibility or resistance of the particular host— factors which are considered in Chapter 8. A virus may not invade the tissues much beyond the point of entry in an animal that has acquired specific immunity from previous infection or is naturally insusceptible. For example, in children who have suffered from measles subsequent exposure may result in local lodgement of virus on the respiratory mucosa without extensive invasion of the tissues. Indeed, immunity may be reinforced by some degree of local multiplication on repeated reexposure of such children. But here we are concerned mainly with the spread of virus within a susceptible host. In such a host the extent of tissue invasion will depend very largely on the intrinsic property of the virus, which is implied in the term virulence. Virus may produce clinical manifestations mainly by local multiplication with only limited extension to neighbouring tissues, as in the common wart; it may spread along mucous surfaces, as in the common cold and influenza; spread may occur to deeper tissues by lymph pathways or to distant organisms by means of the blood-stream or by nerve pathways to the central nervous system. Each of these routes of spread will be considered in turn.

A. LOCAL EXTENSION TO TISSUES AT THE SITE OF ENTRY

Of those viruses that produce lesions near the site of entry but do not spread to distant tissues, transfer to neighbouring cells may occur through direct cell contact or in intercellular fluid. The skin would seem to be particularly suitable for such spread, owing to intercellular bridges in the deeper epithelial layers, and it is possible that the viruses of warts, skin papillomas and molluscum contagiosum, which produce hypertrophic changes but little obvious cell necrosis move from cell to cell in this way. Even in tissues where no such intercellular bridges can be demonstrated, transfer between contiguous cells would seem to occur readily. Electron-microscopic studies of organized tissues or cells in tissue culture demonstrate the close apposition of contiguous cells, and in cell culture virus may spread directly from cell to cell. This has been clearly shown with the viruses of varicella and cytomegalic inclusion disease (Weller 1953; Weller et al., 1957). Cytopathic changes can be shown to spread slowly from the original focus of infection

outward by cell-to-cell infection, and no free virus may be detectable
in extracellular culture fluid. However, in varicella in children, extracellular virus is readily demonstrated in vesicle fluid (Taylor-Robinson,
1959). Indeed, it would be very difficult to understand the pathogenesis of varicella without postulating the liberation of virus in considerable amounts from the cells in which it multiplies during the
incubation period—unless transfer from sites of secondary multiplication to the skin occurred solely within leucocytes in the circulation, and
no direct evidence on this point is available. In the local lesions of
recurrent herpes simplex infections, virus spread occurs in spite of a
considerable titre of antibody in serum and tissue fluid; it may be that
in this instance, spread of virus from cell to cell by intercellular bridges
avoids inactivating contact with antibody, although antibody may
prevent generalization from the local lesion. It has long been known
that the presence of immune serum in tissue culture may retard
growth of virus (Andrewes, 1929) but may fail to prevent slow local
extension of infection within the cultured tissue (Downie and
McGaughey, 1935). Recent observations have suggested an alternative
explanation for the local spread of infection by herpes simplex virus in
immune subjects. This depends on the demonstration of the infectivity
of virus nucleic acids (see Colter and Ellem, 1961). Single HeLa cells
infected with herpes virus and incubated for 30 hours did not release
infective virus on freezing and thawing although capable of producing
virus plaques when placed on monolayers (Stoker, 1958). This finding
and the early production of focal necrotic lesions in HeLa cell monolayers by herpes virus in the presence of strong immune serum, suggests
that cell-to-cell spread may be due to a virus precursor rather than to
fully formed virus (Ross and Orlans, 1958). Infective nucleic acid
without the antigenic protein covering would be insusceptible to the
action of neutralizing antibody. It is still uncertain whether infective
nucleic acids play a part in natural infection, but it has been suggested
that they might be the cause of the long period of infectivity of the
blood in serum hepatitis and in lymphocytic choriomeningitis of mice
and the general absence of particulate infective agents in tumours
(Herriott, 1961).

B. SPREAD OVER MUCOSAL SURFACES

In the local infection of mucous membranes, exemplified by the
common cold and influenza, the mode of extension of the process along
the respiratory epithelium is not precisely known. It seems possible
that direct cell-to-cell infections might occur, although the rapid
involvement of extensive areas of mucosa would seem more compatible

with the spread of virus in the surface film of fluid, which is being constantly moved through ciliary action, or in intercellular fluid. As it has been shown that leucocytes readily phagocytose influenza virus (Boand, Kempe and Hanson, 1957) spread of virus on the surface of the mucosa might also be effected through such cells.

While it is generally believed that the enteroviruses infect through the intestinal mucosa, we have no information on the extent of mucosal involvement which may occur, nor whether virus is moved along the surface to infect susceptible cells or spreads in subepithelial tissues. As enteroviruses are now known which infect domestic animals, it is possible that experimental study of these infections may throw light on the sequence of events in enterovirus infections in man.

C. Spread by Lymphatic Pathways

Perhaps the most obvious clinical evidence of spread of virus by lymphatics is the involvement of the axillary lymph nodes that follows a few days after cutaneous vaccination on the upper arm for the prevention of smallpox. Axillary adenitis following primary vaccination usually becomes apparent about the sixth day, when the vesicle is forming, suggesting that virus spreads to the lymph nodes soon after multiplication in skin epithelium has begun. In the older accounts of variolation, a similar sequence of events was observed. But whereas in *variola inoculata* the virus passes from the lymph nodes to the blood-stream with secondary localization in the skin, this only rarely happens in vaccinia. In most cases when generalized vaccinia follows vaccination, the clinical illness is not unlike that seen in mild smallpox infection and there is evidence of a delayed antibody response following vaccination in these cases (McCarthy, Downie and Bradley, 1958). The regular occurrence of generalization following variolation is probably the result of greater rate of growth and cell necrosis and more rapid involvement of mesodermal tissues by the more virulent variola virus.

The infection of tonsils and adenoids with the adenoviruses seems most likely to result from spread of virus by lymphatic channels from the overlying mucosa. In other exanthemata, especially measles and rubella, enlargement of lymph glands may be apparent several days before the onset of illness. This enlargement may not obviously be associated with the portal of entry in these diseases and is more likely to be concerned with the proliferation of virus which has been disseminated by the blood stream. While lymph glands in the neck are commonly enlarged in rubella, those most markedly affected are the occipital glands (Pitt, 1961) and these do not receive lymph drainage from oropharyngeal or upper respiratory mucosa, which are likely portals of entry. The finding of typical multinucleated cells in lymphoid tissues in the appendix and elsewhere in the incubation period of measles, suggests that in lymphoid tissue, infected through the bloodstream, multiplication of virus precedes the secondary viraemia which is present at the onset of illness.

In experimental infection of animals with pox viruses, the spread of virus from the point of entry to draining lymph glands has been frequently demonstrated (ectromelia: Fenner, 1948a; myxomatosis: Fenner and Woodroofe, 1953; rabbit pox: Bedson and Duckworth, 1963). In these infections, virus is rarely detected in lymph glands until 12–24 hours have elapsed. Quantitative virus titrations have shown increase in virus concentration in the draining lymphatic glands before it spills over to the blood, by which generalization occurs. The virus increase in the lymph nodes might result from accumulation of virus draining from the initial sites of multiplication, although the histological and cytological changes suggest active multiplication in gland cells. In ferrets infected by the intranasal route, distemper virus was plentiful in reticulum cells of sinuses of the cervical lymph nodes after two days, although none was detected in the overlying mucosa by fluorescent antibody at this time (Liu and Coffin, 1957). In this instance the lymph nodes appeared to be the primary site of multiplication of virus prior to general dissemination.

There seems little available information as to whether virus transported in the lymph is free in the fluid or is associated with cells. The observations of Yoffey and Sullivan (1939) indicated that in their experiments virus in lymph was within or adsorbed to lymphocytes. Following intranasal instillation of vaccinia virus in rabbits, they collected lymph by cannulating the vessels draining from the superior cervical lymph node. Virus was found in the lymph 12 hours after instillation of virus, and most of the virus could be recovered from the cells and none from the fluid part of the lymph.

Thus, lymph nodes may be infected and serve as secondary sites of multiplication in various generalized virus infections. They may indeed provide the most susceptible cell type for the growth of some viruses. For example, in lymphogranuloma venereum, although generalized infection may occasionally be evident from the occurrence of meningitis (Sabin and Aring, 1942), infection of inguinal and pelvic lymphatic tissue is responsible for the main features of the disease. Lymphoid tissue would seem to be the main target of attack in fowl and mouse leukaemias. Such selective localization in lymphoid tissue is evidently a specific characteristic of individual viruses, for it is not shown by the virus of psittacosis or other members of the psittacosis–lymphogranuloma group.

D. Spread by the Blood-stream

In many generalized virus infections, the symptomatic phase of illness is associated with involvement of organs or tissues at a distance from the portal of entry—for example, the skin in the exanthemata, salivary glands in mumps, the liver in yellow fever and the muscles in epidemic myalgia. The localization and multiplication of virus in these sites of predilection must, in most instances, follow dissemination of virus by the blood-stream, and virus can usually be demonstrated in the circulating blood in the early days of illness. In some diseases, at least, virus is disseminated by the blood before the rise in temperature which usually heralds the onset of clinical malaise. In serum hepatitis, for example, virus has been found to be present in the serum collected from blood donors who subsequently developed symptoms of hepatitis (Rightsel *et al.*, 1961). In children infected by spraying mumps virus into the back of the throat, virus was first detected in the saliva 11 days later—several days before the onset of clinical parotitis (Henle *et al.*, 1948). As the parotids would appear to be infected from the blood-stream—and viraemia has occasionally been demonstrated in the early stages of illness—the findings of Henle and her colleagues indicate that blood dissemination of virus occurs in the incubation period of mumps. That this kind of evidence is not available in other acute diseases of man may be because there is rarely occasion for such examination to be made. However, in smallpox, the date of onset of eruption in babies born to mothers who suffered from the disease some days before labour, suggests that transplacental infection occurred at the time of onset of illness in the mother or at most only a day or two before (Marsden and Greenfield, 1934). On the other hand, as mentioned previously, the widespread involvement of lymphoid tissue in rubella and measles during the incubation period suggests that in some diseases spread of virus, presumably by the blood, occurs some time before the rise in temperature which marks the onset of illness.

Little information is available from observations on human disease as to the way in which virus reaches the circulation from the initial sites of entry and multiplication, but studies on infections in animals provide some clues as to the mechanisms involved. It would appear that virus may gain access to the circulation in several ways: (*a*) by lymph pathways via the thoracic duct, (*b*) within leucocytes passing from local sites of virus multiplication into blood capillaries, or (*c*) from direct involvement of vascular epithelium near the site of initial entry. The first of these is probably the most important.

In pox virus infections, the involvement of lymph glands draining the site of entry has been already mentioned, and in experimental studies a regular sequence of events in the spread of infection can be readily demonstrated. Figure 1, showing the findings in rabbits infected with rabbit-pox virus by the respiratory route (Bedson and Duckworth, 1963), illustrates the kind of results obtained. The strain of virus was highly virulent for the breed of rabbit used, and the progressive spread of infection was faster than that observed by Fenner in his earlier studies of mouse pox (Fenner, 1948a). The sequential spread of virus to various tissues and organs was, however, similar. In rabbit-pox as in ectromelia, multiplication in lymph nodes preceded infection of the

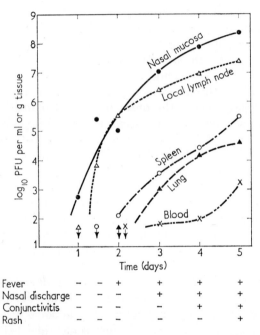

Fig. 1. Intranasal infection with rabbit–pox virus (Utrecht strain). The concentration of virus in various tissues at intervals after infection, in relation to the development of abnormal physical signs.

spleen and other internal organs. The latter were presumably infected via the blood-stream, and multiplication in the internal organs preceded the appearance of skin rash by one or two days. It seems likely, as suggested by Fenner (1948b), that a similar spread and multiplication of virus occurs in smallpox and other exanthemata in man, and such observations as have been made on the incubation period of human infections support this view. In summary then, the sequence of events would appear to be as follows. Virus infecting by the respiratory route quickly passes to lymph nodes draining the site of entry. After multiplication of virus in these lymphatic tissues, virus passes into the circulation but not in such amounts as might be readily detectable by blood culture. This virus is rapidly removed from the circulation by cells of the reticulo-endothelial system throughout the body, including those in the spleen and in the sinuses of lymph nodes. Multiplication proceeds in these secondary sites of localization; this may account for the evidence of virus activity indicated by changes observed in lymphatic tissue in the incubation period of measles and rubella. Only when multiplication has proceeded in these tissues is there a further viraemia, which occurs at the onset of illness and is sufficiently extensive to be detected by laboratory examination. At this time, too, virus in the circulation localizes in the skin and mucous membranes, where the focal lesions of the exanthem and enanthem are to appear a few days later. In patients whose illness runs a favourable course, the viraemia at onset of illness is terminated by the appearance of antibody. In severe and fulminating infections such as haemorrhagic smallpox (*purpura variolosa*), viraemia increases in degree up to the time of death.

1. Presence of virus in circulating leucocytes

At some stages of the viraemic infection, most of the virus seems to be within leucocytes. This has been demonstrated in fowl plague (Todd, 1928), vaccinial infection in the rabbit (Smith, 1929) and other experimental pox infections in animals. In the experiments of Fenner (1948a), Liu and Coffin (1957) and Bedson and Duckworth (1963), the early localization of virus in the spleen was probably due to the removal from the blood of infected leucocytes by that organ. The leucocytic layer from acute measles blood is highly infective (Papp, 1959), and it has been suggested that the leucopenia which is a feature of the acute stage of many virus diseases may be due to the destructive action of virus on circulating leucocytes and on haemopoetic tissues. Virus has been found within leucocytes in the blood in experimental poliomyelitis in monkeys (Verlinde and Beem, 1952), and recently Köhler (1960) has reported the isolation of virus from the leucocyte layer of blood taken from six patients 5–20 days after the onset of paralytic illness. Virus may, however, also be present in blood plasma; high titres are to be found in the serum of animals infected with Arbor viruses and the virus of hepatitis may be found in plasma or serum from blood donors.

2. Multiplication of virus in reticulo-endothelial cells and vascular endothelium

As noted above, in some generalized infections virus from the circulation appears to accumlate in special phagocytic cells in the spleen, in cells in lymph node sinuses and Kupfer cells in the liver etc. In some infections, however, vascular endothelium generally seems to be involved in virus multiplication. In rabbits infected with myxomatosis virus, Hurst (1937) described a peculiar proliferation of vascular and reticular endothelium, and Niven has noted similar reactions of capillary endothelium in various tissues of mice infected with mouse hepatitis virus. In this disease the vascular lesions are focal, the affected cells are shed into the blood stream and their debris can be recognized in the spleen. The endothelial lesions are observed during the incubation period of the disease: by the time symptoms of illness appear, they have disappeared (Niven, personal communication). In mice infected by intracerebral injection of the virus of lymphocytic choriomeningitis, the primary attack of the virus appears to be on endothelial and lymphocytic cells in the spleen, followed by similar evidence of destructive lesions in lymph glands and later in vascular endothelium elsewhere. These lesions may precede signs of involvement of the brain and meninges (Lillie and Armstrong, 1945).

In measles and smallpox, two or three days elapse between the viraemia, present at the onset of illness, and the appearance of the focal eruption in the skin and mucous membranes. In smallpox, the first change detectable in the skin is swelling of the endothelial cells of the capillaries in the *cutis vera* and the accumulation of mononuclear cells around these capillaries. The appearance would suggest that virus multiplies in the capillary endothelium and from these cells is released to infect the neighbouring cells of the epidermis. The numerous haemorrhages in the dermis, characteristic of fulminating cases of smallpox, is consistent with widespread destruction of capillary endothelium consequent on virus growth. The susceptibility of the vascular endothelium to the related cowpox virus is readily demonstrated by the finding of typical inclusions in vascular endothelium of rabbit and chick embryo tissue (Downie, 1939).

The Arbor virus infections depend for their continued propagation on viraemic infections. In certain animal hosts, these viraemic infections may be asymptomatic, but are nevertheless of sufficient intensity to infect the insect vector probing for its blood meal. The infected mosquito presumably deposits virus in or near small blood-vessels. The rapid appearance of viraemia in the animal host suggests infection of vascular endothelium and multiplication of virus in this cell type. In the occasional symptomatic Arbor virus infection in man, the clinical picture is usually one of a generalized febrile illness with viraemia. In severe cases of yellow fever, liver cells are invaded, although it seems likely that this is preceded by multiplication of virus in the endothelial lining of the sinusoids. The spread of virus from

Kupfer cells to parenchymal cells may be more easily effected because there is no basement membrane between the two cell types. In the encephalitis that may complicate infection with certain of the Arbor viruses, the pathological changes found in fatal cases suggest that the primary attack of the virus is on the vascular endothelium in the brain and appears not dissimilar to the lesions found in certain rickettsial infections. Rickettsial infections, like Arbor virus infections, depend for their continued propagation on the presence of the infective agent in the blood of the animal host; in both instances, multiplication in vascular endothelium ensures the high blood concentration necessary for infection of the vector.

It would seem, therefore, that vascular endothelium is extremely susceptible to attack by certain viruses. Our information on the exact location and cell types involved in the spread of virus infections is, however, scanty. A study of the early stages of virus dissemination in experimental infections by careful histological and cytological methods, using fluorescent-antibody and other techniques, seems called for to fill in the many gaps in our knowledge.

3. Localization of virus in target organs

In generalized virus infections, dissemination usually occurs by the blood-stream—the spread of virus by nerve pathways will be considered in the next section. From the blood, virus may localize for the final phase of multiplication in different tissues or organs, damage to which may determine the clinical picture of severe forms of the infective process. The factors which determine such localizations are almost completely unknown. The possible importance of metabolic requirements or metabolic barriers and hormonal factors are discussed in Chapter 8.

In the exanthemata the predilection for the skin might suggest that ectoderm provides a particularly favourable environment for virus multiplication. But, prior to seeding of virus in skin capillaries, the viruses have been multiplying in mesodermal tissues during the incubation period. It has recently been shown (Bedson and Dumbell, 1961) that in chick embryos and in tissue culture the human pox viruses (variola major and minor) have a lower ceiling temperature for growth than the other animal pox viruses; the human viruses will not grow in the chick chorioallantois at a temperature of 39°C or higher. Localization in the skin after the rise in temperature in the human disease might be a consequence of the increased internal body temperature at this time. The tendency of the eruption to be more profuse on the extremities, on the extensor rather than on the flexor aspects of the limbs, and the sparseness of the eruption in the flexures, such as the axillae and groins, might be in keeping with such a notion. But in natives living in the tropics and scantily clothed, the distribution of the eruption is similar to that in the European living in temperate climates (Dixon, 1962). The tendency for lesions to be profuse over points of pressure, areas of friction or recent trauma, may be dependent on stagnation of the capillary circulation, as suggested by Ricketts and Byles (1908). A similar concentration of lesions at such sites is observed in chickenpox. But no obvious explanation is available to explain the different distribution of the skin eruptions in chickenpox and smallpox —a difference sufficiently constant to be of clinical diagnostic value. The centripetal eruption of chickenpox suggests a subtle difference in the conditions of multiplication required by the viruses of varicella and variola.

Experimentally, the localization of intravenously injected virus has been often demonstrated in areas of skin subjected to trauma or irritation, which alters permeability of vascular channels. However, Platt's experiments with foot-and-mouth virus in guinea-pigs led him to conclude that localization of this virus at particular skin sites following intraperitoneal injection was related to the hyperplastic state of the epithelium, as well as persistent local irritation; the metabolic activity of the epithelium was probably more important than increased capillary permeability (Platt, 1960).

The localization of Coxsackie and other viruses in muscles, including cardiac muscles, has at the moment no obvious explanation, although it has been shown by Pearce (1950) that experimental procedures, such as the intravenous injection of gum acacia, pitressin or epinephrine hydrochloride, which tend to cause cardiac anoxia, favour the production of lesions in the heart by viruses inoculated peripherally. This, however, does not serve to explain the selective localization of particular viruses in special tissues not subject to such stresses; for example, the liver in viral hepatitis, the salivary glands in mumps, and the central nervous system in rabies. This localization may ultimately be shown to have a biochemical basis, but the nature of the relevant biochemical differences in various kinds of cells and tissues is at the moment obscure. We are equally ignorant of the explanation for the tissue affinities shown by bacteria; for example, the gonococcus or the leptospira of Weil's disease. Indeed, only recently has a chemical explanation been suggested for the selective localization of one bacterial species in a particular tissue—the localization of Brucella abortus in the foetal placenta of bovines. Smith et al. (1962) have recently provided good evidence that this depends on the presence of a growth-stimulating carbohydrate, erythritol, in the placental cotyledons of cow, sheep, pig and goat, animals in which infection with Br. abortus is commonly followed by abortion. Erythritol was not found in the placenta of rat, rabbit, guinea-pig, or human, species which are not prone to abortion when infected with this organism.

The study of viruses in tissue culture has so far provided no clues to the factors which may be concerned in their localization in the intact animal. Many viruses grow *in vitro* in tissue cells derived from animals which are themselves insusceptible to infection; for example, the virus of mouse-pox may grow in chicken cells, although chickens are not susceptible to infection. The rapidly destructive effect of poliovirus on fibroblasts or epithelial cells in culture has no parallel in the pathology of poliomyelitis seen in either man or monkey; the virus of cytomegalic inclusion disease grows better in human fibroblasts than in epithelial cells in culture (Weller *et al.*, 1957), although in infected humans the inclusions characteristic of this disease are commonly found in epithelial cells of salivary glands, bronchi and kidneys. The ready growth of many viruses in tissue culture and the exceptional susceptibility of embryonic tissue in culture suggest that cell susceptibility may depend on intracellular biochemical reactions associated with rapid cell growth. In the intact animal, cell multiplication and metabolism may be subject to the control of factors, many unknown, which do not operate *in vitro*.

4. Spread from blood to central nervous system

Many systemic virus infections may occasionally involve the central nervous system; mumps, Coxsackie and Echo infections in man and distemper in dogs may be cited as examples. Most of the arthropod-borne viruses produce generalized infections; these are frequently inapparent both in man and in their reservoir animals, but occasionally they result in encephalitis. In most virus encephalitides there is no evidence of passage of virus by nervous pathways to the central nervous system. There is usually no specific localization of lesions within the central nervous system, and, as viraemia is a common feature of these infections, it seems likely that spread to the brain or meninges is secondary to infection of vascular endothelium in the vessels of the brain.

By the use of fluorescent antibody, involvement of blood vessels in the brain has been demonstrated in certain experimental infections. In young mice inoculated intraperitoneally with the virulent Asibi strain of yellow fever virus, visceral multiplication is followed by the appearance of virus in the brain after two days; but it seems to reach all parts of the brain at the same time (Mims 1957). In the ferret, distemper virus inoculated intranasally or intramuscularly produces a generalized infection which kills in about a fortnight. In the later

stages of the process, viral antigen is detected in many organs, but in
the brain it appears to be confined to vascular endothelium (Liu and
Coffin, 1957). In naturally infected dogs which showed symptoms only
of systematic disease, virus in the brain was confined to the blood-
vessels (Coffin and Liu, 1957). In dogs which showed cerebral symptoms,
however, virus was detected by fluorescent antibody throughout the
brain, within neurones, in the walls of small blood-vessels and in
endothelium of capillaries. These studies provide evidence for the
spread of virus to brain tissue from infected endothelium of cerebral
capillaries.

It seems clear that in systemic virus infections characterized by virus
attack on capillary endothelium generally, as, for example, in smallpox
and chickenpox, encephalitis rarely occurs. It is not known whether in
such diseases the capillary endothelium in the brain is spared or whether
the block to spread occurs either at capillary basement membranes
or between these and brain substance. This last possibility seems unlikely, for electronmicrographs indicate that foot-like processes of
astrocytes or glial cells are closely applied to the basement membrane
of capillaries in the brain.

There are certain factors known to favour localization of blood-borne
virus in the central nervous system, among them those favouring
increased dilation and permeability of cerebral vessels (Field, Grayson
and Rogers, 1951; Trueta and Hodes, 1954). Peripheral trauma may
apparently cause increased blood flow through vessels in those parts of
the spinal cord or medulla from which the site of trauma is innervated.
It has been suggested that the apparent spread of virus from sites of
peripheral injection by nerve routes to the cord may, in fact, be the
result of this mechanism operating to localize blood-borne virus in the
central nervous system (Field, 1952). It has recently been shown that
inhalation of 10–30% CO_2 may determine the occurrence of poliomyelitis following intravenous injection of type II virus in mice
(Sellers and Lavender, 1962). In this case, however, the determination
of infection of the brain may not have been entirely due to the effect
of CO_2 inhalation on the vessel walls; for electron micrographs showed
changes in intercellular ground substance and limiting membranes of
cells in the vicinity of the cerebral capillaries. The conditions and factors
concerned with the settling of virus from the blood in brain tissue are
largely unknown and the intrinsic properties of the virus must play a
decisive role in determining this occurrence.

E. SPREAD WITHIN THE NERVOUS SYSTEM

The notion that the noxious agents of certain diseases involving the central nervous system might reach that system by passage along nerve trunks is an old one and seemed to provide an explanation for the sequence of events in tetanus and rabies, where the characteristic symptoms of disease followed infliction of a wound (see Wright, 1953). A great deal of experimental work has been done in the investigation of this problem; many of the earlier studies were devoted to the passage of tetanus toxin, but in the last 40 years the spread of viruses along nerve pathways has also received a good deal of attention. Nonetheless, the exact mode of spread of virus from the portal of entry to the central nervous system, as well as within it, is still in dispute, especially in relation to poliomyelitis. Evidence bearing on this problem is available from epidemiological and clinical observations, from the distribution of virus in the blood, on mucous surfaces and excreta during life and from pathological changes found *post mortem*. Experimental infections of animals have the added advantage that the progress of infection may be followed by examination of animals killed at various stages after exposure to virus. However, the results of such experiments may do little to elucidate the sequence of events in natural disease because of the methods used. For example, the spread of virus following the injection of large doses of viruses intracerebrally or into nerve trunks can bear little resemblance to the early stages of infection in the natural host.

In this section the spread of viruses to the central nervous system by nerve trunks will be considered first. Poliomyelitis will be discussed separately, for in this disease evidence of spread both by blood and along nerves has led to differences of opinion as to the relative importance of the two.

1. Spread in nerve trunks

It has been established by experimental work presently to be discussed that certain viruses may travel along nerves to the central nervous system; but in most there remains doubt as to the tissue compartment within the nerve trunk by which virus travels. The possibilities are that spread occurs (a) in lymphatics within the trunks; (b) in tissue spaces in the epineurium, perineurium or between nerve fibres, (c) along the nerve, through progressive infection of the cells in the connective tissue or Schwann sheath of the fibres, or (d) within the protoplasm of the axons. A combination of two or more of these mechanisms is, of course, possible.

While lymphatics are known to be present in the epineurium of large trunks like the sciatic, such lymph channels do not pass with the nerve into the cord but drain to lymph glands lying in front of the vertebral column. The lymph therefore does not provide a means for direct transport of virus from the periphery to the cord or brain. The interstitial spaces in nerves, however, continue with nerve fibres to the central nervous system, and, like the axons themselves, provide a direct route to the central nervous system. It has been shown by Wright, Morgan and Wright that if a small volume of radioiodinated rabbit serum protein is injected into the calf muscles of a rabbit the subsequent ascent of the radioactive material may be traced along the sciatic trunk (Wright, 1953). While these experiments did not differentiate between possible travel in the lymphatics or in tissue spaces within the nerve, they showed that the pressure of tissue fluid in the muscle provided sufficient propulsive force to move the material along the nerve. Causey (1948) has shown that a pressure of 80 mm Hg. will reduce the cross-sectional area of the nerve to the gastrocnemius of the rabbit by about 28% and of the individual fibres by more than 10%. As the pressures within contracting muscles are often much greater than 80 mm Hg. it is obvious that muscular contraction may readily facilitate centripetal movement of tissue fluid—and virus in it—along nerves within the muscles.

A good deal of doubt has been expressed about the possible movement of virus within the axons. These structures are protoplasmic extensions of nerve cells in the sensory ganglia or of motor nerve cells within the cord, and may be hundreds of times greater in volume than the perikaryon from which they arise. Their nutrition is provided and controlled by the perikaryon, but movement of protoplasm within the axon usually occurs outward from the nerve cell at a rate of about one millimetre a day (Weiss and Hiscoe, 1948). The observations of Causey on the effects of pressure on individual nerve fibres mentioned above, suggests, however, that muscular contraction might, by compression, tend to move axonal protoplasm contripetally. Doubt has, however, been expressed about the possibility of transport of virus within axons, because of the viscuous nature of that protoplasm (Wright, 1953).

(a) *Spread of tetanus toxin.* Observations on tetanus toxin transfer have had considerable influence on the experimental study of neurotropic viruses and are relevant to any discussion of spread of viruses by nerve paths. When small doses of toxin are injected into the gastrocnemius of the hind limb of a rabbit or other animal, local tetanus follows in the injected limb. This may be prevented by section of the sciatic trunk or by injection into it of a small amount of antitoxin. The injection of toxin intramuscularly into one of a pair of parabiotic rats induces ascending tetanus only in the rat injected (Schellenberg and Matzke, 1958). It has also been repeatedly demonstrated that a greater dose of antitoxin is required to protect animals against toxin injected intramuscularly than against the same amount given intravenously. These and similar experiments indicate that tetanus toxin can travel to the central nervous system by nerve trunks and the occurrence of local tetanus in man, and the frequency with which this form occurred in wounded men given prophylactic tetanus antitoxin in World War I, suggests that this mode of spread is operative in the human disease. The exact pathway by which the toxin travels in the nerve trunk was a matter of controversy for many years. Although the axon was at one time believed to provide the direct continuous pathway to the central nervous system, the viscous nature of axoplasm and the absence of any demonstrable centripetal movement within it seemed to make this unlikely. The most direct evidence that would seem to exclude axonal carriage of tetanus toxin has been provided by Baylis and his colleagues (1952). By injection of ethanolamine oleate into the sciatic nerve, they produced a form of sclerosis which left most or all of the motor fibres still functional. When toxin was injected into the calf muscles 15–33 days after the sclerosis had been induced, no local tetanus was produced, although local tetanus developed in all the control rabbits. Injections of a similar dose of toxin into the sciatic nerve above the sclerosis, produced 6–10 days later, typical local tetanus. As a result of these findings and other experimental observations referred to above, it is now generally accepted that tetanus toxin travels from the periphery to the central nervous system in tissue spaces in nerve trunks rather than along axis cylinders of nerve fibres.

(b) *Movement of virus along nerve trunks.* The evidence for travel of virus along nerves has been obtained by experimental work with neurotropic viruses and viruses of the herpes simplex group. Direct transport of herpes simplex virus inoculated into the foot-pads of mice up the sciatic nerve to the lumbar cord has been demonstrated by Wildy (to be published); by infectivity tests he showed its progressive movement up the sciatic nerve and from the lumbar cord upwards to the brain. Similar experiments on the movement of mouse encephalo-myelitis virus up the sciatic nerve of mice have been made by Sanders (1953). The virus was inoculated into the gastrocnemius muscle, and titrations of virus were made at intervals thereafter from ten segments into which the nerve was divided. The spread of infection along the nerve is shown in Fig. 2. In other experiments the virus was inoculated into the tongue and the titre of virus determined in the hypoglossal nucleus in the medulla oblongata. Virus was first detected in small quantity in these nerve cells 20 hours after injection, and was only found irregularly thereafter until multiplication began at 60 hours. Paralysis of the tongue appeared when virus had attained its maximum concentration 100 hours after inoculation. Sanders suggested that the

virus had travelled via the axons of the hypoglossal nerve, but here, as
in the experiments on sciatic transmission, other pathways within the
nerve could not be excluded.

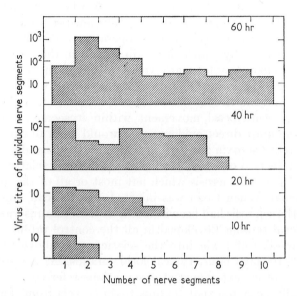

FIG. 2. GD VII virus. Virus content at different levels in the sciatic nerve at intervals
after injection of a standard dose of virus into the gastrocnemius muscle.
Muscle to the left in each case. (With permission.)

Goodpasture believed from his experiments with herpes simplex virus
in rabbits that the virus travelled from the peripheral sites of inoculation to the central nervous system in the axons of the nerves supplying
the site of inoculation (Goodpasture and Teague, 1923; Goodpasture,
1925a). He based this belief on histological studies of animals killed
early in the symptomatic phase of infection. Lesions in the central
nervous system were related to the central nuclei of the nerves supplying the site of inoculation. However, the possibility of transport of
the virus in the tissue spaces of the nerves rather than the axis cylinder
of the fibres was not excluded by his data. Field (1952), repeating the
experiments of Goodpasture with a different strain of virus, got rather
different results; from these he was inclined to favour the views of
Marinesco and Draganesco (1923) on the movement of herpes along
tissue spaces of the nerve trunk.

2. Spread in tissue spaces of the central nervous system

Evidence in support of the view that herpes simplex virus in the rabbit
spreads to the spinal cord and brain stem in tissue spaces in the nerve

trunk and cord is provided by the observations of Boyse *et al* (1956a). They inoculated virus in minute volumes of fluid into either the median, sciatic or first lumbar nerves. When injection was made into the median or sciatic nerve, paralysis of the corresponding limb developed after five or six days. At this time, or next day, rabbit plasma labelled with ^{131}I was injected intravenously, and the rabbits were killed 20 hours later. The spinal cord and brain were fixed and divided into segments; the amount of the radioactivity provided a measure of the severity of myelitis and corresponded generally with the severity of histological changes. The experiments showed that, while the level of radioactivity was greatest in the segment where the injected nerve entered the cord, in animals injected into the median nerve, radio-activity spread caudally down to the lumbar sections and was higher in the lumbar region than in the brain stem. Since the zone of inflammation extended to segments much below the lowest extremity of the descending sensory collateral axons, Boyse *et al*. concluded that the virus became dispersed from its level of entry into the spinal cord through the highly oriented tissue spaces rather than intracellularly along axonal pathways. They have suggested that constantly repeated and asynchronous fluctuations of pressure, due to the impact of the arterial pulse, throughout the cerebrospinal axis may be a factor in dispersal of virus particles through the extracellular compartment of the central nervous system (Boyse *et al*., 1956b).

3. The behaviour of certain neurotropic viruses

(a) *Herpes virus simiae* (B virus) appears to spread in the rabbit by the same nerve pathways as herpes simplex. In the nerve trunks of animals inoculated at a peripheral site, typical intranuclear inclusions are found in Schwann cells and in interstitial cells in nerve trunks (Sabin and Hurst, 1935). This virus does not produce neurological symptoms in the monkey, its normal host. However, in monkeys showing only local lesions on the lips and in the mucous membrane of the mouth Keeble *et al*. (1958) observed histological lesions in the roots of the facial and trigeminal nerves, in the ascending tract of the trigeminal and in the solitary tract of the medulla. The virus of pseudorabies shows many similarities in its apparent mode of spread to that of virus B. In experimentally infected animals, Hurst (1933) observed lesions in nerves similar to those in animals infected with virus B. Here also the natural animal host (the pig) has a relatively mild illness with no symptoms of involvement of the CNS, although lesions in this system may be observed histologically. These observations and similar findings in monkeys inoculated with poliomyelitis virus (Sabin and Ward, 1941b) indicate that virus infection of the central nervous system may frequently be asymptomatic. The histological studies on animals infected with viruses of the herpes group indicate that, in passing along the tissue spaces of nerve trunks, Schwann cells and cells of the interstitial tissue may be involved in the progressive spread of infection.

(b) *Rabies.* It is generally believed that rabies virus reaches the central nervous system from the site of entry by nerve paths. The localization of early symptoms of pain, spasm of muscles or paralysis near the portal of entry would support this view. Goodpasture (1925b), on the basis of experiments in which virus was inoculated into the masseter muscles of rabbits, believed that the virus travelled to the medulla along axons of the fifth cranial nerve, although by the time symptoms developed, lesions were fairly widespread in the central nervous system. Field (1951) in similar experiments failed to find any evidence of early involvement of the motor nucleus of the fifth cranial nerve, and, because of widespread distribution of lesions in spinal root ganglia and elsewhere in the CNS together with signs of early paralysis in the hind limb, he suggested that spread of virus to the CNS might be by the blood-stream. On the other hand, Schindler's experiments in mice indicated that rabies virus spread from the periphery to the cord by the sciatic nerve. After intramuscular injection, virus was first found in the cord, and the sciatic nerve on the injected side showed virus one day before that in the opposite leg (Schindler, 1961). The late appearance of virus in muscles at the injection site suggested that virus spread outwards from the cord along nerves to the periphery. This mechanism is usually held to be responsible for infection of the salivary glands in rabies.

In dogs, virus may be recovered from the saliva before symptoms of nerve involvement appear, although it seems likely that virus may be widely distributed in the brain in the incubation period of the disease. Virus has been recovered from the brains of individuals dying from intercurrent disease within a month of being bitten by rabid dogs (Nikolitsch, 1959). Whether infection of the central nervous system occurs in man without clinical illness is unknown. The fact that patients with symptomatic illness do not recover, may merely indicate that symptoms only occur when infection in the brain is so extensive that recovery is impossible. Virus has rarely been found in the blood of rabid animals, but experimental results may vary according to the animal species and strain of virus used. It has been suggested that the virus is perpetuated in nature in animals which do not suffer from encephalitis, but in which salivary glands, breast tissue and kidneys may be infected (Johnson, 1959).

(c) *Herpes zoster.* The one exclusively human disease in which spread of infection by peripheral nerve routes seems likely is herpes zoster.

In this disease, as in rabies, there would appear to be centrifugal movement of virus along nerves towards the periphery. As the causal virus—varicella—will not infect laboratory animals, evidence is only available from clinical and pathological observations in man. The occurrence of one-sided segmental pain several days before the appearance of skin eruptions suggests that virus activity starts in sensory root ganglia or corresponding sensory ganglia of cranial nerves. Indeed, histological examination of material from zoster patients dying of intercurrent disease confirms this impression by the demonstration of marked inflammatory changes in the ganglia and typical intranuclear inclusions in ganglion cells (Cheatham *et al.*, 1956). The occurrence of subjective symptoms of zoster without the appearance of the skin eruption suggests that virus multiplication in sensory ganglia may not always be followed by spread of virus to the skin (Lewis, 1958). Pathological examination has shown that inflammatory changes may occur in the posterior roots, involve the meninges locally and extend to the posterior and anterior horns of the cord (Denny-Brown, Adams and Fitzgerald, 1944). Virus has been isolated from the cerebrospinal fluid (Gold and Robbins, 1957). The muscular paralysis which may be associated with zoster is explained by spread of infection from affected sensory ganglia to the anterior horns along nerve pathways. The area of skin showing vesicular eruption corresponds closely to the distribution of the sensory nerve derived from the affected posterior root ganglion, and it seems likely therefore that virus spreads to the skin along the sensory nerves. Inflammatory changes found in peripheral nerves related to the affected ganglia would support this view (Denny-Brown *et al.*, 1944; Head and Campbell, 1900).

Goodbody (1953) and Cheatham (1953) considered that virus reached the sensory ganglia by nerve paths from a peripheral point of entry. Epidemiological considerations, however, make it likely that zoster is due to reactivation, by stimuli unknown, of a virus latent in the tissues. It seems strange that a virus which in a fresh non-immune host produces the generalized infection which we recognize as chickenpox, should on reactivation produce the localized syndrome of zoster. However, the occurrence of rare cases of chickenpox complicated by root pain, skin hyperaesthesia and a zoster-like eruption (Cheatham *et al.*, 1956; Taylor-Robinson, 1960) indicate a tendency for varicella virus to localize in sensory nerve ganglia in the primary infection. Zoster, then, is to be regarded in most instances as a localized infection with varicella virus in a person who suffered primary infection many years before, and in whom virus has remained latent in the intervening period. Just as prophylactic antitetanic serum may prevent general tetanus, so in zoster residual immunity is sufficient, in most cases, to prevent generalization of virus but is unable to prevent spread of virus from sensory ganglia along nerves to the skin.

Although it is commonly accepted that virus spreads to skin from affected ganglia along sensory nerves, virus has not yet been demonstrated in the nerves supplying the area of skin affected, and another mechanism to explain the distribution of the skin eruption in zoster was put forward by Wohlwill (1924). He suggested that the lesion in the sensory ganglia resulted in abnormal vasomotor innervation in the related body segment and so enabled the specific virus—presumably derived from the blood-stream—to produce the typical vesicular skin eruption. This suggestion is rather similar to that put forward by Field (1952) to explain the localization in the central nervous system of certain viruses inoculated peripherally. Actual demonstration of virus in the sensory nerves would, of course, be strong evidence in support of the more generally accepted view, and with modern techniques this may prove to be possible.

(d) *Poliomyelitis*. The modes of spread of virus to the central nervous system as discussed on the previous pages are relevant to the present diversity of views about the route taken by poliomyelitis virus.

The demonstration of virus in the blood during or just before minor illness in contacts of poliomyelitis cases, and the successful cultivation of virus in various types of cells, has led to modification of the older view that the virus was strictly neurotropic and travelled to the central nervous system from the portal of entry along the axis cylinders of peripheral nerves. In the chimpanzee, feeding of virus reproduces most of the features of the human infection in that animals may become symptomless excretors or may develop paralytic infections. From his studies on the course of infection in these animals, Bodian (1956) suggests that ingested virus first multiplies in the tonsil or Peyer's patches, from which virus may be excreted in the throat or into the intestines. From the primary sites of multiplication, virus passes to lymph nodes where secondary multiplication occurs, and then by lymph vessels to the blood, from which the central nervous system is infected. Sabin (1956), on the other hand, expresses the view that infection reaches the central nervous system by neural routes from peripheral nerve ganglia which are themselves infected by nerve pathways either from the oropharyngeal or intestinal mucosa or from other susceptible extraneural tissues infected by blood-borne virus.

It is impossible to review here the large amount of experimental work which has been devoted to the elucidation of this problem. The view that the central nervous system is infected directly from the blood stream has been based chiefly on (a) the demonstration of virus in the blood of persons before the appearance of paralysis or in close contacts who fail to develop paralysis, and (b) the occurrence of a period of viraemia in cynomolgous monkeys (Wenner et al., 1959) and in chimpanzees (Bodian, 1956) several days after feeding virus and before the development of paralysis. Numerous particles resembling the virus of poliomyelitis were seen in electronmicrographs of the endothelium of cerebral capillaries of a rhesus monkey killed three days after intramuscular injection of virus (von Mannweiler and Palacios, 1961). This observation would seem to favour infection of the central nervous system directly from the circulation, but in the experiment the dose of virus inoculated was very large (10^7 tissue cultures doses), and the results of such an experiment may have little relevance to the sequence of events in natural infections. The view that virus infects the central nervous system by nerve pathways from the periphery is supported by the demonstration of high concentrations of virus in the sciatic nerve and its early presence in the lumbar cord following intramuscular injection of virus in monkeys (see Wenner and Kamitsuka, 1957) and by the occasional finding of virus in peripheral nerve ganglia before the onset of viraemia in monkeys given virus by mouth (Wenner et al., 1959).

The occurrence of provocative poliomyelitis, i.e. paralysis of muscles of an arm following immunizing injections, and the incidence of bulbar paralysis following tonsillectomy, have been interpreted as evidence of spread of virus to the central nervous system along nerve pathways. In provocative poliomyelitis, it has been suggested, virus temporarily in the circulation of individuals who might, but for the injection, have had an inapparent infection, localizes at the site of trauma and there enters damaged nerves along which it passes to the cord. On the other hand, the view has been expressed that the trauma, by reflex effect on the circulation in the related region of the cord, favours localization of virus from the blood-stream at that site. Such an explanation, although conceivable, seems less likely to explain the occurrence of bulbar poliomyelitis following tonsillectomy, where ready access of virus to damaged nerves and transport of virus along these nerves to the medulla seems likely.

It has been widely accepted that spread of virus in the central nervous system takes place within nerve fibres. It has been shown, however, by Liu and his colleagues (1958, 1959) that hyperimmune rabbit serum injected intravenously into monkeys that had been given virus by the intraspinal route 24–48 hours previously, greatly lessened the mortality and severity of paralysis. This observation would suggest that in these experiments virus moved from cell to cell in intercellular spaces rather than exclusively within axons from one area of the central nervous system to another. If transport of virus within axons from the periphery to the central nervous system is unlikely on anatomical and physiological grounds, it is not obvious why such a route of spread is acceptable within the central nervous system.

It is apparent from a survey of the recent literature that opinions on the mode of spread of poliomyelitis virus in man are not unanimous. It may well be that virus reaches the central nervous system from the periphery either by the blood or by spread in tissue spaces along nerves, and that it multiplies in the mesodermal cells as well as in the epithelial cells of the alimentary tract. The use of newer techniques, such as fluorescent-antibody and autoradiography, may clarify the issues still in dispute.

4. General comment

To summarize very briefly the evidence relating to virus spread within the nervous system, it can be stated that in experimental animals certain viruses can spread from peripheral sites of entry to the central nervous system via the nerves, while other viruses are carried to the central nervous system by the blood. Transport of virus centrifugally from central nervous system to peripheral loci, via the sensory nerves, also undoubtedly occurs in some instances.

The exact mechanism of virus transport within the nerves is still unknown in many cases, but there is good evidence that, in some instances at least, spread may occur in the tissue spaces; and the same is true of the spread of virus within the central nervous system itself. Convincing evidence that viruses may travel within the axons has not been produced, though further work with the modern techniques now available is clearly desirable.

In naturally infected animals, and in man, clinical and pathological findings are compatible with the view that spread of viruses along nerves takes place in ways similar to those demonstrated in experimental animals.

IV. Release of Virus from Host

The mode of spread of virus to fresh hosts, on which survival of virus depends, will usually be related to the route by which virus leaves the body of infected hosts. Viruses which produce lesions on the skin or mucous surfaces will obviously be disseminated from the exudates or secretions from such surfaces. Where a virus may be excreted by more than one route, one may be of primary importance; for example, herpes simplex virus may occasionally be excreted in the faeces, but spread of infection is believed to occur through direct or indirect contact with mouth secretions; similarly in mumps, saliva is the vehicle by which infection is spread, although virus may frequently be demonstrated in the urine in the clinical stage of infection (Utz, Szwed and Kasel, 1958). For the purposes of discussion, it will be convenient to consider release of virus from infections which remain local and those which show more extensive spread in the tissue or generalization by means of the blood stream.

A. Local Infections

In those infections which remain localized at the sites of entry in skin, conjunctiva or mucous surfaces, the release of virus from local lesions would appear to be a relatively straightforward matter. In warts and molluscum contagiosum, where proliferative rather than necrotic changes occur in the affected skin, virus is likely to be released on the surface slowly, perhaps over a long period of time. Where local lesions are associated with rapid necrosis, as in cowpox and fowl pox, there is rapid release of virus over a shorter period. The possible removal of virus from such lesions by biting insects and the importance of such vectors in mechanical transfer of infection to fresh hosts has been mentioned previously. The necrosis of superficial cells of the conjunctiva and genital tract infected with the virus of inclusion blenorrhoea, and of cells in the respiratory mucosa infected with common cold or influenza viruses, releases virus on surfaces from which fresh hosts may be readily infected. The relatively brief duration of excretion of these viruses may result from rapid destruction of susceptible cells, the production of interferon or the development of antibody. Excretion of virus from infections of the intestinal mucosa is considered below.

B. Generalized Infections

The excretion of virus from generalized infections will depend largely on the target organs in which virus proliferation finally takes place, for only in arthropod-borne diseases is virus in the circulation directly concerned in the further natural transmission of infection.

1. Excretion in saliva and sputum

In a few diseases, virus may be excreted in the saliva because of localization of infection in the salivary glands, as in mumps, rabies and salivary gland disease of animals. The presence of virus in the saliva several days before the onset of clinical parotitis (Henle et al., 1948) suggests that epithelial cells in the glands release virus some time before damage to those cells evokes the inflammatory response which gives rise to symptoms. The propagation of rabies depends upon the excretion of virus from the salivary glands of rabid carnivores or symptom-free vampire bats. Virus may also be present in the saliva because of focal lesions in the mucosa of the mouth; in herpes simplex, measles, chickenpox and smallpox, for example. In these diseases, the mouth secretions are an important source of infection, for the lesions of the enanthem discharge virus to the mucous surface early in the disease.

Excretion of virus in sputum would appear to be important in the infection of new hosts only when the upper respiratory tract is involved. When the infection localizes in pulmonary tissue, as in psittacosis, the patient is not highly infectious. Most human infections with this virus are derived from avian sources, and spread from man to man has only occasionally been recorded (see Meyer, 1959). The failure of the virus to pass from man to man is usually attributed to lack of adaptation of the virus to the human host, but it may depend upon the amount of virus excreted, much more being available from the diseased bird.

2. Excretion in faeces

As their name indicates, enteroviruses are frequently present in faeces. Although this may result from an infection confined to the intestinal mucosa, the occasional occurrence of disease involving other tissues and organs justifies their consideration among generalized infections.

From recent reports it appears that the proportion of healthy young children excreting enteroviruses varies with the locality and season. In a survey by the Public Health Laboratory Service covering the two-year period 1957–1959, 28,797 specimens of faeces from apparently healthy children under the age of five years were examined. The virus isolation rates over the whole period were 7·7% for poliomyelitis virus, 9·8% for Coxsackie, 6·5% for adenovirus and 3·6% for Echo viruses. The frequency of isolation varied with the season of the year, Coxsackie and poliovirus being more common in the second and third quarters, adenovirus in the first two quarters and Echo viruses from June to December (Spicer, 1961). The site of multiplication of viruses found in faeces has not in most instances been determined. They may be derived from the tissues of the intestinal wall, from the upper alimentary or respiratory tracts, or may reach the lumen of the gut in bile or possibly in pancreatic secretions.

It has been noted previously that poliovirus is frequently recovered from the tonsillopharyngeal region in the acute phase of disease. This virus has been shown to survive in gastric juice at pH 2·0 for 30 minutes at 37°C (Barski et al., 1954) and might readily survive passage through the stomach to appear in the faeces without multiplication in the intestine. However, the finding of virus in the wall of the ileum and colon in fatal cases (Sabin and Ward, 1941a), and the frequency and duration of intestinal excretion in persons fed attenuated strains, suggest that multiplication readily takes place in the intestinal wall; whether this occurs chiefly in the superficial epithelium or in deeper cells is unknown.

Evidence has recently been accumulating that various types of Echo virus may be associated with gastroenteritis in children (Eichenwald et al., 1958; Ramos-Alvarez and Sabin, 1958; Sommerville, 1958) and in adults (Klein et al., 1960). This type of illness is usually mild. Echo viruses may also cause generalized illness, with or without involvement of the central nervous system, but in these patients, too, virus can be readily recovered from the faeces. It seems likely, therefore, that the generalized infection may arise from sites of primary multiplication in the alimentary tract. The same sort of considerations apply to the faecal excretion of Coxsackie viruses. These also may be found in a proportion of healthy children, and may occasionally give rise to generalized disease or aseptic meningitis, and group A strains produce clinical infections of the mouth and pharynx in the form of herpangina.

The finding of adenoviruses in the faeces of healthy children seems at first a little surprising, as these viruses have usually been associated with mild infection of the conjunctiva and upper respiratory tract. Virus from this region might reach the lower alimentary canal in swallowed secretions but at least some adenovirus strains may multiply in the intestinal wall, as evidenced by the occurrence in children of gastroenteritis (Gardner, McGregor and Dick, 1960; Duncan and Hutchison, 1961) and mesenteric adenitis (Ross, Potter and Zachary, 1962).

The excretion of virus of infectious hepatitis in faeces has been established by experiments on human volunteers (Neefe, Stokes and Reinhold, 1945) and more recently by recovery of virus in tissue culture (Rightsel et al., 1961). There is, however, no evidence known to the author to show whether virus in faeces is derived from the liver or from the bowel wall. The fact that viraemia may be demonstrable up to 11 days before the onset of infectious hepatitis following transfusion (Harden et al., 1955) suggests multiplication in some extrahepatic tissue from which virus reaches the blood to infect liver cells. Whether the primary sites of virus multiplication are in alimentary mucosa and associated lymph nodes is unknown. The importance of faecal excretion in spreading the disease is illustrated by the occurrence of explosive water-borne outbreaks such as that recorded by Anderson (1957), in which a school water supply was contaminated with the effluent from a septic tank.

In other generalized virus infections, secondary lesions may occur in the intestines; for example, in severe cases of smallpox and chickenpox in man, in ectromelia in mice and psittacosis in birds. Faecal excretion of virus in such diseases may be of secondary importance in their spread—except in psittacosis, when nestlings may acquire infection from the droppings of their parents (Burnet, 1953).

3. Excretion in urine

Few viruses appear to produce specific pathological lesions in the kidney, although histological evidence of viral lesions has been observed in smallpox, chickenpox and cytomegalic inclusion disease. Nevertheless, it seems likely that in generalized infections, virus is excreted in the urine during the viraemic phase. The absence of information in certain instances may merely indicate that virus has not been sought by adequate techniques. Virus excretion in the urine has been detected in mumps (Utz et al., 1958), measles (Gresser and Katz, 1960), rubella (Weller and Neva, 1963), Coxsackie infections (Utz and Shelokov, 1958; Hinuma et al., 1962) and in men suffering from a rubella-like illness apparently due to adenovirus (Gutekunst and Heggie, 1961). Cytomegalic inclusion virus has also been found in the urine of young children in the absence of symptoms (Rowe et al., 1958a). In measles, the virus was found in the urine only in the first few days of illness. In the young children studied by Rowe et al., however, cytomegalic inclusion virus was found in urine and in mouth swabs over a period of months and at a time when neutralizing antibody was present in the blood. The presence of virus in the urine in acute generalized infections may merely be the result of spillover from the circulation. However, where urinary excretion is more persistent, it is likely that virus is multiplying in cells of the kidney or elsewhere in the urinary tract. Evidence of such infection is available in cytomegalic inclusion disease of infants (Weller and Hanshaw, 1962) and in distemper of dogs (Liu and Coffin, 1957). In both these diseases, cells with virus inclusions may be demonstrated in the urinary sediment.

In none of the diseases mentioned above is it likely that the urinary excretion of virus is important in the spread of infection. In each case there are other sources from which virus is more readily dispersed.

4. Insect-borne infections

In infections spread by blood-sucking insects, excretion of virus from skin, mucous surfaces, in the urine or faeces is of little importance in propagating infection from one host to another. Thus, although the conjunctival secretion in the rabbit with myxomatosis is infective, it appears to play no great part in the spread of the disease. In Arbor virus infections the insect vector provides a suitable host for further virus multiplication as well as a means of introducing virus to a new host—surely an economical method of providing for continued survival of these viruses in nature.

The recent resurgence of interest in tumour viruses has thrown some light on the propagation of these viruses and their excretion from mammalian hosts. Many years ago the mouse mammary tumour virus was shown by Bittner to be transmitted in the milk. More recently the virus has been shown to be transmissible from males to females during copulation (see Gross, 1961). Polyoma virus in mice is excreted in the urine and faeces, and it has been suggested by Rowe, Huebner and Hartley (1961) that whereas suckling mice may be highly infective during the first few weeks of life, only few adults in an infected colony excrete virus. The maintenance of infection would appear therefore to depend on the size of a mouse colony and the degree of overcrowding within it.

C. DURATION OF VIRUS EXCRETION
AND ITS RELATION TO THE DEVELOPMENT OF ANTIBODY

In the acute generalized virus infections it is usual for virus to be excreted during the acute phase of the disease and sometimes during convalescence, but in many instances excretion ceases soon thereafter. In certain infections, however, virus may continue to be excreted, perhaps intermittently, from localized sites for months or years; in herpes simplex, for example, or lymphogranuloma venereum.

In general, antibody in the serum prevents dissemination of virus within the body, although occasionally virus and antibody may co-exist in the blood. The experiments of Smith (1929) with vaccinia in rabbits suggest that in this latter state the virus is present within leucocytes in the circulation. More commonly, as in measles and small-pox, virus is demonstrable in the blood during the acute stage, before antibody appears. Only when there is no antibody response to virus infection, as in the immunological tolerance shown by Traub's mice to the virus of lymphocytic choriomeningitis, and as in some cases of hepatitis in man, is virus continuously demonstrable in the circulating blood. In smallpox patients who are to recover, antibody can be found in the blood by the fifth or sixth day of illness. This does not, however, coincide with cessation of virus excretion, for virus often in high titre is present in crusts which may not separate until the third week or later. Virus in the pustule and in the crust which later replaces it, is not affected by antibody in the patient's serum or tissue fluids. Antibody, however, is not demonstrable in the fluid of pustules, and it would appear that the dense cellular infiltration at the base of the pustule prevents the passage of antibody into it or that antibody becomes bound by the large amount of soluble antigen in pustule fluid. In chickenpox, however, virus cannot be recovered from crusts (Weller *et al.*, 1958; Taylor-Robinson, 1959). This may be because the methods available for the detection of this virus are less sensitive than those for variola virus. However, the chickenpox vesicle does not show the underlying dense cellular infiltration of the smallpox vesicle, and it is possible that antibody diffuses more readily into it. The fact that extracts of chickenpox crusts, in comparison with those from smallpox, are very much more "anticomplementary" suggests that antibody may be present along with antigen in the dried exudate of which these crusts are largely composed.

Poliomyelitis is a good example of a disease in which serum antibody would appear to terminate viraemia, for in most recorded instances virus has been detected in the blood only in the early stages of non-paralytic infections or before paralysis appears. The continued excretion of virus in the faeces several weeks after the development of an antibody response seems to be due to persistence of infection in the wall of the alimentary canal. The presence of cytomegalic inclusion virus in the mouth secretions and urine of children long after the appearance of antibody would also appear to be due to the persistence of virus in superficial cells in the mucosa of the mouth or urinary tract.

In warts, virus papillomas of animals and molluscum contagiosum where there is little cell necrosis, virus persists in the tissues and no sharp antibody reaction appears to be evoked. On the other hand, in certain acute infections of mucous membranes, particularly in the common cold and influenza, virus excretion does not seem to persist very long after the acute phase of infection. It may be that where virus multiplication is rapid and leads to early death of infected cells, these are rapidly shed; and extension of infection ceases because of lack of susceptible cells together with the local appearance of antibody in the inflammatory exudate promoted by the nature and speed of cell necrosis.

CHAPTER 4

Mechanisms of Cell Infection
I. Virus Attachment and Penetration

A. COHEN

*Department of Bacteriology, University College Hospital
Medical School, London, England*

I. Introduction

Viruses replicate exclusively in the interior of the host cells. To gain
this interior, virus particles must first negotiate the cell membranes of
animal tissues, or the more rigid cell walls of plant tissues and bacteria.
Plant viruses, which are not included in the scope of this chapter,
invade through traumatic injury applied to the host-cell wall at the
time of infection. Except possibly in a few rare instances, bacterial
and animal viruses do not penetrate cells in this way. Instead they use
mechanisms of specific attachment to cell surfaces and of cell penetration, which detailed study of certain viruses has shown may be highly
complex.

The most clearly understood mechanisms of attachment and penetration are those by which the T-even bacteriophages infect their host
bacterium, *Escherichia coli*. These have already been discussed in
Chapter 2 and here need only be recapitulated briefly. T2 phage, the

one most thoroughly studied, attaches by its tail fibres to specific receptor sites on the cell wall, first reversibly by electrostatic attraction and then irreversibly. Weakening of the cell wall by a hydrolytic enzyme, present in the phage tail, is followed by injection of the infective principle (DNA) into the interior of the cell. The protein coat of the phage, which acts as a microsyringe, remains extracellular and can be seen, by means of the electron microscope, attached to the cell wall (Anderson, 1953).

The clear picture of cell attachment and penetration, exhibited by the T-even bacteriophages, has no parallel in the sphere of animal viruses. Enough information is, however, available to suggest a marked similarity in the basic mechanisms of attachment, if not of penetration, between some bacterial and animal virus systems.

Until recently, our knowledge of the early stages of animal virus infection was almost confined to one group, the myxoviruses. The reason for this stems from the observations of Hirst (1941) and McClelland and Hare (1941), who, independently, described the phenomenon of influenza-virus haemagglutination. The later demonstration by Hirst (1943) that many of the reactions between influenza viruses and red cells occur also with host-tissue cells led to the adoption of the virus–erythrocyte system as a model for elucidating the reactions between influenza viruses and susceptible host cells. Other viruses have received less attention because of the absence of suitable virus-haemagglutination systems, and other technical difficulties. In recent years, however, the introduction of *in vitro* tissue-culture techniques has facilitated the study of virus–cell interactions and allowed investigation of some non-haemagglutinating viruses.

The extensive use of the virus–erythrocyte model for the study of virus–cell attachment necessitates a full discussion of the reactions between viruses and erythrocytes before reviewing the interactions between viruses and host cells.

II. Virus–erythrocyte Interaction

The interaction between viruses and erythrocytes is usually manifested by the occurrence of haemagglutination. Many viruses exhibit this phenomenon, but of these only influenza, Newcastle disease (NDV), fowl-plague and mumps viruses are unequivocally known to depend on the presence of specific receptor sites at the red-cell surface. Because these viruses share the same red-cell receptors, and by reason of their common affinity for mucins, they form a distinctive group, the members of which are now known as myxoviruses (Andrewes, Bang and Burnet, 1955).

A. MYXOVIRUSES

1. Haemagglutination

Red blood cells from a wide variety of species are agglutinated by myxoviruses, but the ones most commonly employed in experimental work are those of fowls, humans, and guinea-pigs. Virus particles adsorb on to red cells by means of specific combining sites, a number of which are distributed over the surfaces of both virus and red cell. Many virus particles may become attached to each red cell, and some particles attach simultaneously to more than one. The disparity of size between virus and red cell, however, makes it unlikely that attachment to more than two red cells could occur simultaneously. Nevertheless, in this way a "lattice" of red cells, held together by virus particles, is formed which eventually becomes sufficiently large to be visible to the naked eye.

With some type A strains of influenza virus, the passage history determines the species of cell agglutinated. Strains freshly isolated in the chick amniotic cavity agglutinate human and guinea-pig cells to a higher titre than fowl cells, which in some cases are not agglutinated at all. Such viruses are said to be in the O phase, and grow poorly in the allantoic cavity. Repeated amniotic passage at low dilution leads to selection of a variant which agglutinates fowl cells to the same titre as human and guinea-pig cells. This mutant form, the D phase, which grows rapidly in both the amniotic and allantoic cavities, quickly supplants the parental O-phase form (Burnet and Bull, 1943). Although the phenomenon is not demonstrable with influenza B strains (Hirst, 1947), its occurrence serves to emphasize the highly specific nature of the virus–cell linkage. Where it occurs, agglutination of fowl cells by D-phase virus suggests that one of the mechanisms of adaptation to a new host species may be the selection of variants having a greater affinity for the cell receptors of the new host, thereby facilitating cellular attachment.

(a) *Virus–red cell adsorption.* Adsorption of virus to red cells takes place in suitable ionic environments over a wide temperature range. Above 4°C, adsorbed virus is released from erythrocytes which are then no longer agglutinable by this or other virus preparations. The eluted virus is unchanged and will undergo repeated cycles of adsorption and elution with fresh red-cell suspensions (Hirst, 1942). The enzymic nature of the reaction whereby the cell receptors are destroyed when virus elutes was soon recognized by Hirst.

The specificity of adsorption, its virtual independence of temperature, and its dependence on electrolytes and pH, suggest that it results from an electrostatic interaction between the charged surfaces of virus and red cell. There is much experimental evidence in support of this hypothesis, in particular, the absence of haemagglutination in electrolyte-free media. In those media where haemagglutination occurs, removal of electrolytes from the system sometimes results in dissociation of virus from red cells (Davenport and Horsfall, 1948; Lowell and Buckingham, 1948; Flick, Sandford and Mudd, 1949; Burnet and Edney, 1952). The role which attractive forces between charged surfaces play in virus adsorption is further emphasized by the attachment of viruses to charged surfaces of non-biological origin. Viruses, which carry a net negative charge, adsorb to positively charged surfaces, such as aluminium or anion exchangers, in the absence of salt. Attachment to negatively charged surfaces, such as glass or cation exchangers, takes place only in ionic conditions similar to those demanded by the cell surface (Puck, Garen and Cline, 1951; Puck and Sagik, 1953; Valentine and Allison, 1959). These conditions are not, however, identical, since attachment of some viruses to cells, but not to non-biological surfaces, is inhibited by high ion concentrations (Puck *et al*, 1951; Allison and Valentine, 1960). This lack of identity is, perhaps, not surprising in view of the specificity of cell attachment.

The specific nature of virus–cell linkage suggests that attachment is by active sites on the surfaces of virus and red cell which have complementary configurations. These sites, like the surface of any other biological macromolecule, may be considered as a network of positively and negatively charged atomic groupings, each exerting a localized electric field force. If the approach of virus to cell is close enough, fields of opposite sign will attract. Since both virus and red cell carry net negative charges, the electrostatic repulsion set up between them, in a non-ionic environment, would be sufficient to prevent close enough contact for oppositely charged fields to attract. The presence of cations in suitable concentrations, by the formation of an electrical double layer or by binding on to some of the negative charges, presumably reduces the repulsive forces sufficiently to allow close enough contact for oppositely charged sites to attract. The inhibition of virus–cell attachment by high ion concentrations suggests that beyond a critical concentration net charges of positive sign become manifest on both virus and cell, resulting in the re-establishment of electrostatic repulsion. The charge distribution of non-biological surfaces, being more uniform, is more difficult to alter, and hence will continue to attach virus in the presence of high ion concentrations.

The localized electric fields set up by the network of positively and negatively charged atomic groupings at virus and cell surfaces will exert strong attractive forces where the approach of combining sites is close enough to allow sufficient points of contact between them.

Complementary spatial configurations at the surfaces of virus and cell would not only provide these conditions but also account for the marked specificity of virus–cell attachment. In addition, their inter-action would result in the close fitting of large areas of the opposing surfaces, thereby strengthening the attraction by means of van der Waals forces, which operate effectively only at very close distances. These forces are locally weak, but the large surface areas in close approximation when complementary configurations interact would result in an effective attractive force by summation of effect. The possibility that oppositely charged carboxyl and amino groups provide the main attractive forces is indicated by the minimal adsorption of both phage and myxoviruses at pH 4·0 and 10·0, under which con-ditions these groups are, respectively, un-ionized (Tolmach and Puck, 1952; Sagik and Levine, 1957). The recent demonstration that the negatively charged sialic-acid molecule is the important functional group of the myxovirus cell receptor (vide infra) further suggests that attachment may take place through the carboxyl radical of this mole-cule. However, the recovery of adsorption efficiency at pH 3·0 indicates that other or alternative mechanisms may be involved.

The fact that not all investigators have been able to recover ad-sorbed virus from erythrocytes by removal of electrolytes (Davenport and Horsfall, 1948; Tamm, 1954) and that the recovery, when it does occur, is sometimes incomplete (Lowell and Buckingham, 1948; Flick et al, 1949) suggests the possibility of a mode of linkage other than that determined by non-specific short-range forces. The rate at which virus is adsorbed is virtually independent of temperature, indicating that the energy of activation required by any mode of linkage must be low. Hydrogen-bonding, characterized by its low energy of activation, may therefore be considered as a possible additional means of holding virus and red cell together.

(b) Kinetics of adsorption. Attachment of virus to red cells is dependent on Brownian movement and thus on the concentration of virus and red cells in the system. These conditions may be defined by the equation:

$$\frac{-d\,V}{d\,t} = K\,V\,C \tag{1}$$

where V is the concentration of free virus, C the concentration of cells and K the velocity constant of adsorption. If the ratio of virus to cells is kept sufficiently low, the term C may be considered a constant and the reaction then approximates to first order kinetics, the velocity constant K of which may be defined by the equation:

$$K = \frac{2\cdot3}{Ct} \log \frac{V_0}{V_t} \tag{2}$$

where V_0 and V_t are the concentrations of unattached virus at the beginning and end of the time interval t, respectively. Experimentally this is confirmed by the linear logarithmic relationship which is found in cell–virus systems when unattached virus is plotted against time. K, the attachment velocity constant, may be calculated from the slope so obtained. (Delbrück, 1940a; Puck *et al.*, 1951; Sagik, Puck and Levine, 1954).

The rate of attachment will be limited by the collision efficiency of the system, i.e. the number of collisions which result in binding. The actual collision rate can be calculated theoretically from kinetic theory. If every collision results in attachment, the experimentally observed attachment-velocity constant should be in agreement with the theoretical maximum value based on kinetic theory. The correct alignment of virus and cell demanded by the use of complementary receptor sites suggests that the actual proportion of collisions which results in binding must be low. It is surprising therefore that some authors have sought to prove that the efficiency is in fact high and from this deduced the electrostatic nature of virus–cell attachment. These conclusions have been based on comparison of experimental values with theoretical maximal values for the attachment velocity constant derived from diffusion theory (Schlesinger, 1932a,b; Delbrück, 1940a; Sagik *et al.*, 1954). It is unlikely, however, that diffusion theory supplies a valid model of virus adsorption, since the number of particles near the cell is probably insufficient to define a continuous concentration gradient which the theory requires. Moreover, the use of diffusion equations is unnecessary, since the actual collision rate can be calculated from kinetic theory. Comparison of this value with experimental values would give a correct estimate of collision efficiency. A rough estimate of the collision rate, derived from kinetic theory, of the influenza virus–red cell system gives a value approximately 10^6 times larger than the experimental value of $6 \cdot 6 \times 10^{-9} \, \text{cm}^3 \text{min}^{-1}$ obtained by Sagik *et al.* (1954). This indicates that the collision efficiency is probably low. The assumption that binding takes place by electrostatic forces is not thereby invalidated. The collision efficiency itself can tell us nothing of the nature of the physico-chemical bond involved in binding. This can only be obtained by measurements of the thermodynamic functions of the virus–red cell reaction which have not, so far, been made.

(c) *Elution.* Above 4°C, spontaneous elution, which results in destruction of the cell receptors, follows the stage of adsorption. Hirst's conception of the enzymic nature of this reaction was substantiated by the discovery of an active principle in filtrates of *Vibrio cholerae* cultures which reacts with the red-cell surface to produce effects which are almost identical with those produced by active virus (Stone, 1947).

This active principle, originally referred to as receptor-destroying enzyme (RDE) but now known to be a neuraminidase, has recently been obtained in a highly purified crystalline form by Ada and French (1959).

It is believed that the apposition of specific sites on the virus surface to complementary ones on the cell surface, during the stage of adsorption, orientates the active enzyme groups so that they are correctly aligned to react with their substrate. Chemical evidence, reviewed below, has revealed that the split product after virus enzyme action, free N-acetylneuraminic acid, is a part only of the cell receptor. Its removal is, nevertheless, sufficient to break the attractive forces between virus and cell receptors.

The action of different members of the myxovirus group, and even of different strains of influenza virus, on red cells is not identical but reflects differences in affinity for the cell receptors. After adsorption and elution of one virus strain, erythrocytes remain agglutinable by some members of the group but not others, including the original virus. On this basis viruses can be arranged in sequence according to their capacity for agglutinating red cells which have been previously treated with other members of the group. This sequence, called the receptor gradient, can also be demonstrated by graded treatment of the cells with RDE (Burnet et al., 1945; Burnet, McCrea and Stone, 1946). Thus, such RDE treatment destroys sequentially the capacity of the red cells to be agglutinated by mumps virus, NDV, various strains of types A and B influenza and swine-influenza virus.

Receptor inactivation by myxoviruses or RDE is now known to result from release of N-acetylneuraminic acid, the negatively charged carboxyl group of which is very probably the site to which positively charged groups on the virus surface attach. The number of these attachment sites which are required for firm adsorption is not known, but the sequence in which viruses lose their capacity for agglutinating red cells, which have been treated with various viruses or graded doses of RDE, indicates that it differs for each virus. Thus, viruses such as mumps, which fail to haemagglutinate after minimal enzyme treatment of erythrocytes, probably require more than those which are still capable of haemagglutinating after more complete enzyme treatment. If so, some correspondence between release of N-acetylneuraminic acid by each virus, or its equivalent in terms of soluble enzyme, and the point at which it fails to agglutinate erythrocytes should be demonstrable. Since the carboxyl group of N-acetylneuraminic acid is the dominant ionogenic group at the red-cell surface, its removal results in a reduction of the cell's net negative charge and hence electrophoretic mobility towards the anode (Hanig, 1948; Cook, Heard and Seaman,

1961). Some measure of the release of N-acetylneuraminic acid may therefore be obtained from the change in electrophoretic mobility of red cells produced by enzyme treatment. In general, there is close agreement between the change in red-cell electrophoretic mobility produced by each virus and the sequence in which the capacity for haemagglutination is lost (Ada and Stone, 1950; Stone and Ada, 1950). There are, however, some exceptions to the rule. NDV and swine-influenza virus, in particular, reduce the electrophoretic mobility more than would be expected from their position in the sequence. Possibly these viruses are capable of releasing some molecules of N-acetyl-neuraminic acid normally inaccessible to other members of the myxo-virus group.

It is significant that treatment of cells of the allantoic membrane *in vivo* with graded doses of RDE alters sequentially their susceptibility to infection with various strains of influenza virus (Stone, 1948a). Although this sequence differs from that obtained with red cells, the phenomenon does indicate that viruses may vary in their receptor requirements for the initiation of infection.

The differences of haemagglutination and enzymic behaviour which are brought to light by the receptor-gradient phenomenon are reflected also in the rates at which viruses elute from red cells. Not only do different strains vary in this respect but even virus particles of a single strain in the same infected allantoic fluid are heterogeneous in their elution behaviour. These differences of enzymic activity are not explicable on a simple quantitative basis (Smith and Cohen, 1956). Possibly the efficiency of elution is determined by the accessibility of the virus enzyme to its substrate. Alternatively, the more rapidly eluting viruses may be those which require a large number of cell receptors for firm adsorption. It seems possible that variations of attachment of this type may influence the infectivity of a virus preparation. The absence of any correlation between the elution rate from human red cells and the infectivity of a virus preparation in the allantoic cavity (Smith and Cohen, 1956) does not invalidate this hypothesis. The activity of the virus enzyme on human red cells is not necessarily an indication of its activity on the substrate presented by susceptible host cells, particularly when these are of a different species. Indeed, the rates of elution from fowl red cells of allantoically adapted viruses do not differ nearly as much as those from human cells (Smith and Cohen, 1956). To establish a relationship between enzymic activity and the infectivity of a preparation, combined studies using the same susceptible host cells are needed.

The rate of elution is determined not only by the virus enzymic activity but also by the amount of virus adsorbed on to each individual red cell (Sheffield, Smith and Belyavin, 1954). Anderson *et al.* (1948) suggested that, following release from one receptor, the virus makes contact with another until all the receptors available to it are destroyed. In this way virus migrates or "browses" over the red-cell surface. This hypothesis implies the mediation of forces of attraction greater than the short-range non-specific forces believed to operate in virus adsorption. Theoretically, it is unnecessary to invoke any other concept than the probability of readsorption to the same or other cells following virus release. Where many unaltered cell receptors are available there is greater probability of readsorption by means of random collision. As the reaction proceeds, the number of available receptors decreases with the consequent decrease of the probability of readsorption and increase in the amount of free virus.

(*d*) *Irreversible red-cell adsorption and haemolysis.* Mumps virus and NDV react with erythrocytes in a way exceptional among myxoviruses. Below 30°C with fowl cells and 24°C with human cells, the reactions are similar to those of influenza viruses and are characterized by the normal cycle of adsorption and elution with receptor destruction. Above these temperatures, a proportion of particles in virus preparations of these strains proceeds to a more intimate association with the red-cell receptors, resulting in irreversible adsorption, resistant even to the action of RDE (Burnet 1946, 1950; Anderson, 1947; Burnet and Lind, 1950). Under the conditions in which irreversible binding occurs, the cells undergo haemolysis. Heating the virus to 54°C or above destroys the capacity for irreversible adsorption and haemolysis but leaves that for reversible adsorption intact (Morgan, Enders and Wagley, 1948; Kilham, 1949; Burnet and Lind, 1950; Chu and Morgan, 1950a,b). It is probable, therefore, that the mechanisms of irreversible adsorption and haemolytic activity are closely related. Since both reactions are dependent on the haemagglutination receptors and are abolished by prior treatment of the red cells with RDE, it may be assumed that virus particles which exhibit these properties do so by entering into a more intimate association with the cell receptors than that represented by adsorption and elution.

Irreversible adsorption, but not haemolysis, is exhibited by influenza viruses which have been rendered enzymically inactive by heat at 56°C for 30 minutes. Although unable to elute spontaneously, this heated virus can be released by the action of RDE. When the heated virus–erythrocyte complex is incubated at 37°C, however, virus can no longer be released by the action of RDE (Burnet, 1952). It follows that interaction between specific receptors of myxoviruses and red cells may, under appropriate conditions, lead to four different types of union, manifested by adsorption and elution, adsorption without spontaneous elution but reversible by the action of RDE, irreversible adsorption insusceptible to RDE, and finally haemolysis.

The loss of virus enzymic activity on heating probably results from an alteration of the enzyme's specific three-dimensional structure without affecting the integrity of the receptor configuration responsible for adsorption. After adsorption of enzymically inactive virus, the enzyme substrate, now known to be the glycosidic linkage between sialic acid and an adjacent sugar residue, remains not only unoccupied but also accessible to RDE. Following incubation at 37°C, however, the enzyme substrate becomes inaccessible to RDE, indicating that some further stage in the interaction between the specific receptor sites of virus and cell has taken place. The temperature-dependence of the reaction suggests that some more firm chemical linkage, possibly in the form of covalent bonding which requires a high energy of activation, has replaced the short-range, non-specific forces which are responsible for initial adsorption.

The reactions of mumps virus and NDV with erythrocyte receptors, above 30°C, suggest an interaction not unlike that of heated influenza virus. If so, some of the receptors on the surface of these viruses must differ from the normal myxovirus receptor, possibly by some minor variation in structural configuration, similar to that produced by heat on the normal receptor. This difference is reflected in their altered biological activity; they are enzymically inactive against neuraminidase substrates, more heat-labile, and capable of entering into a more intimate chemical linkage with the cell receptor at 37°C. The mechanism of haemolysis, however, remains unknown. The interaction of receptors peculiar to mumps and NDV with myxovirus cell receptors may result in an enzymic reaction independent of neuraminidase, or the more intimate chemical linkage may result in weakening of the cell wall.

It is not known whether reactions comparable to irreversible adsorption and haemolysis occur with susceptible host-tissue cells, and the relevance of these reactions to any mechanisms of attachment and penetration in host cells remains questionable. Nevertheless, these reactions do possess some similarity to the irreversible adsorption which is a necessary stage of phage infection of the bacterial host cell. Irreversible adsorption of NDV, like that of phage, is temperature-dependent and results in loss of infectivity (Rubin, 1957). Likewise some authors have drawn attention to the analogy between haemolysis and the phenomena of cell leakage and lysis-from-without which occur in the phage–bacterium system (Tolmach, 1957).

2. Inhibitors of haemagglutination

(a) α-*Inhibitors*. The observation of Francis (1947) that haemagglutination by a type B strain of influenza virus, heated at 56°C for 30 minutes, is inhibited by normal human and animal sera was the starting point of a line of investigation which has resulted in the elucidation of the nature of the red-cell receptor substance. The close relationship between this substance and the serum inhibitor was disclosed when the latter was found to be inactivated by treating the serum with either enzymically active virus or RDE (Anderson, 1948a). Subsequently, the recognition of receptor analogues in soluble form greatly simplified the task of chemical identification of the receptor material.

McCrea (1948) located the inhibitory activity in the serum mucoid fraction and from its heat stability, and its inactivation by proteases and potassium periodate, concluded that it was mediated by a muco-protein or mucopolysaccharide component. This conclusion was sub-stantiated by the subsequent demonstration that a number of mucoid substances are potent inhibitors of haemagglutination and are inacti-vated by the virus enzyme or RDE (Burnet, 1948). Inhibitors of this type are now referred to as α (alpha)-inhibitors (Smith and Westwood, 1949; Smith, Westwood and Belyavin, 1951). Typical of these are the ovomucin fraction of eggwhite (Lanni and Beard, 1948; Gottschalk and Lind, 1949a), ovarian cyst mucin (Burnet, 1948), human meconium (Curtain, French and Pye, 1953), extracts of bovine and sheep sub-maxillary glands (McCrea, 1953a; Curtain and Pye, 1955) and urinary mucoprotein (Tamm and Horsfall, 1952).

Most influenza viruses heated at 56°C for 30 minutes cease to be enzymically active but retain their haemagglutinating properties (Briody, 1948). Haemagglutination inhibition by α-type inhibitors is demonstrable only with heated viruses and is commonly assumed to result from irreversible adsorption of enzymically inactive virus to the inhibitor substrate. This assumption is not wholly supported by the experimental facts. Ether-treated virus which is fully active enzymic-ally is inhibited by α-inhibitor (Smith *et al.*, 1953). Furthermore, at 0°C, a temperature at which enzymes are virtually inactive, unheated virus is no more susceptible to the inhibitor than at higher temperatures. Finally, Smith and Westwood (1950) showed that both heated and unheated preparations of PR8 virus combine with α-inhibitor at the same rate and exhibit the same combining capacities. The increased susceptibility of heated virus to haemagglutination inhibitors cannot therefore result simply from destruction of the virus enzyme. It is more likely to be explained by distortion of the virus surface which facilitates occlusion of haemagglutinin receptors by attached inhibitor molecules (Smith and Westwood, 1950).

Attachment of inhibitor molecules to unheated virus without affecting its capacity for haemagglutination indicates that inhibitor and receptor substance are not identical. Their points of resemblance are probably confined to specific prosthetic groups which act as the enzyme substrate. Similarly, quantitative and qualitative differences exhibited by inhibitors from various sources when tested against a number of virus strains (Stone, 1949) suggest that here, too, chemical relationship is limited to specific determinant groups.

(b) *β–Inhibitor*. Another type of inhibitor with distinctive properties is found in normal sera of various animal species (Ginsberg and Horsfall, 1949; Chu, 1951; Smith *et al.*, 1951). The inhibitory component, generally referred to as β–inhibitor, differs from α in its thermolability, insusceptibility to RDE and periodate, and by its inhibition of unheated virus to the same, or higher, titre as heated virus. It is active mainly against types A and A prime strains which have not been mouse-adapted. It is present in high titre in bovine serum (Brans, Herzberger and Binkhorst, 1953) and in lesser amounts in rabbit and mouse serum (Chu, 1951; Smith *et al.*, 1951). β–Inhibitor neutralizes the infectivity of sensitive strains as well as inhibiting haemagglutination.

Chemically, β–inhibitor is not a mucoid substance, and there is no evidence of any relationship with the red-cell receptor. It is found in the globulin fraction of rabbit serum and has been obtained separate from α by ammonium sulphate fractionation and electrophoretic techniques (McCrea, 1946; 1946; Tyrrell, 1954; Cohen and Belyavin, 1961).

(c) *γ–Inhibitor*. Recently a third type of haemagglutination inhibitor, active almost exclusively against Asian (A2)-type strains of influenza virus has been described (Shimojo *et al.*, 1958; Cohen and Belyavin, 1959; Takatsy and Barb, 1959). This inhibitor, which may be referred to as γ, inhibits haemagglutination of both heated and unheated Asian strains, is inactivated by periodate but not by RDE, and is heat-stable. It is present in high titre in normal horse serum which contains little or no α– or β–inhibitor, and is also found in guinea-pig, rabbit, human and ferret sera. Inactivation of γ–inhibitor by periodate suggests that its activity is dependent on polysaccharide prosthetic groups. It is, however, easily distinguished from α–inhibitor by its characteristic properties and by its potent neutralizing activity.

Some A2 strains and variants of A2 strains are partially or completely insensitive to γ–inhibitor (Shimojo *et al.*, 1958; Choppin and Tamm, 1959; Cohen and Belyavin, 1959; James and Fiset, 1959). It is now established that this is due to the existence of sensitive and resistant virus particles, the relative proportions of which determine the inhibitor sensitivity of the particular virus preparation (Cohen and Biddle, 1960).

The adsorption of γ–inhibitor from horse serum by sensitive and insensitive A2 strains (Cohen and Biddle, 1963) suggests that in-hibitor attaches to both types of virus. Only in sensitive strains, however, is haemagglutination inhibited. This indicates that the inhibitor does not unite directly with the virus haemagglutinin recep-tors but exerts its effect by occluding them where the surface con-figuration of the virus particle allows. This is in line with the hypothesis of steric hindrance put forward by Smith and Westwood (1950) to explain the greater sensitivity of heated viruses to α–inhibitor. They suggested that distortion of the virus-surface configuration, by heat, facilitates the occlusion of the haemagglutinin receptors by attached inhibitor molecules.

The wide variety of surface patterns revealed by the study of virus–inhibitor interactions (Cohen and Belyavin, 1959) must reflect the spatial distribution of virus-haemagglutinin receptors. The over-whelming evidence of the part these play in the initiation of infection (*vide infra*) implies that variation of surface structure may affect the probability of initiating infection. In order to determine if this is so, the number of virus particles per infective unit of inhibitor sensitive and insensitive strains should be compared. So far, this comparison has not been made.

Takatsy, Barb and Farkas (1959) have described a new kind of red-cell receptor, specific for inhibitor sensitive Asian strains, and similar to γ–inhibitor in its resistance to destruction by RDE. In their hands, both γ–inhibitor and the new cell receptor are unaffected by periodate. Biddle and Cohen (1962) in this laboratory have failed to confirm the existence of such a receptor. Any difference in the agglutin-ability of RDE-treated cells by inhibitor-sensitive and -insensitive A2 strains has been shown to be a manifestation of the receptor-gradient phenomenon. Adequate RDE treatment of red cells from humans, fowls, and guinea-pigs, renders them inagglutinable by inhibitor-sensitive A2 strains. This discrepancy is probably due to the fact that in the experiments of Takatsy *et al.* treatment of the cells with RDE was limited to one hour's duration, whereas in those of Biddle and Cohen enzyme treatment was continued for four or seven hours. Similarly, the amount of periodate which will prevent haemagglutina-tion is critical. Certainly the use of different concentrations of periodate for inactivation of γ–inhibitor has resulted in the contradictory results which have been reported by different authors (Shimojo *et al.*, 1958; Takatsy *et al.*, 1959).

3. Chemistry of the red-cell receptor and its analogues

Attempts to isolate the receptor substance from red cells have been made by de Burgh *et al.* (1948) and McCrea (1953b) among others. The substance isolated by de Burgh and his colleagues was found in the lipoprotein elinin fraction of human red-cell stromata. It was a highly active haemagglutination inhibitor, susceptible to the action of virus enzyme, but did not behave as a homogeneous substance in the ultracentrifuge. Chemical analysis showed it to contain 50% polysaccaride, 2·6% nitrogen and no phosphorus. McCrea's substance, prepared by treatment of human-red-cell stromata with pentane, followed by extraction with 50% ethyl alcohol, was a less active haemagglutination inhibitor but homogeneous in the ultracentrifuge. Electrophoretic analysis, however, revealed more than one peak, of which only one was associated with inhibitory activity. This activity was destroyed by virus enzyme, RDE and periodic acid, but not by trypsin. More recently Kathan, Winzler and Johnson, (1961) have obtained a potent glycoprotein inhibitor from human-red-cell stromata, which is homogeneous on both electrophoretic and ultracentrifugal analysis and is believed to be the receptor substance. McCrea's analysis of the receptor substance is compared with that of Kathan et al. in table I.

TABLE I

Chemical Analysis of Human Red-Cell-Receptor Substance

Reference	Nitrogen (%)	Phosphorus (%)	Sulphur (%)	Reducing Sugar (%)	Hexosamine (%)	Sialic acid (%)
McCrea (1953b)	10	0·5	2·6	14·7*	9·5 (as glucosamine HCl)	‡
Kathan et al. (1961)	10·1	0·25	‡	13·52†	12·1 (as glucosamine)	22·7

* Calculated as glucose.
† Protein-bound hexose (as galactose) 12·4%
  Fucose 1·12%
‡ Not tested.

The difficulty of preparing a purified, homogeneous receptor substance from red cells has rendered the direct approach unsuitable for elucidation of its chemical structure. The study of the viral enzyme substrate in the form of soluble haemagglutination inhibitors has proved more profitable. The first conclusive chemical evidence of the enzymic nature of virus–inhibitor interaction was obtained by Gottschalk and Lind (1949b). They treated ovomucin with active virus at

38°C until 95% of its inhibitory potency had been destroyed, and then isolated by dialysis a low-molecular-weight compound which had the properties of a carbohydrate–peptide complex. The carbohydrate moiety proved to be an oligosaccharide with unusual chemical properties. The recovery of a similar product by the action of RDE, and its absence after treatment with heat-inactivated virus, confirmed that it was indeed the product of enzymic activity. Later a similar substance was obtained by the action of virus on an electrophoretically homogeneous preparation of urinary mucoprotein (Gottschalk, 1951). Odin (1952) was the first to recognize that Gottschalk's split product may be related to sialic acid, a substance originally isolated by Blix from bovine-submaxillary-gland mucin (Blix, 1936), and that sialic acid is an important constituent of α-type haemagglutination inhibitors. The split product obtained from urinary mucoprotein by the enzymic action of influenza virus was finally identified by Klenk, Faillard and Lempfrid (1955) as N–acetylneuraminic acid (NANA). Odin's suggestion of the close relationship between the split product and Blix's sialic acid, now known to be diacetyl neuraminic acid, was thus confirmed.

From a series of chemical studies by Gottschalk and others, recently summarized in a monograph and two review articles (Gottschalk, 1959a, b, 6, 1960), Gottschalk was able to assign to N–acetylneuraminic acid the formula:

$$
\begin{array}{c}
\text{CHOH} \\
\overset{(4)}{} \\
\text{H}\diagdown \\
\quad \text{C}_{(3)} \quad \text{HCNHCOCH}_3 \\
\text{H}\diagup \quad \quad (5) \\
\text{HO}\diagdown \quad \quad \diagup \text{H} \\
\quad \text{C} \quad (6)\text{C} \\
\text{HOOC}\diagup \, (2) \diagdown \text{O}\diagup \quad \text{HCOH} \\
\quad (1) \\
\quad \quad \quad \quad \text{HCOH} \\
\quad \quad \quad \quad \text{CH}_2\text{OH} \\
\quad \quad \quad \quad (9)
\end{array}
$$

All subsequent studies have confirmed this structure, and conclusive proof has been provided by the synthesis of N–acetylneuraminic acid which is identical in every way with the naturally occurring product (Cornforth, Daines and Gottschalk, 1957; Cornforth, Firth and Gottschalk, 1958). In nature a number of substituted neuraminic acids occur, and the term sialic acid is now used as a group name for all acetylated neuraminic acids. In the form N–acetylneuraminic acid, sialic acid is present in a number of mucoprotein inhibitors and may be split off by the action of virus enzyme or RDE (Böhm, Ross and Baumeister, 1957; Faillard, 1957; Zilliken et al., 1957). The recovery of N–acetylneuraminic acid by treatment of human red cells with RDE

(Klenk and Lempfrid, 1957) and virus enzyme (Howe, Rose and Schneider, 1957) has demonstrated unequivocally the chemical relationship between the red-cell-receptor substance and α-inhibitory mucoproteins.

In urinary mucoprotein and bovine-submaxillary-gland mucoprotein the sialic acid is located in polysaccharide prosthetic groups (Gottschalk, 1952, 1957b; Odin, 1952), and its liberation by RDE or acid hydrolysis indicates that it is in the terminal position (Gottschalk, 1956; Faillard, 1957). By mild alkali treatment the main carbohydrate prosthetic group of bovine-submaxillary-gland mucoprotein has been split off and shown to be 6–α–N–acetyl–D–neuraminyl–N–acetylgalactosamine with the formula:

Disaccharide prosthetic group of bovine submaxillary-gland mucoprotein
(Gottschalk and Graham, 1958).

The same oligosaccharide prosthetic group was found in ovine submaxillary mucoprotein by Graham and Gottschalk (1960). The site of action of the virus enzyme or RDE is at the ketosidic linkage of NANA to the adjacent sugar residue, and the name neuraminidase has been suggested for this enzyme by Gottschalk (1957a).

Although there is little doubt that the inhibitory potency of α-type mucoprotein inhibitors depends on the presence of sialic acid, their inactivation by trypsin indicates that the protein moiety is also important. Sialic acid itself is not a haemagglutination inhibitor even when it is ketosidically linked to an adjacent sugar residue. Neither the disaccharide prosthetic group of bovine-submaxillary-gland muco-protein nor the trisaccharide neuramin–lactose, obtainable from rat mammary glands, inhibits haemagglutination, although both are split by neuraminidase (Trucco and Caputto, 1954; Gottschalk, 1956, 1957a, 1959b). Moreover, there is no direct relationship between the amount of sialic acid in a mucoprotein molecule and its inhibitory potency. Bovine-salivary-gland mucoprotein, which has a high sialic-acid content, is a poor inhibitor. Clearly, the inhibitory potency of a molecule must depend on the molecular configuration as a whole, that part of the molecule consisting of sialic acid ketosidically linked to an adjacent sugar residue acting as the enzyme substrate only. It is well known that α–inhibitors from various sources differ in the range of heated viruses they inhibit (Stone, 1949), and recently Gottschalk and Fazekas de St. Groth (1960) have presented good evidence that in-hibitors whose polysaccharide prosthetic groups have similar carbo-hydrate compositions exhibit similar patterns of inhibitory activity. As more knowledge of the exact chemical and physical structure of inhibitory mucoproteins becomes available, its correlation with bio-logical activity will lead to a more detailed understanding of inhibitory and receptor mechanisms at the molecular level.

Chemical analysis of McCrea's receptor substance isolated from erythrocytes showed it to be a mucoprotein closely related to urinary mucoprotein and bovine-submaxillary-gland mucoprotein (McCrea, 1953b). Like these, the red-cell receptor may be regarded as a muco-protein, the carbohydrate prosthetic group of which is an oligo-saccharide terminating in sialic acid linked ketosidically to an adjacent sugar unit. Sialic acid may be regarded as the keystone of the receptor molecule; its removal by enzymic action inactivates the receptor probably by alteration of its charge distribution, which in turn may alter the shape of the receptor molecule.

The receptors responsible for attachment of virus to red cells and for virus–inhibitor reactions may be synonymous with the functional enzyme groups and their now chemically defined substrate. There are valid reasons, however, for supposing that enzyme and substrate form only part of larger receptor areas on virus and red cell, or inhibitor, respectively. The behaviour of heated virus has been interpreted as the result of modification of the enzyme groups so that they no longer function enzymically but retain their structural configuration suffi-ciently to adsorb. The lack of any strict correlation between the activity of the enzyme and sensitivity to α–inhibitor casts doubt on this inter-pretation. If true, simple enzyme substrates such as neuramin–lactose would be expected to be inhibitory. Moreover, it is significant that heat-inactivated virus may be removed from red cells by RDE or active virus, indicating that the enzyme substrate is unoccupied and still accessible. In view of these difficulties, specific receptors of which enzyme and substrate form only a part are more likely models.

4. Summary of virus–red cell interaction

The specificity of virus adsorption to red cells leads to the assumption that union is due to complementary steric configurations on the surfaces of both virus and red cell. Since both are negatively charged, the presence of cations is necessary for adsorption to take place. The cations reduce electrostatic repulsion between virus and red cell sufficiently to allow an approach close enough for specific reversible binding to occur. When the virus is specifically bound, sialic acid is released by enzymatic action and the virus subsequently freed.

B. OTHER VIRUSES

There is little doubt that myxoviruses attach to both red cells and host cells by means of specific receptors. This raises the question of specific receptor mechanisms for other viruses. The success of the virus–erythrocyte model in elucidating the surface reactions between myxoviruses and their host cells has naturally turned attention to the haemagglutination phenomena of other viruses. Many viruses do, in fact, haemagglutinate, and the limited range of erythrocytes agglutinated by different viruses, together with the critical conditions of temperature and ion concentration required, indicate that the reaction is mediated by specific receptor sites on the erythrocyte surface. In a few cases only, however, is the myxovirus receptor utilized. In still fewer cases can the relevance of haemagglutination to virus–host cell interaction be established. Indeed, in two virus groups, the pox viruses and the psittacosis–lymphogranuloma venereum group, the haemagglutinin is readily separable from the infective virus particle, which does not participate directly in the reaction. Because of its smaller size, the non-infective haemagglutinin remains in the supernatant fluid after deposition of the virus by centrifugation; it is therefore referred to as soluble haemagglutinin.

1. Soluble haemagglutinins

Since the infective virus particle does not haemagglutinate, it is extremely unlikely that haemagglutination by soluble haemagglutinins is based on mechanisms which are concerned in the processes of cell infection. However, the probability that the production of soluble haemagglutinins results from interaction of viral and host-tissue components does not allow us to rule out the possibility that it is released as a result of virus–host cell interaction during the course of attachment or penetration.

Although they differ in the range of red cells agglutinated, the pox-virus and psittacosis haemagglutinins appear to be chemically similar and are characterized as phospho-lipo-proteins. (Stone, 1946a; Gogolek and Ross, 1955). The phospholipid moiety is the active haemagglutinating agent on which the protein moiety confers serological specificity. In the psittacosis group the serologically reactive protein of the haemagglutinin can be identified in the viral particle, although this does not haemagglutinate. The fact that tissue lipids haemagglutinate non-specifically (Stone, 1946b) suggests that the lipid moiety of soluble haemagglutinins may be of host origin, and that soluble haemagglutinins result from interaction of virus and host material either during virus synthesis or as a result of virus degradation. If the latter, this may even occur at the cell surface during the early stages of infection.

2. Viral haemagglutinins

With the exception of the above-mentioned viruses, haemagglutination is the function of the infective virus particle itself. A more direct relationship between haemagglutination phenomena and virus–host cell interaction might therefore be expected. In only two groups, however, the enteroviruses and the encephalomyocarditis group, has any such relationship been experimentally demonstrable, and only the latter uses a receptor similar to that of myxoviruses.

(a) *Enteroviruses.* Some types of ECHO virus and Coxsackie B3 agglutinate human group "O" cells (Goldfield, Srihongse and Fox, 1957; Lahelle, 1958). The cell receptors are quite distinct from the sialomucoprotein receptor of myxoviruses and are probably protein in nature (Philipson, 1959). A relationship between the mechanisms of attachment to red cells and host cells is indicated by the inactivation of both haemagglutinin and infectivity after treatment of virus with reagents reacting with sulphydryl groups (Philipson and Choppin, 1960; Choppin and Philipson, 1961). Other viruses tested, with the exception of eastern-equine-encephalitis virus, were unaffected by sulphydryl reagents, indicating a distinct mode of attachment for the sensitive viruses which is worthy of further investigation.

(b) *Encephalomyocarditis viruses.* These viruses agglutinate sheep red cells and to a lesser extent human, rat and guinea-pig cells under specified conditions in the absence of potassium (Olitzky and Yager, 1949; Hallauer, 1951; Horvath and Jungeblut, 1952). Treatment of the cells with cholera filtrate renders them inagglutinable by these viruses and indicates a cell receptor similar to, if not identical with, that of myxoviruses. Moreover, cholera filtrate administered intraperitoneally protects mice against infection with Columbia–SK virus (Verlinde and de Baan, 1949; Jungeblut, 1950; Verlinde *et al.*, 1951), indicating that the same type of receptor is utilized in the initiation of infection by this virus.

Some evidence that attachment to a receptor similar to that of myxoviruses is an essential step in infection with viruses of this group is obtained from the experiments of Kodza and Jungeblut (1958) with encephalomyocarditis (EMC) virus. They found that HeLa cells were protected from infection with this virus by treatment with cholera filtrate. Furthermore, they showed that RDE adsorbed on and eluted from HeLa cells, after which EMC virus failed to adsorb. After four days the cell receptors had regenerated sufficiently to restore the susceptibility of the cells to virus. When L cells were used as host cells no protection against EMC infection was obtained by the use of RDE, nor was there any evidence that attachment to an RDE-sensitive receptor was an essential stage in the mechanism of infection of these cells. This raises the interesting possibility that a virus can use alternative receptors or mechanisms of infection with different host cells. For this reason it is dangerous to assume that virus behaviour under artificial or experimental conditions necessarily reflects host–virus interaction in natural infection. This is particularly so when red blood cells, which are not true host cells capable of sustaining virus growth, are used.

(c) *Pneumonia virus of mice (PVM)*. A good example of how experimental results may be misleading is provided by the haemagglutination phenomena encountered with PVM. Untreated mouse-lung suspensions do not haemagglutinate, and it was only after the reactions of heated suspensions were studied by Mills and Dochez (1944) that the haemagglutinating activity of the virus became evident. The virus, in normally prepared suspensions, is firmly bound to an inhibitor released by disruption of the tissues. Heating at 80° for 10 minutes, or alteration of the ion concentration of the medium, frees the virus particles, which then readily agglutinate mouse and hamster cells (Curnen and Horsfall, 1946; Davenport and Horsfall, 1948). Virus prepared from infected mouse lungs by non-traumatic techniques is also free from the inhibitor and therefore haemagglutinates without prior heating (Curnen and Horsfall, 1947).

The presence of a haemagglutination inhibitor in the tissues, as distinct from the body fluids, of susceptible hosts suggests that it may have some significance in the mechanism of infection. The similarity of conditions which dissociate virus from red cell and from inhibitor further suggests a relationship between the red-cell receptor and inhibitor. Blockage of the virus haemagglutinin receptor does not, however, prevent infection in susceptible animals (Curnen and Horsfall, 1947), so that if the inhibitor does represent a cell-surface receptor substance it is necessary to postulate dissociation of the virus–inhibitor complex *in vivo* in order to free the virus receptors for their attachment to susceptible cells. The haemagglutination receptor, however, may not be the receptor responsible for attachment to the host cell surface.

(d) *Miscellaneous.* Haemagglutination of two other virus groups is of interest, because with at least some of their members red cell attachment is by the sialomucoprotein receptors utilized by the myxoviruses. Some adenovirus types agglutinate human group "O" red cells through receptors which are destroyed by RDE or influenza viruses, although they do not themselves possess the eluting enzyme (Kasel, Rowe and Nemes, 1960). The natural host cells of these viruses are those of the upper respiratory tissues, which are known to possess myxovirus receptors. It is likely therefore that these adenoviruses utilize sialomucoprotein receptors for attachment to their natural host cells and initiation of infection, but, so far, experimental proof is lacking.

Also of interest is the demonstration that a tumour virus, the polyoma virus, agglutinates red cells of guinea-pigs, hamsters and humans by attachment to myxovirus receptors, although it lacks the eluting enzyme (Eddy *et al.*, 1958; Hartley *et al.*, 1959). No evidence that this receptor forms part of the mechanism of infection is yet available.

None of the other haemagglutinating viruses, the arthropod-borne encephalitic viruses (Casals and Brown, 1954) or the GD VII strain of murine poliomyelitis (Lahelle and Horsfall, 1949) provide any clues to the mechanisms of infection from their reactions with erythrocytes.

III. Interaction between Viruses and Susceptible Host-tissue Cells

A. MYXOVIRUSES

1. Phenomena demonstrable in vitro

The demonstration of influenza-virus adsorption and elution with host-tissue cells, rendered non-viable by excision or by treatment with formalin or sodium azide (Hirst, 1943; Fazekas de St. Groth, 1948a; Stone, 1948a), soon established that the reactions which occur between myxoviruses and red cells occur also with host cells. The close similarity, if not identity, of the receptors through which these reactions take place was confirmed by the destruction of host-cell receptors by RDE and their modification by periodate (Fazekas de St. Groth, 1948a;

Stone, 1948a; Fazekas de St. Groth and Graham, 1949). There is thus cogent evidence for the presence of specific myxovirus receptors on the surface of host cells. However, the use in these experiments of non-viable host cells, incapable of supporting virus replication, did not allow any conclusions regarding the function of these receptors in the initiation of infection. This could only be determined by observations on viable host cells.

2. In vivo interaction

Experimental work *in vivo*, both in intact animals and tissue cultures, has left little doubt that attachment to the specific receptors, so clearly demonstrated in *in vitro* systems, is an essential first step in the process of infection. The significance of virus elution, however, is much more doubtful. The role of the virus enzyme is discussed in a subsequent section; suffice it to say here that attachment to cells *in vivo* is not followed by elution, or, if it is, only to a small extent (Hirst, 1943; Stone, 1948a). This is, perhaps, not surprising when we consider that for infection to occur virus must penetrate the cell membrane and gain the interior of the cell.

Although enzymically active virus does not elute from viable host cells to any great degree, there is no doubt of the susceptibility of the host receptors to the neuraminidase enzyme. Treatment of cells lining the allantoic cavity of the chick embryo with RDE prevents completely, or delays, the onset of infection with several influenza-virus strains, and mumps virus. RDE applied locally to the site of infection, prior to virus inoculation, is equally effective in protecting mice against infection (Stone, 1948b; Cairns, 1951). The effect is more marked with some strains than others, indicating a difference in the number of receptors required for the initiation of infection. Such differences in receptor requirements for the initiation of infection are analogous to those responsible for the receptor-gradient phenomenon where they are reflected in the haemagglutination behaviour of various viruses.

After treatment of viable host cells with RDE, the cell surface is not irreparably damaged or permanently insusceptible to infection with influenza viruses. In both eggs and mice, receptors destroyed by RDE undergo a process of regeneration (Fazekas de St. Groth, 1948b; Stone, 1948a, b; Finter *et al.*, 1954). In mice, regeneration of receptors begins from eight to 30 hours after RDE inoculation and is complete in six days. With large doses of RDE, more receptors are present after regeneration than before (Fazekas de St. Groth, 1948b).

The use of the same or closely similar sialomucoprotein receptors for attachment to red cells and host cells *in vivo* suggests that attachment in the two systems may be the same in other respects. It is not surprising, therefore, that Levine and Sagik (1956) found the characteristics of NDV adsorption to red cells and chick-embryo cells in monolayers to be identical in their salt requirements, velocity constants, relative independence of temperature and response to variations of pH. However, only a minimal amount of virus was eluted from the chick-embryo cells compared with that eluted from red cells.

Some observations by Ackerman and his colleagues on the effect of an antimetabolite α-amino-p-methoxyphenylmethane sulphonic acid (AMPS) on the early stages of cell infection by influenza virus led them to suggest the possibility that for the successful initiation of infection, attachment by more than one type of receptor may be necessary. They followed the processes of infection in pieces of chick chorioallantoic membrane, maintained in a suitable medium, in the vessels of a Warburg respirometer (Ackerman, 1951). Addition of AMPS to the medium reversibly inhibited the growth cycle of influenza virus when administered within 30 minutes of virus inoculation. After this time growth was no longer inhibited, but the yield was reduced owing to impairment of virus release. An inhibitory reaction occurring so soon after virus inoculation suggested some interference with the processes of attachment or penetration (Ackermann and Maassab, 1954a). In the experiments of Ackermann, Ishida and Maassab (1955) the ability of the chorioallantoic membrane to bind virus effectively was impaired to some extent but not lost in the presence of AMPS or by pretreatment of the membrane with RDE. If, however, the membrane was first treated with RDE and then exposed to virus in the presence of AMPS, effective binding was completely prevented. From this the presence of two types of cell receptor was postulated by these authors, one sensitive to RDE and one to AMPS. Since either of these substances alone prevented infection, attachment to both types of receptor was considered necessary for the initiation of infection. An alternative explanation is, however, possible which obviates the introduction of another type of receptor for which there is no other evidence. The failure of RDE to prevent virus attachment completely may be a quantitative effect, and AMPS may act by blocking penetration. It is well known that attachment to cells impenetrable by virus is followed by elution. This is the sequence of events in both red cells and non-viable host cells. Attachment to cells in which penetration has been prevented by AMPS may thus be followed by elution, with an apparent decrease in the efficiency of effective binding. The reversibility of the inhibitory effect of AMPS by excess of potassium, added before or at the same time as the inhibitory substance, lends some support to this hypothesis, since potassium is believed to have some effect on virus penetration (Levine et al., 1956).

B. Other Viruses

In comparison with myxoviruses, little is known about the mechanism by which other viruses attach to host cells. On *a priori* grounds, efficient attachment to the cell surface must be an essential prerequisite for cell infection. The clear evidence that attachment to host cells of such diverse viruses as myxoviruses and bacteriophages is effected by means of specific receptors suggests the possibility that a similar mechanism may be operative for other viruses. A certain amount of evidence has now been adduced which is consistent with this hypothesis.

With some viruses, attachment to red cells, from only a limited number of species under specific conditions, suggests the presence of specific erythrocyte receptors. However, with few exceptions, it has not been possible to establish a relationship between these and any similar structures on the surface of host cells. The difficulty of demonstrating specific host-cell receptors has been twofold. First, the absence of any receptor-destroying enzyme, comparable with neuraminidase, makes their demonstration or chemical characterization particularly difficult. Secondly, the lack, until recently, of host-cell systems suitable for the kind of experimental investigation required, militated against successful exploration of the problem. The introduction of tissue-culture methods has now filled this gap, so that the adsorption mechanisms of more viruses can be investigated.

With each particular type of virus only a limited range of cells, adapted to tissue culture, can be infected. For this to occur, the cell must be capable not only of adsorbing virus and allowing penetration but also of supporting virus replication once this has been achieved. Insusceptibility to infection may therefore depend on inability to carry out any one of these functions. In culture, cells from a variety of tissues obtained from primates adsorb poliovirus whether they are susceptible to infection or not (Hsiung and Melnick, 1958; Vogt and Dulbecco, 1958; Darnell and Sawyer, 1960). With the exception of bovine-embryo tissues (Warren and Cutchins, 1957), cells from non-primate species, which are not susceptible to infection with poliovirus, fail to adsorb it to any great extent (Kaplan, 1955a; McLaren, Holland and Syverton, 1959), although they are fully competent to support virus replication if intact virus or its infective RNA principle gets into the interior of the cell (Holland, McLaren and Syverton, 1959b). The assumption is that the difference in susceptibility of primate and non-primate cells, in culture, depends on their capacity to adsorb virus, and it is reasonable to suppose that this, in turn, depends on the presence or absence of specific surface-receptor sites. The extraction from cells susceptible to infection with enteroviruses, WEE, NDV, and vaccinia viruses, but not at all or only in very small amounts from insusceptible cells, of substances which bind to and inactivate these viruses *in vitro* supports this view (Holland and McLaren, 1959; Holland, 1961; Quersin-Thiry, 1961; Quersin-Thiry and Nihoul, 1961). The extraction of an active substance is not, of course, proof that it is the surface-receptor material, nor can such proof be obtained until the isolation of "pure" cell membrane, if such an entity exists, allows us to investigate the question directly. Until then, evidence that the active cell extract is the surface-receptor material will have to be circumstantial. Some evidence of this type is available. Thus, the extraction of material from susceptible human-amnion cells, which inactivates polio virus, is correlated with the capacity of intact cells to adsorb virus (Holland, 1961). Furthermore, the conditions required for enterovirus inactivation by cell extracts are similar to those required for virus attachment to intact cells (Holland and McLaren, 1959). Certain similarities between these conditions and those required for cell attachment of myxoviruses are apparent. Thus, adsorption to cell suspensions is markedly affected by the ionic environment and is independent of temperature (Bachtold, Bubel and Gebhardt, 1957; Holland and McLaren, 1959), suggesting an electrostatic mechanism of attachment not unlike that of myxoviruses. It must be admitted, however, that adsorption to cell monolayers is temperature-dependent and not, therefore, consistent with this hypothesis, although it is possible that differences in the technique used for assaying virus adsorption in cell monolayers and suspensions may account for the discrepancy (Holland and McLaren, 1959).

The acquirement of susceptibility to enterovirus infection by cells in tissue culture which in organized tissues of the intact animal are resistant to infection (Evans *et al.*, 1954; Kaplan, 1955a) has long been a puzzling feature. The demonstration that this change is associated with the production of receptor material (Holland, 1961; Quersin-Thiry, 1961) suggests that the resistance of these cells *in situ*, or before adaptation to tissue culture, is due to their inability to carry out the essential first stage of infection, namely, attachment of virus to the cell surface. It is possible that the more strict tissue tropism of poliovirus infection in the intact animal may be similarly explained. With the occasional exception of liver cells, only those tissues from humans and monkeys which are known to be susceptible to poliovirus infection *in vivo* produce cell-receptor material capable of inactivating virus (Holland, 1961). Furthermore, the attenuated LSc strain of type-1 polio, which is characterized by its decreased ability to infect nerve cells of the brain and spinal cord in primates, is not inactivated significantly by cell homogenates from these tissues, in contrast to virulent strains of this type (Sabin, 1957; Holland, 1961). Its undiminished ability to infect cells of the alimentary tract, however, is matched by its inactivation with cell homogenates from this tissue. Adsorption of the LSc strain to the intestinal "receptor" material, but not to that of nervous tissue, suggests some slight difference between them. The possibility that passage of virus in different hosts may alter its receptor affinity is not unlikely; indeed the O → D change of influenza viruses is a classic example.

The persistent appearance of "receptor" material in susceptible cells is sufficiently striking to suggest that it plays an essential role in the mechanism of infection. All the evidence favours the view that one, at least, of its functions is to provide a mechanism by which virus can attach to the cell surface. In this connection it is of interest to note that cells susceptible to myxovirus infection, the only ones for which we have direct evidence of specific surface receptors, yield receptor material on extraction, which is probably an integral part of the cell cytoplasm and not confined to the cell surface (Schlesinger and Karr, 1956a).

Using a completely different approach, Habel et al. (1958) and Quersin-Thiry (1958) obtained some evidence to support the view that some viruses, other than myxoviruses, attach to the cell surface by means of specific receptors. They found that pretreatment of HeLa and monkey-kidney cells with sub-agglutinating doses of homologous anticellular serum protected them against infection with some viruses but not others. If, as is assumed, anticellular serum acts by blocking surface receptors, the protective effect should be associated with some decrease of virus adsorption. With poliovirus this has, in fact, been demonstrated (Quersin-Thiry, 1958; Holland and McLaren, 1959). Furthermore, with the exception of ECHO 1 virus, the serum is active only when added before or at the time of virus inoculation (Habel et al., 1958; Holland and McLaren, 1959), which is good evidence that one of its mechanisms of action, at least, is the blockage of virus adsorption. If so, the site of action must be at the cell surface, and the recent electron-microscopic observations of Easton, Goldberg and Green (1962) on the reaction between ferritin-labelled anticellular serum and intact Krebs-ascites-tumour cells has provided direct confirmation of this.

If anticellular serum acts in this way, what is the mechanism of its action? The specific receptors themselves may be antigenic, and simple attachment of homologous antibody molecules to these antigens would then be sufficient to prevent virus attachment. Alternatively, antibody molecules may attach to antigenic sites on the cell surface which are independent of the specific receptors and thus exert their effect by steric hindrance. Blockage of receptors would then depend on their spatial configuration and their distribution over the cell surface. Such a hypothesis would more adequately explain the partial or complete resistance of some viruses to the action of anticellular serum. More support for it is obtained from the finding that serum prepared against the microsomal fraction of susceptible cells does not protect them against virus infection (Habel *et al.*, 1958), although receptor material is found in this fraction (Holland, 1961; Holland and McLaren, 1961).

IV. Cell Penetration

Passage of virus particles from the cell surface to the interior necessitates transmission across the cell membrane. In contrast to the bacterial-cell wall, the animal-cell membrane is a very much less rigid and more dynamic structure. It is believed to be a bimolecular lipid layer with a coating of protein on either side, the whole being about 30–150Å thick. The mechanism of penetration might, therefore, be expected to differ from that evolved by the T2 bacteriophage to negotiate the thick, rigid bacterial-cell wall of *E. coli*. Whatever this is, energy is still required to overcome the resistance of the cell membrane, and must be provided by the virus or cell. With T2 phage the energy-producing mechanisms reside in the phage particle, and consist of a succession of complex physico-chemical reactions triggered by inter-action between the phage and the cell surface. These reactions, reviewed by Garen and Kozloff (1959) allow the phage particle to inject its DNA, by a syringe mechanism, through an enzymic weakening of the cell wall. So far, with the possible exception of myxoviruses, there is no evidence of any energy-producing mechanism residing in the animal-virus particle which would allow it to overcome the resistance of the cell-membrane barrier. Although the enzymic destruction of specific receptors by myxoviruses, after adsorption, suggested originally that this was a necessary step in the penetration of the cell membrane, there is now little doubt that penetration may occur without it. In the absence of any evidence that the energy requirements of penetration are provided by the virus particle, it must be assumed that the cell itself plays an active part. Nevertheless, any discussion of the mechanism of cell penetration would not be complete without a consideration of the function of the myxovirus enzyme.

A. ROLE OF THE MYXOVIRUS ENZYME

Convincing evidence that enzymically inactive virus can penetrate the cells of the allantoic cavity has been obtained by many authors.

Fazekas de St. Groth (1948c) was the first to show that enzymically inactive, heat-killed virus was taken up by these cells at approximately the same rate as enzymically active virus. The interference experiments of Isaacs and Edney (1950) confirmed that enzymically inactive virus can achieve an intracellular position, and the production of interferon in cells of the chorioallantoic membrane by heat-killed virus (Isaacs and Lindenmann, 1957) is further evidence of this.

Virus not only penetrates the cell after inactivation of its enzyme but can infect although the cell receptors are rendered insusceptible to the action of neuraminidase. Cells whose receptors are thus altered by treatment with critical amounts of potassium periodate, retain their adsorptive capacity for virus and susceptibility to virus infection. There is little doubt that under certain experimental conditions virus is capable of penetrating the cell and initiating infection without enzymic destruction of receptors.

The absence of any correlation between the neuraminidase activity of virus particles and their ability to penetrate has recently been questioned by Rubin and his colleagues. Using ^{32}P-labelled NDV, Rubin (1957) showed that the properties of infectivity and enzymic elution from red cells were inactivated by immune serum at almost identical rates, suggesting a close relationship between them. From theoretical treatment of his experimental results he calculated the number of sites on the virus particle responsible for enzymic activity and for infection, and found them to be of the same order of magnitude, thus supporting a role for the enzyme in the initiation of infection. A numerical correlation between two properties is not necessarily evidence of a causal relationship. Indeed, the fact that both enzymic activity and the first stage of cell infection are dependent on the same site on the virus surface, namely the haemagglutinin receptor, may well be sufficient explanation of Rubin's results. Nevertheless, Rubin (1957) and Rubin and Franklin (1957) on the basis of their studies of the neutralization of NDV by immune serum, attribute to the enzyme a role in penetration. Their results suggested that although several antibody molecules attached to a virus particle prevent its adsorption to cells, attachment of a single molecule allows adsorption but may prevent enzymic activity and cell penetration. From the agreement of his experimental results with a theoretical model, Rubin (1957) postulates that virus particles adsorb by any one of a number of sites mediating both enzymic activity and infectivity. When each of these sites is occupied by several antibody molecules, adsorption is completely prevented. A site occupied by a single antibody molecule, however, can still effect attachment of the virus particle to the cell surface, but in this case the antibody will block enzymic activity and hence prevent virus penetration. Thus, with small amounts of antibody the chance orientation of virus particle to cell surface will determine whether adsorption is followed by penetration and infection.

The effect of small amounts of antibody in allowing adsorption to host cells but not penetration, obtains not only with NDV but also with poliovirus (Mandel, 1958). It is not unreasonable therefore to assume a common mechanism of action. Since poliovirus does not possess any receptor-destroying enzyme, it seems unnecessary to invoke it to explain the action of antibody on NDV. With both viruses the data suggest adsorption to the cell by the same site to which antibody is attached. If so, it must be assumed that one antibody molecule is not sufficient to block the receptor as a whole. Possibly, the attached antibody molecule prevents the virus from achieving full mutual orientation with the complementary cell-receptor sites, and the defective virus–cell linkage so formed prevents the onset of penetration. It cannot be said that any of the experiments yet performed has provided unequivocal evidence in support of a role for the myxovirus enzyme in the process of penetration.

If the enzyme plays no part in the mechanism of penetration, it is pertinent to ask what, in fact, its real function could be. It may play some part in virus replication (Schlesinger and Karr, 1956b) or in virus release (Ackermann and Maassab, 1954b). A more widely held view is that the function of the enzyme is to release virus from α–inhibitory mucoprotein, contained in secretions of the upper respiratory tract, which would otherwise prevent access to the cell receptor. What is known of virus-inhibitory reactions does not support this hypothesis. α–inhibitory substances do not neutralize virus infectivity nor do they inhibit haemagglutination of active viruses even under conditions when the enzyme is inactive. It is, therefore, unlikely that mucous, lining the respiratory-tract epithelium, would neutralize infective virus. It is, however, possible that a change in its viscosity as a result of virus enzymic activity may facilitate contact between virus and host cell.

B. Viropexis

Although the function of the virus enzyme has not been established, it is significant that reactions between myxoviruses and non-viable cells are confined to the cell surface without subsequent penetration. This implies that the cell itself plays an active part in the uptake of virus. The mechanism of penetration suggested by Fazekas de St. Groth (1948c) has therefore gained wide acceptance. On the basis of his experiments with enzymically inactive virus, he suggests that virus particles are taken into cells by an active process of ingestion which he refers to as "viropexis". The electron-microscopic observations of Flewett (1953) support this hypothesis, although no other direct observations are available. In its favour is its general applicability to other viruses without reserve or difficulty. It is well known that non-phagocytic cells are able to engulf fluid droplets, a phenomenon described by Lewis (1931) and called by him pinocytosis. It is not unreasonable to suppose, therefore, that a similar mechanism may be employed for the uptake of submicroscopic particles.

In pinocytosis, fluid droplets are engulfed or sucked in by the cell and enclosed in a vesicle of invaginated cell membrane which buds off and enters the interior of the cell. Certain inorganic salts and proteins have the property of inducing pinocytosis, which, it is believed, is initiated by their specific adsorption to the cell surface (Brandt, 1958; Schumaker, 1958; Barnett and Ball, 1960). It is interesting to note here that nucleic acid is not, like some proteins, an inducer. Although material ingested by pinocytosis achieves an intracellular position, it is still enclosed in a vesicle surrounded by part of the cell membrane. How large molecules traverse this membrane to enter the cytoplasm is not yet known. Some digestion of the membrane by cytoplasmic enzymes with release of the vesicle contents is a possibility.

Although most of the observations on pinocytosis have been made with amoebae, the phenomenon does occur with a wide variety of mammalian tissue cells (Holter and Holzer, 1959). Furthermore, it has been observed at submicroscopic levels visible only in the electron microscope (Palade, 1953; de Robertis and Bennett, 1954; Odor, 1956; Barnett and Ball, 1960; Farquhar and Palade, 1960), and NDV particles have actually been seen in pinocytosis vesicles of chick macrophages (Holtz and Bang, 1957). A mechanism of virus penetration similar to that of pinocytosis is, therefore, readily conceivable. The interaction of charged surfaces, following specific adsorption of molecules or ions to the cell membrane, which occurs in pinocytosis, is thought to be an essential prelude to the invagination of the cell membrane and transport of the adsorbed material, together with some of the solvent, into the cell interior (Bennett, 1956; Brandt, 1958; Holter, 1961). Following interaction of the charged surfaces of virus and cell, a similar invagination of the surface at the attachment area could occur. The only difference between the two mechanisms would then be in the nature of the material ingested. Such a mechanism suggests a function for the virus protein coat additional to that of protection, and it is significant that the low infective potency of enterovirus RNA preparations may be due to failure of the RNA to adsorb to host cells (Holland et al., 1960a).

Although there is little direct evidence in favour of the hypothesis of "viropexis", it is a very plausible one. However, the recent demonstration that infective RNA can be extracted from a number of animal viruses, although not yet from influenza (Colter, Bird and Brown, 1957; Alexander *et al.*, 1958; Ada and Anderson, 1959) raises another question. Does the whole virus particle enter the cell or only the infective nucleic acid principle as with bacteriophage?

C. DOES THE WHOLE VIRUS PARTICLE ENTER THE CELL?

There is no direct evidence that animal viruses split into nucleic acid and protein components at the cell surface with entry of only the former component into the cell. However, the clear demonstration that this is the mechanism by which the T2 phage infects its host cell (Hershey and Chase, 1952; Anderson, 1953) has stimulated virologists to search for evidence of a similar mechanism operative for animal viruses. With influenza and polio viruses some evidence which, at least, is compatible with the hypothesis of virus "splitting" has been obtained.

1. Myxoviruses

Applying the technique of radioactive labelling, Hoyle and his colleagues have attempted to follow the fate of viral protein and nucleic acid, labelled with ^{35}S and ^{32}P, respectively, on entry of influenza virus into the cell. From their results, they concluded that within two hours after inoculation the "soluble" antigen component, which has been characterized as a ribonucleoprotein with a particle size of 120Å (Hoyle, 1952; Hoyle, Reed and Astbury, 1953; Hoyle, Jolles and Mitchell, 1954) was released from the virus particle. Most of this ribonucleoprotein became intimately associated with the cell nucleus where free nucleic acid was split off, and the protein moiety hydrolysed into amino acids (Hoyle and Frisch-Niggemeyer, 1955; Hoyle and Finter, 1957). Although the fate of the virus haemagglutinin could not be traced, their results gave some indication of the fate of the virus membrane envelope. This phospho-lipo-protein structure appeared to be broken into low-molecular-weight, water-soluble, phosphorous compounds, and what Hoyle and Finter inferred must be the protein moiety was firmly bound to some cytoplasmic constituent without disintegration. They suggested that the protein of the virus envelope remained at the cell surface, nucleoprotein only gaining entrance to the cell. From their results, however, the envelope protein moiety could equally well have been bound to some cytoplasmic constituent deep to the cell surface. In this respect, the results obtained by Wecker and Schäfer (1957b) from similar experiments with ^{32}P-labelled myxoviruses are of interest. Although they confirmed the disintegration of virus with release of "soluble" antigen, they were able to recover labelled phospholipid unchanged, in soluble form, from cell homogenates. This suggests that the phospho-lipo-protein envelope may enter the cell unchanged and that it does not become bound to any cytoplasmic constituent.

Thus, although all are agreed that disintegration of influenza-virus particles takes place in the course of cell infection, its precise localization has not yet been determined. Indeed, it is doubtful if radioactive-tracer experiments could provide this information in the absence of any method of separating the cell membrane from the cytoplasm. Unequivocal evidence is more likely to come from direct visual observation under the electron microscope, which, with improvements in techniques utilizing electron-dense tracer substances, should soon be possible.

So far, information derived from electron microscopy of virus adsorption and penetration is scanty, but one observation of Adams and Prince (1957) makes it unwise at this stage to rule out the possibility of some break-up of the virus particle at the cell surface before actual penetration. These authors observed the infection of Ehrlich's ascites-tumour cells with NDV. The virus particles appeared as eliptical or circular dense bodies, approximately 140mμ in diameter, which were surrounded by a limiting membrane of two layers. The inner layer, 35–50Å thick, was separated from the outer layer, itself 30–40Å thick, by a less dense zone approximately 40–60Å wide. Where the plane of section passed through the sites of virus–cell adsorption the electron micrographs suggested a disappearance of the outer membrane layer and the subjacent cell membrane at the point of contact. Unfortunately, the virus–cell system used in this investigation did not lead to the production of infective virus but only to "incomplete" virus, which was both structurally and functionally deficient. Some caution is therefore necessary before findings from an atypical virus–cell system of this sort are extrapolated to the normal sequence of infection. Nevertheless, this observation provides a clue to a hypothesis, admittedly speculative, of myxovirus penetration which has the advantage of being compatible with all the experimental observations relevant to penetration. This is that on close apposition of virus and cell surfaces there is fusion of the opposing lipo-protein membranes with the establishment of continuity. In this way the virus-membrane envelope becomes incorporated in the cell membrane and the internal constituents of the virus become extruded into the cytoplasm. It is well known that lipid membranes possess surface-active properties and that some alteration in interfacial tension when they meet may result in their fusion, as occurs with oil droplets in an aqueous medium. A consideration of the pinocytotic mechanism makes it apparent that breaches of continuity with subsequent fusion of opposing areas of the cell membrane itself must occur, otherwise it is difficult to see how continuity could be re-established after budding off the pinocytotic vesicle. The possibility that a common mechanism underlies self-sealing of the cell membrane and its fusion with the virus-membrane envelope, is suggested by the increasing evidence from both dark-field and electron microscopy, that the virus membrane is actually derived from the host-cell membrane in the course of virus liberation. (Hoyle, 1950, 1954; Wyckoff, 1953; Morgan, Rose and Moore, 1956). It is evident, of course, that the cell membrane incorporated with the virus particle acquires additional enzymic and serological properties. But the observations of Hotchin et al. (1958) and Morgan et al. (1961) that the surface membranes of cells infected with influenza virus not only acquire the antigenic characteristics of the virus, but undergo a change which renders them capable of attaching to red cells, strengthens the view that the virus lipo-protein envelope is derived from a modified host-cell membrane. A penetration mechanism of the type outlined here would explain the transport of virus across the cell membrane. It could thus operate in association with pinocytosis, or viropexis, in which no satisfactory explanation of how virus traverses the cell membrane after engulfment has yet been put forward.

It is necessary to emphasize at this point that a hypothesis of virus penetration based on the interaction of lipid membranes must be confined to myxoviruses, with possible extension to other viruses which possess a limiting membrane of lipid composition.

2. Other viruses

So little experimental data concerning the mode of penetration by viruses other than myxoviruses is available, that it is not possible to form any conception of a precise mechanism supported by experimental evidence, direct or indirect. With poliovirus, however, recent experiments by Joklik and Darnell (1961) have provided some evidence relevant to the problem of virus breakdown at the cell surface. Working with radioactively labelled virus, these authors were able to show that 70–80% of poliovirus adsorbed to HeLa-cell suspensions was eluted at 37°C. The eluted virus was grossly altered, and differed from the parent virus in its failure to adsorb to any great extent and its markedly reduced infective potency, although the same amount of infective RNA could be extracted from both parent and eluted virus. These changes suggested that some damage to the surface protein of the virus occurred after attachment to the cell surface. This may be a prelude, as Joklik and Darnell suggest, to the release of RNA and its penetration of the cell membrane. A small amount of RNA sensitive to the enzyme RNAse, and therefore presumably free from protein, was found in the cell, but this does not, of course, constitute proof of its release at the cell surface. Its release in the deeper layers of the cell is just as likely. Furthermore, damage to the virus-surface protein may be the end result of abortive virus–cell interaction only. Nevertheless, these results are sufficiently suggestive to warrant further investigation of the problem both by labelling techniques and electron microscopy.

D. Observations Based on Infectivity and Sensitivity to Antibody

The great difficulty in studying the mechanisms and kinetics of penetration is the experimental isolation of this stage from the rest of the infective cycle. In the almost complete absence of electron-microscopic observations, the position of virus relative to the cell membrane can only be inferred from some change in its reactivity resulting from its invasion of the cell. Two phenomena which occur in the course of infection have been inferred by many investigators to indicate completion of penetration. These are: first, the inability of immune serum to arrest the course of virus replication if it is added to the medium after virus adsorption has taken place; second, the fact that very little of the virus which is adsorbed can be recovered from the cells in infective form.

Andrewes (1929; 1930) first showed that virus initiating infection becomes insusceptible to the neutralizing activity of immune serum. For this reason failure to arrest the course of infection by the addition of immune serum is generally assumed to indicate that virus penetration of the cell has already occurred; the inference being that the cell membrane is impermeable to antibody. The time required for addition of immune serum to become ineffective has therefore been used as a measure of the rate of penetration. Reported penetration times are very variable, ranging from 20 to 40 minutes for poliovirus (Holland and McLaren, 1959; Darnell and Sawyer, 1960), and 15 minutes to three hours for Herpes virus (Scott et al., 1953; Watkins, 1960), but they are not comparable, having been obtained under various experimental conditions. Of course, penetration times of each individual virus particle are widely scattered, and some may penetrate very soon after adsorption.

As a general rule, firm attachment to host cells is accompanied by a decrease in the amount of infective virus recoverable. Conversion to a non-infective form is considered by most workers to be a necessary step in the virus replication cycle, and is referred to as the eclipse phase (for review, see Isaacs, 1959). Usually, a small percentage of attached virus, less than 5%, is recoverable during this phase. Although it has not yet been unequivocally proved that the recoverable virus takes no part in the production of new virus, the neutralization of most of it by treatment with antiserum suggests that it occupies an extracellular position. That part of it not so neutralized is probably also surface virus but protected from the action of antiserum by its position in deep invaginations of the cell membrane, as has been suggested for Herpes virus by Stoker and Ross (1958). Not all virus particles which are adsorbed to the cell surface are, therefore, capable of initiating infection. Probably, the residual infective virus does not progress beyond the stage of adsorption. Its failure to penetrate is unlikely to be due to any incapacity, since it is perfectly capable of initiating infection if transferred to new host cells. It must be assumed that penetration at some adsorption sites is blocked. This could result from some defect in the receptor itself or possibly from faulty orientation of virus and receptor site which prevents their interaction going to completion.

The assumption that virus becomes non-infective and insusceptible to antibody after penetration is consistent with the hypothesis of viral breakdown and release of nucleic acid in the course of its passage through the cell membrane. It is well known that RNA is a very inefficient infective agent and not sensitive to the neutralizing activity of immune serum. However, with Herpes simplex and influenza viruses, there is some evidence that the virus initiating infection becomes converted to the non-infective form at a time when the addition of immune serum is still effective in arresting the course of cell infection. Presumably, such non-infective virus which retains its sensitivity to antibody is both intact and extracellular (Wildy, 1954; Ishida and Ackermann, 1956; Watkins, 1960). In this state, loss of infectivity probably does not represent true eclipse but merely firm combination with cell-surface receptors. The fact that firm attachment of NDV to red cells, which are not penetrable by viruses, results in loss of infectivity (Rubin, 1957) lends some support to this suggestion. The apparent loss of infectivity which may occur on firm binding to cell receptors does not necessarily reflect an irreversible change in the virus particle. Inactivation of enteroviruses by cell debris containing specific receptor material was at first thought to be irreversible, but recovery of infective virus in the presence of the chelating agent EDTA (ethylenediamine sodium tetra-acetate) or at acid pH, later showed this to be incorrect (McLaren, Holland and Syverton, 1960). Although the virus can be recovered from intact cells under these conditions after a two-minute adsorption period, it is no longer recoverable after one hour at 37°C. It is evident that loss of infectivity alone is not always evidence of penetration. In favour of this view is the fact that penetration, indicated by the moment when virus initiating infection becomes insusceptible to the neutralizing activity of immune serum, occurs rapidly at 37°C but very slowly or not at all at low temperatures (Ishida and Ackermann, 1956; Mandel, 1958; Holland and McLaren, 1959; Postlethwaite, 1960), whereas loss of infectivity may occur at 3°C (Ishida and Ackerman, 1956).

E. Direct Cell-to-cell Transfer

If a virus can infect cells only through specific mechanisms of adsorption and penetration, it follows that for spread of the infection to occur, the virus must be released from infected cells into the extracellular environment and gain attachment to fresh cells. With some viruses, however, there is evidence of an alternative mode of spread from infected to neighbouring cells by a mechanism which bypasses the extracellular environment. From the nature and distribution of the lesions which it produced in tissue culture, in the presence of immune serum, Black and Melnick (1955) concluded that Herpes B virus had spread from cell to cell where these were in contact, without release into the extracellular environment. Likewise, varicella and Herpes zoster viruses, now considered to be two phases of a single virus entity, cannot be recovered from the extracellular phase of tissue cultures, and can spread from cell to cell in the presence of antiserum. They are, therefore, believed to spread in this way (Weller, Witton and Bell, 1958), as is Herpes simplex (Stoker, 1959). Although the mechanism is not yet understood, the implication is that these viruses can penetrate without the aid of specific surface adsorption. A clue to the mechanism of penetration is provided by the histology of the lesions which they produce. Thus, multinuclear cells are characteristic of these infections, indicating some dissolution of the membranes of contiguous cells and fusion of their cytoplasm. This type of cellular reaction to virus infection provides a ready explanation for intracellular transfer, particularly if it occurs also on a scale not visible by the light microscope.

Of great interest is the fact that the ability of some viruses to spread in this way seems to be associated with the particular clinical manifestations of the diseases which they produce. Contrary to the usual pattern of infective disease, Herpes simplex is a recurrent condition which occurs in patients with a high level of circulating antibody. Recurrences are believed to be due to reactivation of virus which remains latent in the tissues. Similarly, most cases of Herpes zoster are believed to be due to reactivation of virus which remains latent in nerve cells of the posterior root ganglia after an attack of varicella

(Stokes, 1959). Following reactivation, the virus travels via the nerve fibres. Characteristic of all these infections is the localization of the lesions. Probably, the presence of circulating antibody confines the spread of virus to intracellular transfer by a mechanism similar to that postulated for its spread in tissue culture.

V. Concluding Remarks

Any conclusions concerning mechanisms of virus attachment and penetration must be based on experimental evidence obtained almost entirely from two groups of viruses, the myxoviruses and the enteroviruses, which have been selected as models for investigation because of the relative ease with which they may be studied in the laboratory. Without further study the application of these conclusions to other viruses is not justified and may even be misleading. It should not be forgotten that marked differences of structure and chemical composition of viruses do exist; it would therefore be wiser to defer any generalizations until adequate data are available, especially as myxoviruses, the ones which have been most intensively studied, are unique in their possession of a receptor-destroying enzyme. Nevertheless, both the myxoviruses and enteroviruses have provided models to help us frame common hypotheses of attachment and penetration which can be tested directly on other viruses, as suitable techniques become available. Meanwhile, the beginnings which have been made in the formulation of the myxovirus receptor in chemical terms, besides being one of the most exciting recent advances in virus research, cannot fail to lead to a deeper understanding of the mechanism of attachment and, possibly, also of penetration.

Even with those viruses which have proved such useful models for elucidating the mode of virus attachment, the mechanism by which they penetrate is far from fully understood. The initiation of infection by the nucleic-acid moiety of some of the smaller animal viruses suggests the possibility of penetration by some mechanism similar to that of the T2 bacteriophage. However, the vast difference of structure and function of the barriers which they have to overcome, as well as of the morphology of the virus particles themselves, makes this unlikely. The dissimilarity is reinforced by their apparent difference in energy requirements. Penetration by T2 phage is independent of energy-yielding reactions of the host cell and depends on free energy stored in the structures of the phage particle. Conversely, the impenetrability of non-viable cells indicates that penetration by animal viruses is dependent on the energy-yielding reactions of the host cell. With the possible exception of myxoviruses, there is nothing to suggest any mechanism other than incorporation of the whole virus particle into the cell with subsequent breakdown into protein and nucleic-acid components.

Besides its theoretical interest, an understanding of the mechanisms of attachment and penetration is not without its practical importance. When we know how virus attachment and entry are effected we may be able to devise some means of preventing them. Preventing initiation of infection in the early stages may indeed have some advantage over attempts to block virus replication itself. Virus replication is a process so intimately linked to the host cell's own metabolism that it is difficult to affect the one without the other. With influenza viruses of the Asian (A2) type, non-specific inhibitor, which acts by blocking virus-receptor sites, has been shown not only to prevent infection but also to be a valuable prophylactic agent in experimental animals (Cohen and Belyavin, 1959; Cohen, 1960). The possible prevention and even therapy of virus infections by the use of virus-receptor-blocking agents is an added stimulus in the search for, and chemical analysis of, cell-surface receptors operative in the specific attachment of viruses.

CHAPTER 5

Mechanisms of Cell Infection
II. Intracellular Virus Replication

ALICK ISAACS

National Institute for Medical Research,
Mill Hill, London, England

I. Introduction

This chapter is concerned with the events in virus-infected animal cells from the time that the virus has penetrated the cell until newly formed virus has matured and is ready to be liberated. In the case of virulent bacteriophages this is referred to as the vegetative phase of multiplication, and it is from intensive study of bacteriophage multiplication (see Chapter 2) that most of our ideas about the development of animal viruses arise.

Two important concepts from the bacteriophage field have greatly influenced research on animal viruses. One is the eclipse phase, which was first referred to by Wollman and Wollman (1937) and later investigated in more detail by Doermann (1952). It now seems clear that an eclipse phase is a general characteristic of the multiplication of animal viruses. The second concept derives from the finding of Hershey and Chase (1952) that following adsorption of bacteriophage to the bacterial host cell the phage DNA enters the cell while the bulk of the phage protein remains outside. An important development of this work was the demonstration, first with tobacco mosaic virus (Fraenkel-Conrat, 1956; Gierer and Schramm, 1956) and then with numerous animal viruses, that viral infection could be initiated by nucleic acid, from which the bulk of the viral protein had been removed. A third concept, which seems to apply to many animal viruses, is that production of viral protein and viral nucleic acid are separate events, which may occur at different sites within the cell and at different times during the viral growth cycle.

Until quite recently, much of the accent in the study of the multiplication of animal viruses was on the kinetics of virus growth—adsorption and penetration of virus, the eclipse phase and the rate at which mature virus particles develop and are liberated from cells, as studied by one-step growth curves. Within the last few years the emphasis has shifted from the study of mature virus and whole cells towards the study of individual viral components and their relationship to sub-cellular organelles. There has also been a change in methodology, with more attention being devoted to biochemical techniques. Indeed, in one report (Riley et al., 1960) the only evidence that mice were infected with a particular virus was an increase in lactic dehydrogenase in their sera. Work of this kind may be a pointer to a new area of future virus research. In this chapter discussion is based on work in which serological and biochemical techniques were mainly used; morphological changes in virus-infected cells are considered in more detail in Chapter 7.

In studying a field as broad as that of virus multiplication there is a tendency to search for generalizations. The attempt is made even although the viruses studied range from small RNA-containing viruses to large DNA-containing viruses, and the cells range from embryonic cells in an intact chick embryo to human-cancer cells grown as cell-lines. This introduces an unfortunate bias, since there is a temptation to look for points of resemblance rather than differences in different virus–cell interactions. Again, the changes which are demonstrable in, for example, HeLa cells infected with poliovirus, may have a totally different significance from the changes occurring in virus-infected plant or bacterial cells, where the proportion of the cell which becomes changed into virus may be very much greater than in virus-infected animal cells. There is also a tendency to generalize from the viruses that have been studied most. Fortunately these include small RNA-containing viruses such as poliovirus, the medium-sized RNA-containing influenza group and the large DNA viruses such as vaccinia, so that quite a wide range of virus size and behaviour is well covered.

In considering the range of animal viruses it is not easy to know where the line should be drawn that divides the largest viruses from the smallest bacteria. The psittacosis–lymphogranuloma organisms are referred to as viruses in the daily talk of microbiologists, yet they have four characteristics of bacteria which are not found in true viruses. First, they are sensitive to a number of antibiotics. Secondly, their cell walls contain muramic acid, a hexosamine found particularly in bacteria (Allison and Perkins, 1960). Thirdly, these organisms probably divide by binary fission; although this has not been observed directly as in the case of rickettsiae (Schaechter, Bozeman and Smadel, 1957), the available evidence strongly favours this interpretation (Bedson and Gostling, 1954). And fourthly, they contain both DNA and RNA, as bacteria do, whereas true viruses contain only one or the other nucleic acid. Thus, although the psittacosis–lymphogranuloma organisms resemble viruses in showing an eclipse phase (Girardi, Allen and Sigel, 1952), at the moment the differences from viruses outnumber the resemblances and it seems best therefore to omit them from this chapter.

We shall consider first the eclipse phase and the evidence that the production of viral nucleic acid and protein are separate events, before going on to study the formation of the individual viral constituents and their assembly into virus particles.

II. The Eclipse Phase

With a large number of animal viruses it has been observed that shortly after the initiation of infection the amount of infective virus recoverable from cells is only a small fraction of the amount of virus taken up. However, this still leaves the question unanswered as to whether the virus that has disappeared or the virus which is recoverable, is the parent of the new virus progeny. This question was answered when a more rigid demonstration of the eclipse phase was provided

by Rubin, Baluda and Hotchin (1955). They showed that virus could
not be recovered from isolated chick-embryo cells 30 minutes after
being infected with a high multiplicity of western-equine-encephalitis
virus which would ultimately lead to a high proportion of the cells
becoming virus yielders. The main point is that the number of virus
particles recovered is only a small fraction of the number of cells that
will ultimately yield virus, and similar evidence has been produced
for other viruses, e.g. Rous sarcoma (Rubin, 1955), Herpes simplex
(Stoker and Ross, 1958) and vaccinia (Postlethwaite and Maitland,
1960).

At first the eclipse phase was described as a stage in virus growth
when viral infectivity "disappeared". More recent evidence suggests
that the eclipse phase is better interpreted as a change of state, in
which the viral nucleic acid becomes separated from the protein
capsomeres (i.e. the sub-units of the viral protein coat). The low
infectivity found during the eclipse phase is possibly due to the fact
that the viral nucleic acid has a much lower probability of initiating
infection than mature virus particles. Evidence favouring this interpretation will now be presented.

A. Loss of Integrity of Virus Particles during the Eclipse Phase

There is good evidence that early in the eclipse phase a change of
physical state occurs in a proportion of the infecting virus particles.
Hoyle and Frisch-Niggemeyer (1955) studied infection of chick chorioallantoic membranes by influenza virus labelled with ^{32}P, an isotope
which enters the viral RNA and lipid. When the membranes were
frozen and thawed to disrupt the cells one and a half hours after
infection, about 20% of the adsorbed ^{32}P was found in the supernatant
extract and the remainder in the deposited residual membranes. When
the extracts were then centrifuged at 100,000 g for three hours, the
greater part of the ^{32}P was not sedimented. Further studies were
carried out by Hoyle and Finter (1957) with virus labelled with ^{35}S,
which enters the viral protein and nucleoprotein. Again, a considerable
part of the label in the membrane extract was not sedimentable at
100,000 g for four hours. Schäfer (1959) has reported similar findings
with fowl-plague virus labelled with ^{32}P; in these experiments the
behaviour of extracts of infected chick-embryo cells was compared with
that of extracts of normal cells to which ^{32}P-labelled intact virus
particles were added. Centrifugation experiments showed that 25–61%
of the ^{32}P of the "infected" extracts could not be sedimented by gravi-
tational forces which sedimented 84–93% of the "hot" virus particles

in the controls. This was found with infected extracts prepared 30 minutes after infection as well as at a later time. Part of this non-sedimentable ^{32}P could be precipitated by antiserum to the "soluble" nucleoprotein antigen, whereas this did not occur to any significant extent in the controls. These findings suggest that within 30 minutes of infection a high proportion of the infecting virus particles lose their physical integrity and break down into smaller sub-units, one of which can be recognized as the viral nucleoprotein.

Another viral component that can be recognized in cells during the eclipse period is infective viral RNA. Sanders (1960) found that within 35 minutes of infection of Krebs-mouse-ascites cells with encephalo-myocarditis virus, infective viral RNA could be detected in the cells by treatment with phenol at 4°C, a technique which does not yield infective RNA from encephalomyocarditis-virus particles. Brown, Cartwright and Stewart (1961a) found that infective RNA could be extracted from pig-kidney cells 15 minutes after infection with foot-and-mouth-disease virus. All the extractable infective RNA was in a form that was susceptible to ribonuclease, unlike infectivity of the intact virus particles. At the same time a protein, serologically identical with the 7 mμ non-infective protein, could be extracted from infected cells. The recoveries of infective RNA and 7 mμ protein reported by Brown, Cartwright and Stewart (1961a) are of great interest. They found that 100% of the infective RNA present in the virus inoculum could be extracted from infected cells during the eclipse phase in a form that was inactivated by ribonuclease. Also, by extracting infected cells during the eclipse period with ether they were able to recover 50% of the 7 mμ protein that was obtainable by treatment of the virus inoculum. The 7 mμ protein was also found in infected cells when purified (20 mμ) virus was used to initiate infection. These results suggest that the bulk of the foot-and-mouth-disease virus is broken down into viral RNA and 7 mμ protein within 15 minutes of the initiation of infection.

The site at which release of infectious RNA from protein occurs has not been defined. Holland and McLaren (1959) have shown that the amount of poliovirus RNA that can be obtained from cells is not affected by treating the intact cells with relatively high concentrations of ribonuclease. They conclude that release of RNA from viral protein does not occur at the cell surface. They also found that HeLa cells that were rendered nonviable by heating at 56°, by prolonged starvation or by incubation in high concentrations of sodium azide, were able to "eclipse" poliovirus just as effectively as fully viable HeLa cells.

It seems reasonable to conclude that shortly after virus particles enter cells they are broken down into their protein capsomeres and nucleic acid or nucleoprotein. The fate of the capsomeres is not known, but it is possible that in delivering the viral nucleic acid safely to the cells they have performed their function.

B. Initiation of Infection by Viral Nucleic Acid

Following the demonstration that tobacco-mosaic-virus RNA, from which the bulk of the viral protein had been removed, was able to initiate infection, numerous reports of this kind appeared with reference to animal viruses. Among the many viruses shown to yield infective RNA by the method which Gierer and Schramm used with tobacco mosaic virus were Mengo encephalitis (Colter, Bird and Brown, 1957a), eastern equine encephalitis (Wecker and Schäfer, 1957b), poliomyelitis (Colter et al., 1957b), encephalomyocarditis (Huppert and Sanders, 1958), foot-and-mouth disease (Brown and Stewart, 1959) and Coxsackie and ECHO viruses (Holland, McLaren and Syverton, 1959a). In addition, success has more recently been achieved with the DNA viruses, polyoma (di Mayorca et al., 1959) and bacteriophage (Meyer et al., 1961), as well as with the phage $\phi \times 174$ which contains single-stranded DNA (Guthrie and Sinsheimer, 1960). In all these cases it was shown that viral nucleic acid, from which the bulk of the protein had been removed, was able to initiate infection. Also, in many cases, the infectivity was abolished by treatment with the corresponding nuclease, which does not occur when intact virus particles are treated with enzyme. Furthermore, it has been shown for poliovirus that the virus produced as a result of infection with nucleic acid has the same serological and other marker characteristics as the parent virus (Alexander et al., 1958; Gerber and Kirchstein, 1960).

A most striking demonstration of the chemical basis of the infectivity of viral nucleic acid came from the findings of Gierer and Mundry (1958) and Schuster and Schramm (1959), who treated tobacco-mosaic-virus RNA with nitrous acid. The nitrous acid converts amino groups to hydroxyl groups, and this deamination has the effect of transforming adenine to hypoxanthine, guanine to xanthine and cytosine to uracil, uracil itself remaining unchanged. By determining the rate of the deamination reactions it was shown that the deamination of one base out of 3000 was sufficient to inactivate the RNA molecule. However, under particular conditions, Gierer and Mundry showed that the change of a single base of the RNA can be mutagenic; the maximal mutation rate being found when an average of one deamination has taken place per RNA molecule. Similar production of mutants by nitrous acid was reported by Tessman (1959) for bacteriophages and by Boéye (1959) for poliovirus.

These important findings of the infectivity of viral nucleic acid alone thus provide a basis for regarding the first stage of the eclipse as a separation of the virus particle into nucleic acid and capsomeres, the viral nucleic acid being responsible for the whole of further stages of viral multiplication while the protein capsomeres are no longer required. However, although this may describe events for many of the smaller viruses, the situation for some of the larger viruses is more complex. Two reports have appeared of the production of infectious RNA from myxoviruses (Maassab, 1959, Portocala, Boeru and Samuel, 1959), but this is not the general experience among virologists, and so far it appears that myxoviral infectious RNA cannot be prepared readily in the same way as with enteroviruses or Arbor viruses (Schäfer, 1959). Possibly the RNA in myxoviruses is bound to protein and the whole nucleoprotein is required to initiate infection. Secondly, evidence has been produced that viral protein may be essential in initiating one step in the multiplication of poxviruses. The evidence comes from a study of the phenomenon whereby poxviruses inactivated by heat can be reactivated in cells in which another poxvirus is multiplying (Berry and Dedrick, 1936, Fenner *et al.*, 1959). It is likely that the heat inactivates the viral protein but not the DNA, since the genetic markers of the heated virus are preserved. Joklik, Abel and Holmes (1960) found that rabbit-pox virus inactivated by heat could be reactivated by a variant strain which had been inactivated by nitrogen mustard, which reacts preferentially with viral DNA. It appears that the protein of the nitrogen-mustard-treated virus was assisting the DNA of the heated virus to produce virus particles of the genetic character of the heated virus. The function of the viral protein is not understood, and one theory is that the protein may set off a cellular mechanism whereby viral DNA is released from the virus particle. But whatever its function these reservations do not alter the basic idea of the importance of the separation of viral nucleic acid and capsomeres followed by replication of the nucleic acid, but rather they point to supplementary mechanisms which may be required during the multiplication of the larger viruses.

There is a great deal to be learned about what occurs in the eclipse phase after the time that viral protein and nucleic acid become separated and before synthesis of new viral nucleic acid and protein can be detected. This interval of time may last an hour or longer with different viruses (Cairns, 1960; Darnell *et al.*, 1961; Martin, 1961), and it separates a relatively short interval of time at the beginning of the eclipse period, when the viral nucleic acid is released, from a longer interval of time at the end of the eclipse period, when the viral nucleic acid and protein are synthesized. Presumably it is during this interval that the viral nucleic acid reaches its site of multiplication, and that the energy and enzymes required in synthesizing viral nucleic acid and protein are made available. At the moment it is difficult to say more than this, nor is it likely that progress will be rapid in this particular field.

III. Formation of Viral Nucleic Acid and Protein as Separate Events

One of the most interesting findings about virus multiplication that has emerged during the last few years is that the replication of viral nucleic acid and the production of the protein of the viral coat are two separate events. The evidence for this comes from three different types of investigation: (a) Viral nucleic acid and protein may be produced at different times in the growth cycle; (b) they may be produced at different sites within the cell; (c) inhibitors are known which will block the production of one more than the other.

A. Production of Viral Nucleic Acid and Protein at Different Times in the Virus-growth Cycle

One of the first to suggest that production of viral nucleic acid might precede that of viral protein was Hoyle (1948). He produced evidence that in chick embryos infected with influenza virus the influenzal soluble antigen, subsequently shown to be a nucleoprotein, preceded the protein haemagglutinin in appearance. Essentially similar results were reported by Henle and Henle (1949), and further evidence was obtained in more recent work carried out by similar techniques and by the fluorescent-antibody method (see Section III B). However, the interpretation was criticized, and it was suggested that the fact that the soluble antigen could be detected first was due to the tests differing in sensitivity. Against these criticisms Hoyle (1953) defended his interpretation, which seems to be generally accepted today.

In Krebs-mouse-ascites cells infected with encephalomyocarditis virus Sanders (1960) showed that the production of infective RNA was practically complete at the time that new virus particles began to be formed. In the same system Martin (1961) studied the time after infection at which labelled precursors could be incorporated into viral RNA or viral protein, a technique used earlier by Darnell and Levintow (1960). Martin found by this method that viral RNA was synthesized between the third and fifth hours while viral protein was synthesized between the fourth and seventh hours after infection. These findings demonstrate that the appearance of viral nucleic acid can precede that of viral protein. That this does not always occur is shown by the findings of Darnell et al. (1961) with HeLa cells infected

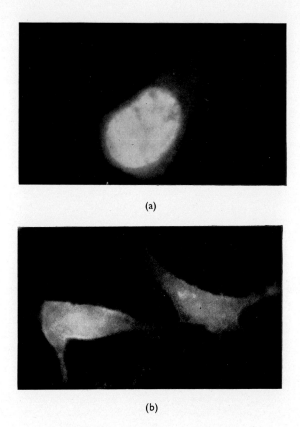

(a)

(b)

PLATE 1. (a) L-Cell infected with fowl plague virus and showing nuclear fluorescence due to nucleoprotein S antigen.
(b) Chick embryo fibroblasts infected with fowl plague virus showing cytoplasmic fluorescence due to viral haemagglutinating antigen.
(Photographs by courtesy of Dr. W. Schäfer, Max Planck Institute für Virusforschung, Tubingen, Germany.)

with poliovirus. By the use of the labelling technique Darnell *et al.* showed that synthesis of viral RNA and protein began at about the same time and proceeded in parallel.

B. Production of Viral Nucleic Acid and Protein at Different Sites within the Cell

During an investigation by means of fluorescent-labelled antibody of the epithelial cells of the nasal turbinates of ferrets infected with influenza virus, Liu (1955) observed nuclear and cytoplasmic fluorescence. Nuclear fluorescence was the chief manifestation with three strains of influenza virus A, and since nuclear staining occurred with antisera to homologous and heterologous virus strains it was suspected that this nuclear fluorescence might be due to the group-specific soluble antigen. Antigen found at the free border of the cell cytoplasm was thought to be the type-specific viral antigen. A more detailed investigation was carried out by Breitenfeld and Schäfer (1957). They observed the growth of fowl-plague virus in chick-embryo fibroblasts in tissue culture by means of fluorescent antibodies which reacted specifically with the soluble nucleoprotein antigen or the viral haemagglutinin. The soluble antigen was found in the nucleus three hours after infection. The haemagglutinin was first detected four hours after infection; it was present throughout the cell but especially in a juxtanuclear position. Later in infection the soluble antigen was found in the cytoplasm. Breitenfeld and Schäfer concluded that the two antigens were synthesized in different parts of the cell and that later the soluble antigen diffused into the cytoplasm, where it combined with the haemagglutinin to form mature virus particles. The separate formation of these two antigens is illustrated in Plate 1.

Essentially similar findings on the separate synthesis of viral soluble antigen and haemagglutinin were reported by Franklin and Breitenfeld (1959) for fowl-plague virus grown in Earle's L cells, and by Holtermann, Hillis and Moffat (1960) for an A2 strain of influenza virus grown in bovine-embryo-kidney cells. However, the latter authors also observed that eight hours and more after infection the nuclei of some cells showed from one to four small well-defined foci of fluorescence caused by haemagglutinating antigen. Another piece of evidence that the distinction of nuclear and cytoplasmic sites of formation of the two antigens may not be absolute comes from the work of Mueller, von Zahn-Ullman and Schäfer (1960). They infected chick-embryo fibroblasts with fowl-plague virus, disrupted the cells at various intervals of time and studied the incorporation of [^{14}C]leucine into the protein of the soluble antigen. For this purpose the cell homogenates were

incubated along with an energy-generating system, and after incubation
the soluble antigen was isolated by precipitation with antiserum, and
the extent of labelling determined. Mueller *et al.* found that homogenates prepared two hours after infection gave rise to significant
labelling, and optimal labelling after three hours. However, a significant
proportion of the labelling of the soluble antigen occurred when virus-
infected homogenates were tested after removal of the nuclear fraction
by centrifugation. This could mean that some cytoplasmic formation
of the protein of the soluble antigen was occurring. Nevertheless, it
seems reasonable to conclude that the viral nucleic acid is made in the
nucleus and that the nucleoprotein antigen is usually synthesized
entirely in the cell nucleus, whereas the bulk of the haemagglutinin is
synthesized in the cytoplasm.

A similar division is suggested by investigations with encephalomyocarditis virus. Bellett and Burness (1960) detected infective RNA
of this virus in the nuclear fraction of cells 30 minutes after infection
at 4°. The amount of infective RNA in the nucleus increased during
incubation at 37° showing a seventyfold increase between three and
four and a half hours. There was only a small increase in the amount
of infective RNA in the mitochondrial fraction during this time. On
the other hand, haemagglutinin was first detected in high concentration
in the mitochondrial fraction at four and a half hours, and it increased
rapidly thereafter; there was only a small rise in haemagglutinin in the
nuclear fraction at this time. It is important to know whether more
examples of this kind can be observed. However, it is clear from work
with vaccinia discussed in Section IV B that in some cases the different
viral constituents may be synthesized at the same site within the cell
(Cairns, 1960), and indeed this may be characteristic of DNA viruses
in general. The conclusion that is justified is that synthesis of individual
virus constituents *can* occur at different sites within the cells.

C. Effect of Inhibitors that Act Preferentially on the Formation of One Viral Constituent

Experiments on infection carried out in the presence of proflavine in
concentrations of 1–10 mg/ml have been reported for polio, fowl-
plague and foot-and-mouth-disease viruses. It is known that when
Escherichia coli is infected with T2 phage and then exposed to proflavine the cells lyse but release non-infective virus. Ledinko (1958)
carried out comparable experiments with poliovirus. She found that
2.5 mg/ml proflavine completely suppressed the formation of infective
type-1 poliovirus but that the cells degenerated completely at the
expected time; the proflavine alone did not affect the cells at this dose.

The treated cells liberated a non-infective complement-fixing viral antigen to the same titre as control cells. Franklin (1958a) investigated the effect of similar doses of proflavine on the growth of fowl-plague virus in chick-embryo fibroblasts. Proflavine in low doses inhibited production of viral haemagglutinin and infectious particles, but did not inhibit production of the nucleoprotein soluble antigen. In pig-kidney cells infected with foot-and-mouth-disease virus, Brown and Stewart (1960) found that low doses of proflavine caused a considerable reduction in the yield of infective virus, but the amounts of infective RNA and 7 mμ protein complement-fixing antigen were not reduced correspondingly. These observations have shown different responses of three virus–cell systems to low doses of proflavine. Proflavine inhibited the production of one or other viral component differentially, or it allowed the formation of both viral components but inhibited their assembly into mature virus particles. Some of the effect might be due to incorporation of proflavine into the developing virus, with subsequent photodynamic action of light on the virus particle. This explanation is suggested by the recent findings of Crowther and Melnick (1961).

Zimmerman and Schäfer (1960) found that p-fluorophenylalanine inhibited the growth of fowl-plague virus in chick-embryo fibroblasts. The effect is a result of inhibition of protein synthesis, and the inhibition is reversible by phenylalanine. If the inhibitor was given two hours after the initiation of viral synthesis, the production of soluble antigen was not inhibited but haemagglutinin and viral particles were not formed. Sanders (1960) studied the effect of 5-fluorouracil at a concentration of 50 mg/ml on the growth of encephalomyocarditis virus in Krebs-ascites cells. The fluorouracil presumably replaces uridylic acid and thus causes the formation of anomalous RNA which is not infective. There was a pronounced inhibition of the production of viral RNA and of infective virus but only a relatively slight effect on the production of haemagglutinin. Sanders also found that euflavine, at a concentration of 0·5 μgm/ml suppressed the formation of infective nucleic acid and infective virus, while the formation of viral haemagglutinin was actually enhanced.

The experiments described in this section all lead to the same conclusion, that the formation of viral nucleic acid and viral protein can be considered as separate events. Their separateness is seen in experiments which show that they may be formed at different times in the growth cycle or at different sites in the cell and that by the use of suitable inhibitors it is possible to prevent the formation of one without affecting the formation of the other. Dulbecco (1960) points out that formation of normal cellular nucleic acid is predominantly a nuclear process, and formation of normal cellular protein a cytoplasmic process, and that we may consider that the virus perpetuates itself by substituting its own nucleic acid for the normal cellular nucleic acid of the same kind. Then, by adopting the same general procedures as obtain in the normal cell, the viral nucleic acid replicates in the cell nucleus and governs the synthesis of protein in the cytoplasm. This is a very useful general formulation, and although vaccinia and adenoviruses provide exceptions that will be discussed in the next sections, the concept nevertheless supplies a useful guide to the understanding of some of the facets of viral synthesis.

Having considered the general characteristics of the synthesis of animal viruses we can next go on to study the production of viral nucleic acid and viral protein, and their assembly to form virus particles.

IV. Production of Viral Nucleic Acid

A proper understanding of the processes governing synthesis of viral nucleic acid and protein will have to await an understanding of the synthesis of normal cellular nucleic acid and protein. A comprehensive review of the vast biochemical literature on these subjects is quite beyond the scope of this book, but Cohen (1959a) has carefully reviewed virus synthesis with reference to the formation of polymers in general. In the next two sections we shall be dealing with what is known of the production of viral nucleic acid and protein, with the sources from which viral macromolecules are built up, and with the gross changes in cellular nucleic acids and proteins that accompany the synthesis of virus. In considering the development of viral nucleic acid it will be helpful to deal with the RNA and DNA viruses separately.

A. RNA Viruses

After the initiation of infection by small RNA viruses it has frequently been found possible to obtain an infective RNA by extraction of the infected cells with phenol in the cold. With some viruses such as eastern equine encephalomyelitis and encephalomyocarditis, extraction with phenol of purified virus particles does not give rise to infective RNA unless the extraction is carried out at 40–50° (Schäfer, 1959). In these cases one can therefore conclude that the infective RNA isolated from cells with cold phenol is not derived from mature virus particles (Wecker and Schäfer, 1957a; Huppert and Sanders, 1958). With other viruses such as poliomyelitis or mouse encephalomyelitis, cold phenol extraction of purified virus particles does yield infective RNA, so that RNA extracted from infected cells by this technique could have been present in the cell either in the form of an RNA-containing viral precursor or as the RNA component of mature virus particles. A decision between these two possibilities may be possible by studying the effect of treatment with ribonuclease or viral antiserum or high-speed centrifugation (all carried out before phenol treatment) on the extractability of infective RNA. It is on evidence of this kind that we can base conclusions about the source of the infectious RNA extracted from cells during the course of viral development.

1. Production of infective RNA in the cell

Holland *et al.* (1960b) followed the appearance of infective RNA in HeLa cells infected with poliovirus at a high multiplicity. The cells were harvested at intervals into either buffer, for assay of virus, or into phenol, for assay of infectious RNA. Between the second and fourth hours after infection the infective RNA rose from its base level to reach its peak. Viral infectivity rose after the third hour and reached its peak shortly after the infective RNA. The rates of production of the two were similar. The fact that the rise of infective RNA preceded that of virus particles suggests that the infective RNA, as extracted from the cell, had not yet been incorporated into mature virus particles, but experiments with ribonuclease treatment, or high-speed centrifugation carried out before phenol extraction, are desirable in order to obtain further evidence. However, very similar conclusions about the time of formation of poliovirus RNA were reached by Darnell *et al.* (1961) by different methods. They infected HeLa cells with poliovirus and then added [8-^{14}C]adenosine to portions of the cells at intervals after infection. The virus yields from the different samples were then isolated and carefully purified, and the specific radioactivity of the adenosine derived from the virus samples determined. The principle of the method is that the longer the addition of [^{14}C]adenosine can be delayed, yet still lead to fully labelled viruses, the later one can infer that synthesis of poliovirus RNA is occurring. Darnell *et al.* found that when the label was added one or two hours after infection the virus that was produced had RNA that was maximally labelled; hence viral RNA could not have been formed to any significant extent during the first two hours after infection. When the label was added at the third hour the resulting virus was only partially labelled indicating the onset of RNA synthesis before this time, and it was possible to show that viral RNA synthesis was completed by from five to five and a half hours, or about one hour before the completion of viral maturation. Owing to the time taken for the adenosine to equilibrate with the intracellular nucleotide pool, these figures are maximal.

In Krebs-mouse-ascites cells infected with encephalomyocarditis virus Sanders (1960) has followed the course of infective RNA synthesis.

With this virus, extraction of virus particles with phenol at 4° does not yield infective RNA; this is only found if extraction is carried out at relatively high temperatures (40–60°). Hence infective RNA extractable from infected cells with cold phenol must be present in a form other than as a constituent of mature virus particles. Sanders found that between one and five hours after infection there was a steady rise in the yield of infective RNA, which was practically maximal at the time new virus particles were being formed. (This commenced at four hours.) Martin (1961) has confirmed these findings by means of the technique (described above) of Darnell *et al.* (1961). He measured the time at which labelled precursors were incorporated into the viral particles, and showed by this means that viral RNA was synthesized between three and five hours after infection, about two hours earlier than the appearance of an equivalent amount of mature virus.

Sanders (1960) also showed that the infective RNA came from a component that was not sedimented appreciably under conditions which bring down virus particles. Bellett and Burness (1961) studied further the state of this component. They found that three hours after infection the non-sedimented component could be treated with ribonuclease without affecting the ability to extract subsequently a full yield of infective RNA with phenol. The infective RNA thus appears to be in some way protected from the action of ribonuclease, but the component was rendered more susceptible to the action of ribonuclease by pre-treatment with up to 10 mg/ml of papain. This suggests that the infective RNA may be coated by protein. However, one puzzling finding was that treatment of the component with a large dose of papain (100 mg/ml) by itself caused a considerable drop in infectivity, and subsequent treatment with ribonuclease then abolished the remainder. Bellett and Burness suggested that the RNA component consists of RNA particles coated with protein and that these represent the vegetative form of the virus. They proposed the name virosome for this component.

The situation seems to be different for foot-and-mouth-disease virus growing in pig-kidney cells. Brown and Stewart (1960) showed that the infective RNA, extractable from cells by phenol, changes in its sensitivity to ribonuclease during the course of infection. During the first two or three hours of infection, if cell homogenates were digested with ribonuclease prior to phenol extraction the infectivity of the RNA was virtually abolished. At a later stage in infection, ribonuclease treatment did not affect the amount of infective RNA recoverable by phenol extraction. Clearly, therefore, the infective RNA is not coated with protective protein in this virus until its incorporation into the virus particle. A similar situation was found by Wecker (1960) for infective RNA extracted from chick-embryo cells infected with eastern-equine-encephalomyelitis virus. If homogenates were treated with ribonuclease before extraction with phenol, no infective RNA was obtained. It is possible, therefore, that the association of infective RNA with protein described for encephalomyocarditis virus may be adventitious, and at the moment it may be better not to use the term virosome until the concept can be more clearly defined. Nevertheless, it is interesting to speculate on whether the RNA of these viruses replicates in one or other of two distinct ways, i.e. in close association with protein or in the absence of such a close association. Myxoviruses and probably encephalomyocarditis virus provide examples of the former, and foot-and-mouth-disease virus of the latter.

Scholtissek and Rott (1961a) used a new technique for following the appearance of viral RNA in chick cells infected with fowl-plague virus. They grew the cells in a ^{32}P-labelled medium, homogenized the cells, separated nuclear from cytoplasmic fractions, digested the RNA with ribonuclease and then characterized the labelled nucleotides obtained. The RNA from infected cells was then compared with normal cellular RNA and with viral RNA similarly treated. This gives a rough measure of the qualitative nature of the RNA formed in terms of its base composition, and it is a less sensitive technique than those described earlier, but the results are nevertheless of interest. Viral RNA could not be detected until two hours after infection and it was then mainly bound to protein and was precipitable by specific antibody to the soluble antigen. When the soluble antigen was first precipitated with antiserum and the remaining newly synthesized RNA characterized, it was found to have a base composition similar to that of normal cellular RNA. This technique may allow changes in both normal cellular and viral nucleic acids to be followed under a variety of experimental conditions.

Wecker and Schonne (1961) have shown that p-fluorophenylalanine, an inhibitor of protein synthesis, blocks the formation of infective RNA by western-equine-encephalitis virus growing in chick-embryo fibroblasts. The block was complete even when the p-fluorophenylalanine was added some time after the onset of viral RNA formation. This shows that protein synthesis is essential for the formation of viral RNA and that the protein is unlikely to be a new type of enzyme required for synthesizing viral RNA. Instead it suggests that the synthesis of viral RNA and of protein are closely related and dependent on one another. Essentially similar findings and conclusions were reported by Brown et al. (1961b) for foot-and-mouth-disease virus.

Scholtissek and Rott (1961b) showed by an application of their

technique (described above) that p-fluorophenylalanine given immediately after infection prevents the synthesis of fowl-plague virus
nucleic acid, presumably by preventing the synthesis of a protein
necessary for the production of viral RNA. They also found that when
p-fluorophenylalanine was given two hours after the initiation of
infection the oligonucleotide pattern of the RNA of infected cells
shifted towards that of the purified virus, just as occurs in cells infected
in the absence of p-fluorophenylalanine. However, nucleoprotein
(soluble) antigen synthesized in the presence of p-fluorophenylalanine
and labelled with [¹⁴C]leucine was not incorporated into the virus
particle. This implies that faulty nucleoprotein antigen, in which
p-fluorophenylalanine is incorporated into the protein instead of
phenylalanine, is still serologically demonstrable, but does not fit into
the intact virus.

2. Sources of viral RNA

Wecker (1957) studied the effect of pre-incubating ³²P-labelled phosphate with chick cells for varying periods of time before infecting with
fowl-plague virus, on the resultant radioactivity of the viral RNA. No
significant differences were found in the labelling of viral nucleic acid
when the ³²P was given along with the virus or for periods up to 48
hours before the virus. The results suggest that viral RNA is not
synthesized from cellular constituents that have a slow turnover of
³²P. At the same time, Wecker studied the radioactivity of viral phospholipid (see Section VII) and this gave results which contrasted
sharply with those for the nucleic acid.

Salzman and Sebring (1961) were able to provide more direct evidence
on the cellular constituents used to synthesize polioviral RNA in
infected HeLa cells. Four hours before infecting the cells they added
[2-¹⁴C]uridine and [8-¹⁴C]adenine to the medium. It is known that
the [2-¹⁴C]uridine is an effective precursor of the uracil and cytosine
of RNA, and [8-¹⁴C]adenine of the adenine and guanine of RNA. The
specific activities were then measured in the acid-soluble nucleotide
pool, and in the bases of the cellular RNA and the viral RNA. At
from six to nine hours after infection the specific activities of the pool
nucleotides were high but those of the cellular RNA bases were only
$\frac{1}{4} - \frac{1}{6}$ of those of the nucleotide pool bases. On the other hand, the
RNA of the virus showed the same degree of specific activity as that of
the pool, suggesting that the latter is the principal source of material
used for synthesizing viral RNA. This conclusion receives indirect
support from the work of Arnoff and Rafelson (1959) who found that
L-azaserine, in doses which completely inhibit biosynthesis of acid-
soluble purine nucleotides, did not affect the yield of influenza virus

in isolated chick chorioallantoic membranes. This shows that fresh formation of purines and their incorporation into RNA are not essential for virus synthesis in this system, and when taken along with the other work it again suggests that preformed components of the nucleotide pool are used for synthesizing viral RNA.

3. Changes in cellular nucleic acids

Conflicting results have been reported on the changes in cellular nucleic acids occurring in the course of viral synthesis. Maassab, Loh and Ackermann (1957) reported that in HeLa cells infected with polio virus there was a considerable increase in cytoplasmic RNA. By the sixth hour this was two and a half times greater than in the controls. There was either no change in nuclear RNA or DNA or a slight decrease. Nuclear RNA and DNA and cytoplasmic RNA showed a greatly increased incorporation of ^{32}P in infected cells, indicating enhanced metabolic activity of nuclear nucleic acids and net increase of cytoplasmic RNA. This result was puzzling in the light of findings by Darnell, Eagle and Sawyer (1959) that HeLa cells synthesized poliovirus when suspended in a buffer containing only glucose, glutamine and salts. In such a medium, net increase of RNA would not be expected to occur. The increases of cytoplasmic RNA reported by Maassab *et al.* (1957) might not therefore be a necessary condition for viral synthesis or a necessary result of virus formation, and the findings of Salzman, Lockart and Sebring (1959) would favour this view. These workers studied HeLa cells growing logarithmically and infected with poliovirus in suspension. Normal cells grown under these conditions showed a net increase in RNA and DNA in a 12-hour period, but infected cells showed no increase. Instead there was a pronounced loss of RNA from the cells. Between six and nine hours after infection, 30% of the RNA was lost, and this preceded any loss of protein from the cells. This finding might be due to the release of cellular ribonuclease, and indeed there was an increase in the acid-soluble nucleotide pool which would support this interpretation. Alternatively, it might suggest normal synthesis but decreased utilization of nucleotides in forming RNA.

The difference between these two sets of findings might be due to different conditions of cultivating the cells. In the experiments of Salzman *et al.* the cells were growing logarithmically, and the uninfected control cells showed an increase in number and a net increase of nucleic acids and protein. In the experiments of Maassab *et al.* (1957) the cells were kept in maintenance medium and the uninfected control cells did not increase in number nor in the amounts of DNA or RNA per cell during the seven-hour experimental period. Whether this will account for the differences in these findings remains to be seen. Ackermann, Loh and Payne (1959) also showed that the newly formed cytoplasmic RNA had a nucleotide composition similar to that of cellular RNA and unlike that of viral RNA.

Goldfine, Koppelman and Evans (1958) investigated the incorporation of [^{14}C]cytidine into the RNA and DNA of HeLa cells infected with poliovirus. During the first 11 hours of infection there was considerable inhibition of incorporation into DNA, whereas incorporation into RNA was only slightly reduced. Very similar findings were reported by Salzman *et al* (1959). Rothstein and Manson (1959) studied cellular RNA by labelling with ^{32}P-orthophosphate added to the medium in the same virus–cell system. The specific activities of nucleotides in infected cells were either the same as, or slightly lower than those of the controls; no net increase in RNA was found.

Martin (1961) has made a very careful study of the changes occurring in the cellular RNA of Krebs-mouse-ascites cells infected with mouse encephalomyocarditis virus. No net changes occurred in total RNA, DNA or protein during the first seven hours of infection. When the cells were infected in the presence of [6-^{14}C]orotic acid, which enters uridine nucleotides of RNA, there was at first an increase of about 20% over the controls in the orotic acid present in the acid-soluble nucleotide pool; presumably this built up as a result of inhibition of transfer to RNA. This inefficient synthesis of RNA occurred in the first four hours, but after that there was an increased turnover, indicating an increase in the rate of RNA synthesis. Normally the greatest RNA turnover occurs in the nucleus. However, in infected cells there was a profound inhibition of the incorporation of precursor into nuclear RNA, which was evident at one hour after infection and continued until the sixth hour. When the virus titre was increasing, at the fifth to sixth hours, there was a large increase in the turnover of mitochondrial and microsomal RNA. This apparently occurs after the time that the infective RNA is increasing (Sanders, 1960) and presumably has a different cause; it may be related to the increase in intracellular haemagglutinin. Martin describes two fractions of nuclear RNA, a fraction soluble in dilute buffer and representing the nuclear cell-sap, and an insoluble fraction which is thought to be nucleolar. The fall in nuclear RNA is confined to the soluble fraction.

It is natural to wonder at the significance of the various changes in cellular RNA which accompany virus multiplication. In discussing this problem it may be useful to consider first the possible role of DNA in the replication of RNA viruses. Two of the reports quoted in the preceding section mentioned that in poliovirus-infected cells there was a decrease in the incorporation of [^{14}C]cytidine into the DNA of the cells but not into the RNA. This suggests that cellular DNA may not play a very important role in the synthesis of poliovirus, but more compelling evidence comes from the behaviour of inhibitors. Salzman (1960) studied the action of 5-fluorodeoxyuridine (10^{-6}M), which inhibits the synthesis of DNA (but not of RNA or protein) by blocking the conversion of deoxyuridylic acid to thymidylic acid. At this concentration 5-fluorodeoxyuridine completely inhibited the growth of a DNA virus, vaccinia, but it did not inhibit the growth of the RNA poliovirus at a concentration 100 times higher. Simon (1961) extended this finding and showed that aminopterin and 5-fluorouracil, in doses that stopped DNA synthesis in HeLa cells, inhibited the growth of vaccinia, but not of Newcastle disease or polioviruses. Similar results with regard to polyoma and encephalomyocarditis viruses were described by Smith et al. (1960). These findings make it clear that DNA synthesis is not required in the reproduction of RNA viruses.

This leaves us to consider what significance the changes found in cellular RNA have for the production of viral RNA and protein. The increase in cellular RNA reported by Ackermann, Loh and Payne (1959) does not appear to be a necessary accompaniment of virus infection but it may be a significant pointer to an unusual biological phenomenon. Various workers have suggested that overproduction of cellular protein or nucleic acid during the course of viral multiplication may point to a disorganization of those cellular mechanisms which normally control the synthesis of protein and nucleic acid. Although this is a very difficult field to investigate in animal cells, it is possible that the virus-infected cell might yield important clues to the question of mechanisms that control cellular synthesis.

From the fact that infection can probably be initiated by viral nucleic acid alone, at least in the case of the smaller RNA viruses, it seems likely that viral RNA can govern its own replication and the synthesis of viral protein. Of these two events there is evidence, reviewed above for influenza, fowl-plague and encephalomyocarditis viruses, and also found for mouse-encephalomyelitis virus (Hausen and Schäfer, 1961), that the replication of viral RNA precedes the synthesis of viral protein. This has not been shown to occur for poliovirus, but it may nevertheless be a general rule. If so, it raises the question whether RNA must first be replicated in the nucleus and then pass to the cytoplasm where it would act as a template for the synthesis of viral protein. Volkin and Astrachan (1956) have found that in phage-infected bacteria there was a high turnover in a minor RNA component of the cells and that this minor component had a nucleotide composition which differed from that of the normal bacterial RNA; this RNA component seems to play an intermediate role in the DNA control of the synthesis of phage protein. Recently, Brenner, Jacob and Meselson (1961) have produced evidence that during the multiplication of bacteriophages, information is transferred from phage DNA to bacterial ribosomes by RNA with a very short life—"messenger" RNA. Presumably this corresponds to that described by Volkin and Astrachan. The production of viral protein in this system depends on an intimate association between messenger RNA and bacterial ribosomes. It is not known whether a similar mechanism is associated with the transfer of information from viral RNA to microsomes for the manufacture of viral protein in animal cells. However, the work of Mueller *et al.* (1960) on the synthesis of the protein of the soluble antigen of fowl-plague virus in cell homogenates gives grounds for hoping that some of these questions can be tackled experimentally within the next few years.

B. DNA VIRUSES

1. Production and sources of viral DNA

The DNA viruses have been less thoroughly investigated than RNA viruses, and until now no studies have been published of the course of formation of infective DNA during virus multiplication. However, Salzman (1960) has followed the synthesis of vaccinia viral DNA by indirect methods. He used 5-fluorodeoxyuridine (or FUDR), which inhibits DNA synthesis by blocking the conversion of deoxyuridylic acid to thymidylic acid. Thus, FUDR inhibits formation of thymidylic acid but not its incorporation into DNA. If it is added at intervals after infection has started, any virus that is formed must contain DNA synthesized before the inhibitor was added. In this way FUDR can be used to obtain an indirect measure of the fraction of viral DNA synthesized up to the time that the FUDR was added. In experiments of this kind Salzman showed that synthesis of vaccinia viral DNA was complete by six and a half hours, when only a small fraction of the mature virus was formed. In fact synthesis of viral DNA preceded that of mature virus by about 4 hours. Indirect support for these findings comes from studies by Magee, Sheek and Burrous (1960) with HeLa cells infected with vaccinia virus. During the period from three and a half to six hours after infection, infected cells incorporated radioactive thymidine much more actively than control cells; this increased activity declined again six hours after infection, at a time when Salzman had shown that production of viral DNA was complete. By means of autoradiographs, Magee *et al.* showed that in infected cells the radioactive thymidine was found in the cytoplasm as well as in the nucleus.

Cairns (1960) has made a most detailed study of the progress of infection of KB cells with vaccinia virus. He used tritiated thymidine and autoradiography in order to follow the synthesis of DNA, and fluorescein-labelled antibody to observe the synthesis of viral protein. Under conditions in which cells were infected with more than one virus particle, a corresponding number of sites of virus synthesis developed in the cytoplasm of infected cells. At each cytoplasmic site, synthesis of DNA and virus protein antigen appeared to start at about the same time. Thus, between five and six hours after infection both viral protein and DNA were found in about half the cells which would ultimately show evidence of infection by these techniques. At this time, and even up to the tenth hour, when the first mature virus particles begin to appear, the newly formed DNA is sensitive to the action of DNAase. If we assume that this cytoplasmic DNA is mostly viral DNA there appears to be quite a long interval of time between the formation of viral DNA and protein and its assembly into mature virus particles. It was also found that with increasing multiplicity of infection there was a more synchronous response of the cells but no change in the minimum time interval between infection and virus synthesis. Cairns concludes from this that in multiply infected cells one virus particle triggers some starting reaction which then sets off a simultaneous synthesis of DNA and virus antigen at all the sites of infection within a cell. The nature of this process of initiation is not known, but it could be the supply of some enzyme, or some source of energy, needed for virus synthesis. DNA synthesis normally occurs in the nucleus, but its occurrence in the cytoplasm need not be surprising since it is likely that the enzymes needed for synthesizing DNA (Kornberg, 1960) are present in the cytoplasm.

Ginsberg and Dixon (1961) have studied HeLa cells infected with type-4 adenovirus in order to determine whether new DNA synthesized as a result of virus infection was derived from host material or from the medium. [^{32}P]Phosphate or [^{14}C]formate was incorporated in the medium 48 hours before infection and then removed by washing at the time of infection. In parallel cultures the isotope was added 21 or 23 hours after infection. Twenty-four hours after infection the nucleic acids were extracted and their specific activities were determined. A high degree of labelling was found in cells labelled for 48 hours before infection, but infected cells showed a lower specific activity of saline-soluble DNA than uninfected cells. In contrast, when the isotope was added after infection a low degree of labelling was found but infected cells showed a much higher specific activity than uninfected cells. These results imply that precursors of the saline-soluble DNA that is synthesized as a result of virus infection were obtained from the medium and from the precursor pool of the cell rather than from the breakdown of cellular DNA. However, experiments with purified virus in line with those carried out for poliovirus by Darnell *et al.* (1961) are required to characterize further the source of viral DNA. The findings of Salzman (1960) on the inhibition by 5-fluorodeoxyuridine of the synthesis of viral DNA imply that *de novo* formation of thymidylic acid is necessary for synthesis of vaccinia virus DNA. This is in contrast to the behaviour reported for RNA viruses and for adenovirus in which, apparently, the normal components of the nucleotide pool are sufficient for virus synthesis.

2. Changes in cellular nucleic acids

Green (1959) found that KB cells infected with type-2 adenovirus showed stimulation of incorporation of [^{32}P]orthophosphate into RNA mononucleotides and into DNA. The stimulation was most noticeable at 9–18 hours after infection and could be due to increased incorporation of medium ^{32}P into the phosphate pool of the cell. Later there was a continued increased uptake of isotope into the DNA of the infected cell, and this might be due to synthesis of a new DNA. Ginsberg and Dixon (1961) found that in HeLa cells infected with type 4 adenovirus there was increased synthesis of a saline-soluble DNA but not of water-soluble DNA. The water-soluble DNA has the "classical" base-pairing of a double-stranded DNA, i.e. the adenine equals the thymine and the guanine equals the cytosine (Watson and Crick, 1953b). However, the newly formed saline-soluble DNA did not show base-pairing, so it might represent single-stranded DNA. When ^{32}P-containing inorganic phosphate was added to the medium an increase in the specific activity of the saline-soluble DNA, but not the water-soluble DNA, was found. Saline-soluble DNA began to increase 10–12 hours after virus infection and 3–4 hours before the appearance of newly formed virus. A large increase in the total DNA and RNA content of cells infected with type-2 adenovirus seems to be due to inhibition by the virus of cell division, so that infected cells increased greatly in mass (Green and Daesch, 1961).

   This effect of adenovirus on cell division may be related to the fact that multiplication of adenovirus is virtually confined to the nucleus. It is interesting to note that Herpes virus, another DNA virus whose multiplication is probably confined to the nucleus, also inhibits mitosis (Stoker and Newton, 1959); this is not a general effect of DNA viruses, e.g. polyoma virus behaves quite differently, but it may suggest some point of resemblance between Herpes and adenoviruses. Herpes-virus infection has been found to increase the DNA content of HeLa cells from six to nine hours after infection or from three to six hours before any increase in virus was detectable (Newton and Stoker, 1958). Kaplan and Ben-Porat (1960) found that the closely related pseudorabies virus caused an increase in the ratio of DNA to protein in primary cultures of rabbit kidney. This increase was observed in nine-day-old cultures which were in a stationary phase of growth but not in actively growing five-day-old cultures. Nine-day cultures also showed on infection a greatly increased capacity to incorporate $[2\text{-}^{14}C]$ thymidine whereas the five-day cultures showed good incorporation of thymidine in the controls but suppression of uptake after infection. It is interesting to recall the findings of Ackermann and co-workers (see section IV A 3) with poliovirus grown in HeLa cells kept in maintenance medium; large increases were found in cytoplasmic RNA, but this was not found by other investigators who studied cells growing logarithmically. Kaplan and Ben-Porat's results with five-day-old and nine-day-old cultures may be another example of the same effect.

Joklik and Rodrick (1959) found increased incorporation of $[8\text{-}^{14}C]$ adenine into the microsomal fraction of HeLa cells infected with vaccinia virus. The increased labelling seems to be confined to microsomal RNA (Joklik, 1959) and no significant increase in RNA or DNA could be found in infected cells. On the other hand, Ackermann and Loh (1960) reported that their results in a similar system depended on whether the cells were growing actively or resting. In growing cells, infection with vaccinia virus resulted in an inhibition of nuclear activity but stimulation of cytoplasmic RNA production. In resting cells there was considerable net synthesis of cytoplasmic RNA which preceded the first appearance of intracellular virus by several hours. The increase was found mainly in the cell-sap and it is suggested that this might consist of low molecular weight RNA associated with the activation of amino acids. These variable results are similar to those found for poliovirus (see Section IV A 3), and it is natural to wonder whether here, too, the increases in cytoplasmic RNA found in vaccinial infection are not a necessary accompaniment of the multiplication of this virus.

It is difficult to generalize about DNA viruses from the limited results available. However, the increases in the amount of cellular DNA after infection with DNA viruses are interesting and may be related to the inhibition of mitosis. When more is learned of the mechanisms controlling mitosis it may be possible to understand how these are affected by the synthesis of large amounts of foreign nuclear DNA.

V. Production of Viral Protein

A. VIRAL PROTEIN DETECTED BY SEROLOGICAL METHODS

Viral protein is normally detected by a serological technique, either alone or in combination with radioactive labelling. Less commonly viral or viral-associated proteins can be recognized by some other property such as the haemagglutination found with many different viruses, or the protein associated with adenovirus particles, which is capable of detaching tissue-culture cells from a glass surface. Some viral proteins found in cells appear to be constituents of the viral coat, which can be detected before they are incorporated into the virus particles. Other proteins such as the lipoprotein haemagglutinin of the pox viruses (Nagler, 1942) or the early cytopathic factor of the adeno-virus (Everett and Ginsberg, 1958; Pereira, 1958; Rowe *et al.*, 1958) are formed during virus multiplication but do not appear to become significantly incorporated into virus particles. Insufficient is known to say whether these are essential factors for some stage of virus multi-plication or accidental byproducts of an abnormal cell metabolism, but the point is clearly of some significance for our understanding of virus-multiplication processes. The work of Breitenfeld and Schäfer (1957) and others on the cytoplasmic site of formation of fowl-plague-virus protein was referred to in Section III B. In general, viral proteins of the capsomeres of RNA viruses seem to be formed in the cytoplasm, but the protein associated with the RNA of myxoviruses to form the "soluble" antigen and the protein of some DNA viruses such as adeno-virus are formed within the nucleus.

Granoff, Liu and Henle (1950) carried out observations on chick chorioallantoic membranes and fluids from eggs infected with Newcastle-disease virus. They found that the membranes, but not the fluids, contained a haemagglutinin antigenically similar to the virus, but smaller (or less dense) and lacking infectivity. Similar findings were reported by Schäfer and Munk (1952) for fowl-plague virus and by Granoff (1955) for influenza virus. These haemagglutinating particles presumably correspond to those found with the use of fluorescent monospecific antibody in a juxtanuclear position four hours after infection of chick-embryo fibroblasts with fowl-plague virus (Breiten-feld and Schäfer, 1957). Their absence from the allantoic fluid implies that they are not liberated from cells along with virus particles but are presumably largely incorporated into the maturing virus particles. They appear to be formed shortly after the viral nucleoprotein. The production of this haemagglutinin can be inhibited by adding *p*-fluorophenylalanine to cells two hours after the initiation of infection.

In encephalomyocarditis-virus infection the viral haemagglutinin was first detected in high concentration in the mitochondrial fraction at four and a half hours after infection (Bellett and Burness, 1960). This is at a time when infective viral nucleic acid has reached its peak and is beginning to pass from the nucleus to the cytoplasm. Martin (1961) measured the time at which labelled precursors were incorporated into the complete virus particle, by the technique of Darnell and Levintow (1960). In synchronously infected cells it was found that viral protein was synthesized at from four to seven hours after infection, from one to two hours later than viral RNA, as measured by the same technique. In poliovirus there seems to be no evidence that formation of viral RNA precedes that of viral protein (Darnell, *et al.* 1961).

HeLa or HEP-2 cells infected with type 5 adenovirus have shown a most striking development—large intranuclear protein crystals visible by light microscopy and reaching up to 30 μ in length (Leuchtenberger and Boyer, 1957; Morgan *et al.*, 1957). The crystals were distinctive for type-5 adenovirus and differed from the virus crystals found in infection with other adenovirus types. They developed only in nuclei which showed virus particles. On electron microscopy the molecules making up the crystal were seen to form a linear pattern spaced at 400 Å. Godman *et al.* (1960) found that 12 hours after infection with type 5 adenovirus a protein matrix appeared within which there developed regular protein crystals with hexagonal faces; these crystals were distinct from other crystals which subsequently gave rise to virus particles. Pereira (1960) has made an interesting suggestion about this protein, based on a study of three non-infectious antigens which were identified in cells infected with type 5 adenovirus. The antigens could be separated by electrophoresis or by chromatography on diethyl-aminoethyl cellulose columns, and two of them were shown to contain DNA and protein (antigens A and C) while the third was protein (antigen B) (Allison, Pereira and Farthing, 1960). Antigen A was serologically distinct from the others but antigens B and C showed partial identity by gel-diffusion. Antigen B appears to be a complex of a trypsin-sensitive protein which is responsible for the early cytopathic effect associated with adenovirus preparations and a trypsin-resistant fraction which is antigenically related to antigen C. Pereira suggests that an antigen present in antigen C can aggregate either with protein to form protein crystals or with DNA or a nucleoprotein to form virus particles. The implication is that these protein crystals are accidental byproducts of virus synthesis for which no obvious function can be found. This type of investigation illustrates the complexity that can appear in the serological analysis of the proteins associated with virus multiplication.

B. Sources of Viral Protein

Darnell *et al.* (1959) showed that HeLa cells producing poliovirus needed only glucose, glutamine and salts when the cells were kept in a concentrated suspension. Under these conditions glutamine is the only

V.I.—H.

amino acid of the pool which falls below detectable levels. At lower cell populations there is more extensive depletion of the pool, and virus formation is reduced but can be restored to normal by addition of amino acids which the cell cannot synthesize. This suggests that virus protein is formed from the free amino acids of the cell rather than from breakdown products of cell protein. Further evidence for this comes from experiments with L-[14C]valine carried out by Darnell and Levintow (1960). By adding the label at different times before infection it was possible to show that the specific activity of valine in the viral protein reflected the specific activity of the amino-acid pool and not that of the host-cell protein. In these experiments it was shown that synthesis of viral protein began about three to four hours after the initiation of infection, i.e. about the same time as maturation of the virus began, but proceeded more rapidly than virus maturation. Nevertheless, on the average, protein synthesis is only about one hour ahead of virus maturation with this virus.

C. Changes in Cell Protein During Virus Multiplication

As was found for cellular nucleic acid, Ackermann and co-workers have reported increases in the cellular protein beginning early in the course of virus multiplication. Increased synthesis of protein in the course of poliovirus multiplication (Ackermann et al., 1959) is not a general finding, however, and Salzman et al. (1959) and Darnell and Levintow (1960) could find no net increase of cell protein. Similarly, Martin (1961) found no changes in the total protein content of Krebs cells infected with encephalomyocarditis virus. As with the changes reported for cellular nucleic acids, these discrepancies may reflect the state of the cells at the time of test. This is suggested by the findings of Ackermann and Loh (1960) that during infection with vaccinia virus, actively "growing" cells showed quite a variable response to infection; an increase in cytoplasmic protein content occurred in control and infected cells but appeared to be slightly greater in infected cells. In "resting" cells, no changes in protein content were found in control cultures, but considerable net increase of cytoplasmic protein occurred in infected cells. The increase in cytoplasmic protein preceded the increase in virus by three or four hours. The authors felt, however, that this protein synthesis might be more incidental than essential for virus production.

D. Reversible Change of State in a Viral Macromolecule

While observing the effects of different temperatures and of heavy water (D$_2$O) on the growth of poliomyelitis virus, Lwoff and Lwoff have revealed a most interesting phenomenon which may have considerable influence on the future study of virus multiplication.

Lwoff and Lwoff (1961a) measured the yield of poliovirus in a single cycle of growth in KB cells. For each virus strain studied there was a range of temperatures within which growth of virus was maximal, and supra-optimal and infra-optimal zones of temperature, in which virus growth was partially or wholly inhibited. If infected cells were maintained at supra-optimal temperatures for three hours and then transferred to normal temperatures, viral development proceeded normally. But if they were transferred to supra-optimal temperatures after the third hour of virus growth, virus development stopped rapidly (Lwoff and Lwoff, 1960). On the other hand, when infra-optimal temperatures were investigated it was found that if infected cells were kept for three hours at 29° and then transferred to 37° virus development was delayed by just three hours. But if virus infection were allowed to proceed during the first three hours at 37°, it would then continue at 29° or even 27°, temperatures at which virus development is normally extremely slow. These results imply that there are two stages in the development of polioviruses. The first stage occurs during the first three hours and is greatly inhibited at low temperatures but proceeds normally at supra-optimal temperatures. The second stage occurs after the third hour. It is greatly inhibited at supra-optimal temperatures but proceeds at only a slightly reduced rate at infra-optimal temperatures. In viral mutants the whole temperature range was shifted, i.e. a virus mutant has supra-optimal and infra-optimal zones of temperature which are either both higher or both lower than those of the wild strain. This suggests that host factors cannot explain these findings and that a single mutation may affect a virus macromolecule which takes part in different reactions in the primary and secondary stages. These reactions could be folding and unfolding of a virus macromolecule.

Further evidence on this phenomenon comes from a study of the effect of heavy water (D_2O) on the growth of poliovirus. This was shown by Carp, Kritchevsky and Koprowski (1960) to increase fivefold to tenfold the burst size of poliovirus. The observations were extended by Lwoff and Lwoff (1961b) who showed that D_2O increased the yield of virus at supra-optimal temperatures but decreased it at infra-optimal temperatures. D_2O in fact had the effect of raising the whole zone range of optimal temperatures. It was also shown by suitable experiments that D_2O increased the duration of the eclipse phase and that at infra-optimal temperatures it acted on the first stage of virus growth. At supra-optimal temperatures, however, D_2O acted on the second stage of virus growth.

It is known that in the presence of D_2O the hydrogen atoms of certain groups are replaced by deuterium, particularly the carboxyl and amino groups of proteins. Lwoff and Lwoff (1961c) assume that temperature and deuterium influence two reversible states of a viral macromolecule which could be nucleic acid or protein. During the first stage of virus growth unfolding of this macromolecule occurs, whereas in the second stage re-folding takes place. Hydrogen-bonding may play an important role in maintaining the structure of this macromolecule, and temperature and D_2O modify the equilibrium of a reversible change of its state.

This work introduces a new concept, that the structural state of a viral macromolecule may play an important role in controlling viral synthesis. It will be important to see whether this macromolecule will be nucleic acid or protein and what is the role played by its change of structural state in the virus-multiplication cycle.

VI. The Source of Energy for Viral Synthesis

The energy for normal cellular synthesis comes mainly from the high-energy bonds in compounds such as adenosine triphosphate (ATP). In normal cells ATP is formed predominantly in the course of oxidative processes, and to a lesser extent as a result of glycolysis. There is no general agreement on the relative importance of these processes in supplying energy for viral synthesis.

Evidence for the importance of oxidative processes comes from studies that show inhibition of virus growth when oxygen is excluded from cultures. This was found for influenza virus grown in chick chorio-allantoic membranes (Magill and Francis, 1936; Ackermann, 1951), for Theiler's virus (Pearson, 1950) and for feline pneumonitis virus (Moulder, McCormack and Itatani, 1953). A similar inhibition occurs if dinitrophenol, or other substance that inhibits oxidative processes, is added (Ackermann, 1951; Eaton, 1952; Ackermann and Johnson, 1953). This behaviour was found in normal cells, but tumour cells frequently show high anaerobic glycolysis and are therefore not dependent on oxidative processes for their supply of energy. As a result tumour cells can support virus growth in anaerobic conditions, or in the presence of dinitrophenol (Gifford and Syverton, 1957; Gifford and Blakey, 1959; Eaton, Jewell and Scala, 1960).

Some cultures of normal cells also show high anaerobic glycolysis, and in addition there is evidence that virus infection stimulates both aerobic glycolysis (Smith and Kun, 1954; Fisher and Ginsberg, 1957) and anaerobic glycolysis (Levy and Baron, 1957). The latter authors have shown that stimulation of glycolysis in monkey-kidney cells occurs within an hour of infection by poliovirus. Thus, in normal cells with high anaerobic glycolysis an important part of the energy for viral synthesis could come from this source, and this may explain the results of Polatnick and Bachrach (1961) that normal bovine-kidney cells supported full growth of foot-and-mouth-disease virus under anaerobic conditions. But this does not seem to be a general rule, and Baron, Porterfield and Isaacs (1961) have shown that different viruses are able to grow in cultures of normal cells kept under different depths of agar. Their experiments point clearly to the conclusion that viruses grown in normal cells have small but definite oxygen requirements which vary from one virus to another.

Cells react to virus infection by producing interferon, a protein which protects cells against the growth of a variety of different viruses (Isaacs and Lindenmann, 1957). Indirect evidence suggests that interferon may act by inhibiting some oxidative process that supplies energy for viral synthesis in normal cells—possibly by an uncoupling of oxidation from phosphorylation. Thus, interferon resembles dinitrophenol (a known uncoupler of oxidative phosphorylation) in showing a much weaker antiviral action in tumour cells than in normal cells (Isaacs, Porterfield and Baron, 1961). The implication is that cells react to defend themselves against virus infection by producing interferon, a protein that inhibits an oxidative process which would normally provide the energy for viral synthesis.

Klemperer (1961) has shown that an early result of infection of chick cells by influenza virus is a stimulation of the direct oxidation of glucose via the pentose shunt. Interferon has the reverse effect. A similar shift towards direct oxidation of glucose via the pentose shunt was found by Kun, Ayling and Siegel (1960) for avian-pox virus and by Fisher and Fisher (1961) for Herpes virus. At the moment, the significance of these observations is not known.

VII. Virus Maturation

After viral protein and nucleic acids have been synthesized they are assembled together to form mature virus particles, a process which is generally referred to as virus maturation. Before discussing normal virus maturation, however, it may be worth while considering those processes in which virus maturation does not occur in the usual way. This happens in certain cell–virus systems, in which viral protein and nucleic acid are formed but the process does not continue beyond this stage. Faults in maturation also occur when cells are infected with a high multiplicity of virus resulting in the formation of incomplete virus, and when cells simultaneously infected with two related viruses

yield phenotypic mixtures. These examples of faulty virus maturation
will now be considered briefly.

A. FAULTY VIRUS MATURATION AS SHOWN BY FORMATION OF INCOMPLETE VIRUS AND PHENOTYPIC MIXTURES

A number of instances have been described in which viral infection of
certain cells does not lead to the production of fully mature virus but
only to the formation of viral nucleic acid and protein. This has been
reported particularly for myxoviruses and was described by Schlesinger
(1950) for infection of the mouse brain; by Isaacs and Fulton (1953) for
infection of the chick chorion, as distinct from the allantois of the same
membrane; by Henle, Girardi and Henle (1955) for infection of HeLa
cells; and by Franklin and Breitenfeld (1959) for infection of Earle's
L cells. In all these cases the production of viral nucleoprotein and
viral haemagglutinin were detected within cells by serological techniques, but maturation of virus did not occur. Franklin and Breitenfeld
studied infected L cells with fluorescent antibody and they showed that
the nucleoprotein antigen appeared in the nucleus as in normal infection, but that it could not subsequently be detected in the cytoplasm.
They concluded that failure of maturation was due in this case to
inhibition of the normal release of nucleoprotein antigen from the
nucleus preventing the union with haemagglutinin to form mature
virus particles.

The formation of incomplete virus may also, to some extent, be
considered as a fault in virus maturation. Incomplete virus was described in a series of studies of influenza virus by von Magnus. However,
there are no examples of other viruses in which a similar phenomenon
has been unequivocally demonstrated. von Magnus (1951) showed that
if cells were infected with influenza virus at a high multiplicity, the
vast majority of the progeny was incomplete, since the virus preparations had a very low ratio of infective to total virus particles. ("Infective", in this sense, implies the ability to initiate and complete a series
of cycles of virus multiplication.) On continued passage of undiluted
seed virus, the extent of this change increased and after from three to
six passages virus was produced with a ratio of about one infective
unit per million virus particles, in place of the ratio of about one in ten
for the starting material. The low infectivity of incomplete virus appears
to be related to the fact that it has a low content of nucleic acid, and
Ada and Perry (1956) found that when different preparations of
incomplete virus were examined there was a linear relation between
the nucleic acid and the logarithm of the infectivity per virus particle.
Lief and Henle (1956) found that incomplete virus showed a low content
of nucleoprotein-"soluble" antigen extractable from the virus particles

by ether. The low relative infectivity of incomplete virus can therefore be ascribed to the fact that the virus particles produced have a low content of viral nucleoprotein enclosed apparently within a normal content of viral haemagglutinin. Presumably, the basic fault is an error in the synthesis of viral nucleoprotein, possibly occurring as a result of the cells being strained by infection at high multiplicity. This faulty nucleoprotein is then incorporated with viral haemagglutinin to form incomplete virus particles.

A third type of error of virus maturation results in the phenomenon of phenotypic mixing which was described independently by Fraser (1953) and Hirst and Gotlieb (1953). In this phenomenon the progeny of mixed infection of cells with two different viruses carry in their protein coats antigens derived from both virus parents. However, these mixed coats are not transmitted to the progeny of such particles, so that it would seem that in these cases one cell may synthesize nucleoprotein of one kind and protein haemagglutinin of two different kinds, both of which then become associated with the single nucleoprotein. Thus, the haemagglutinin of virus particles produced by mixed infection of cells by influenza-A and Newcastle-disease virus is inhibited by antisera to both viruses, showing that its haemagglutinin coat contains antigens of both these viruses (Granoff and Hirst, 1954). This suggests that the association of viral nucleoprotein with the protein coat is not precisely determined, so that protein of a distinctly different type can become associated with viral nucleoprotein in quite a random manner.

In phenotypic mixing there is no interaction in the genetic materials of the two viruses. In other cases, double infection of a cell may result in the formation of heterozygotes, i.e. diploid virus particles containing two different genetic units, which on further passage segregate into both parent types (Gotlieb and Hirst, 1954). Thirdly, double infection can result in the formation of virus recombinants (Burnet, 1959; Fenner et al., 1959; Hirst, 1959) in which part of the progeny have a distribution of properties not found in either parent. The genetic aspects of heterozygosis and recombination will not be considered here.

B. Normal Virus Maturation

The examples of faulty virus maturation show that in viruses such as myxoviruses, where viral nucleoprotein and haemagglutinin are formed at different sites within the cell, normal maturation requires release of nucleoprotein into the cytoplasm, followed by an association between nucleoprotein and protein molecules that is not too precisely determined. For many viruses this step is followed by a covering of lipid from the cell surface, and evidence suggests that the lipid is normal lipid from the cell periphery and not lipid synthesized as a result of virus infection. This was shown by Wecker (1957), who studied the labelling of viral nucleic acid and phospholipid in chick cells infected with fowl-plague virus and incubated with ^{32}P-labelled phosphate for different intervals of time before infection. His results for nucleic acid have already been described in Section IV A 2, and the findings for viral phospholipid are that the longer the period of incubation with ^{32}P the higher the radioactivity of the viral phospholipid. This is the reverse of what was found for viral nucleic acid and it implies that viral phospholipid comes directly from preformed cellular lipid, in contrast to viral nucleic acid, which is newly synthesized from its nucleotide components. This cellular coat of lipid is presumably applied near the cell surface where the viral nucleoprotein and haemagglutinin are aggregating together to form virus particles. Electron microscopy confirms that myxoviruses are found only close to the cell surface (Morgan and Rose, 1959).

Many myxoviruses show filamentous forms of very variable size in addition to the spherical forms. The filaments appear to be fully infective and to have haemagglutinin along their entire length (Donald and Isaacs, 1954). This great variability in the shape of the myxovirus particles confirms the evidence from the experiments with phenotypic mixtures that the maturation process in myxoviruses is of a rather random nature, and is not as precisely defined as in the case of other animal viruses.

Franklin (1958b) has pointed out that animal viruses can be divided into two groups: ether-sensitive viruses which contain lipid as an essential component of their coat, and ether-resistant viruses which do not contain surface lipid. He concludes that, in the former, virus maturation occurs close to the cell surface; whereas, in the latter, maturation occurs within the cells. Franklin also suggests that there are differences in the manner of release of viruses of the two groups from cells, and this is discussed in Chapter 6. In addition to myxoviruses, the Arbor and Herpes groups of viruses are ether-sensitive and have been shown or are believed to contain surface lipid, whereas enteroviruses and pox viruses are resistant to ether and are presumed to be free from surface lipid.

The evidence that lipid-free viruses mature within the cell is both biological and based on electron microscopy. Henry and Franklin (1959) found that mouse-encephalomyelitis virus, which is ether-resistant and resembles poliovirus, gave rise to high titres of virus infectivity which was associated with the cells. This cell-associated virus is not affected by treating the cells with large doses of viral antiserum, suggesting that the virus had completed its maturation within the cells. The electron-microscopical evidence comes from studies such as those with adenoviruses (Kjellén *et al.*, 1955; Morgan and Rose, 1959), which show maturation of virus particles within the cell nuclei. The striking feature of the maturation of these and a number of other viruses is the regular crystalline arrays of virus particles found within cells. This regularity is in striking contrast to the irregularity of formation of myxovirus particles.

Crick and Watson (1956) made a prediction that has turned out to be very accurate: that many "spherical" viruses would be found to consist of a core encased in a shell of similar subunits packed in accordance with cubic symmetry. Their reasoning was based on the fact that many RNA viruses have an RNA content with a molecular weight of about 2,000,000, and that on the basis of existing theories of protein synthesis there is insufficient "information" in RNA of molecular weight 2,000,000 to code the synthesis of more than very small numbers of distinct protein molecules. The most economic method of putting together a virus particle would then be to pack large numbers of protein sub-units symmetrically around a nucleic-acid-containing core. Many electron-microscopic studies of animal and plant viruses by the negative-staining technique of Brenner and Horne (1959) have revealed particles whose surfaces show sub-units arranged symmetrically in just the manner predicted by Crick and Watson. It is clear, therefore, that for these viruses with regular architecture maturation implies aggregation of protein sub-units (or capsomeres) around the core in accordance with cubic symmetry. The question of what determines the precise size and shape and symmetry of different viruses is a very interesting one, and it has been postulated that given sub-units of a certain size and shape only one pattern of aggregation is possible.

A consequence of the regularity in the assembly of these virus particles is that under suitable conditions they can pack together to form the crystals that have been demonstrated by electron microscopy. With some viruses, such as adenovirus, polyoma and a strain of Herpes virus, crystal formation occurs within the nucleus. With others, such as some enteroviruses, crystalline arrays of virus particles are found in the cytoplasm, and Stuart and Fogh (1961) suggest that maturation of these viruses may occur, in general, in close association with the cellular membranes of the ergastoplasm. In those viruses that form crystalline arrays it would seem likely that the protein of the capsomeres and the viral nucleic acid are synthesized close together. The relationship between the structure of the two constituents that allows the formation of virus particles showing cubic symmetry will form a subject of growing interest.

VIII. Conclusion

In this chapter we have considered the events that occur when an actively multiplying virus infects cells, from the time that the virus particle has entered the cell until the newly formed progeny virus has matured. This has left out of account those latent virus infections, such as infection of man with Herpes simplex virus, in which the virus can remain dormant for long periods of time, to become active on some particular stimulus. The analogy that comes to mind is lysogenic infection, in which the phage genetic structure is replicated during the course of bacterial multiplication, but can lead to the formation of virulent bacteriophage and death of the host bacterium under specific inducing stimuli (Lwoff, 1953). So far, no examples of latent virus infection of animal cells have been found that correspond strictly to the model of lysogeny. Yet, with the extensive use of monkey-kidney cells for making poliomyelitis vaccines, many examples of latent virus infections are being observed, and an explanation of the mechanism by which these virus infections are held in check is greatly needed (cf Chapter 7). Interferon may play a role here, as it has been proposed as an important factor in maintaining chronic virus infections *in vitro* (Ho and Enders, 1959; Henle *et al.*, 1959). It seems likely that both in the case of latent virus infections and virulent infections, a most profitable field of investigation will be an analysis of the cellular factors that normally keep the synthesis of nucleic acid and protein in check, and the methods by which these controls can be released.

CHAPTER 6

Mechanisms of Cell Infection
III. Virus Release

D. A. J. TYRRELL

Harvard Hospital, Salisbury, Wiltshire, England

I. Introduction

Most vertebrate viruses cannot coexist indefinitely with the cells in which they grow; the cell may die or may simply cease to supply all the factors required for continued virus multiplication. Such viruses must therefore spread from one cell to another or become extinct. In order to spread, infectious particles leave the confines of the cell in which they have matured and enter an uninfected cell. The mechanisms of release on maturation vary considerably, as one would expect from the fact that animal viruses vary so greatly among themselves and also parasitize a large variety of species and types of host cells. The very efficient and dramatic release of bacterial viruses by the sudden lysis of the bacterial cell finds no parallel amongst the animal viruses, though in some cases there is a superficial resemblance. Neither do any of the animal viruses, so far as we know, display such perfect parasitism as do certain bacterial viruses (temperate phages) which survive by the transmission of their genetic material along with the genetic material of the host cell at each cell division. Some of them, however, do pass directly from cell to cell without being released into the medium.

In order to study virus release adequately, it is necessary to use a variety of techniques. Certain techniques cannot be applied to certain viruses; for example, haemadsorption will work only if the virus agglutinates red cells. However, much basic information about virus release can be obtained in almost every case by means of growth curve experiments.

Refined growth-curve techniques, which were originally developed during studies on bacteriophage, have now been adapted to the study of the replication of animal viruses. They reveal when infectious virus particles are assembled from precursors in the cells of a culture and when and to what extent they are released into the medium. However, only when growth curves have been co-ordinated with other studies can a picture of the release process be built up. It may then be possible to deduce the mechanism by which the virus escapes from the cell. It is important not to draw conclusions from results obtained by one technique only and to recognize clearly the particular contribution that each method of study can make. Therefore, before going on to describe how viruses of various groups escape from cells we shall consider in more detail the basis of the techniques usually used in the study of such problems.

II. Techniques for the Study of Release Mechanisms

A. GROWTH CURVES

1. Some basic parameters

The object of a growth-curve experiment is to infect a mass cell culture so uniformly that all the cells react in unison and various phases of virus reproduction can therefore be detected because the whole culture behaves as one large cell. To do this a large number of similar host cells are exposed simultaneously to a known amount of virus. The unadsorbed inoculum is removed, and thereafter at regular intervals groups of cells are tested for the presence of virus or virus antigen. If the conditions are carefully controlled and if an accurate method of virus assay is available, results are usually reproducible within acceptable limits of experimental error. The virus contents of the medium and of washed cells are assayed separately. "Virus release" in such an experiment is shown by the appearance of newly completed virus in the medium fraction. In some cases there is such a short interval between the maturation of a virus particle and its release that the appearance of demonstrable virus in the medium virtually coincides with the end of the latent period. In other cases almost all the new virus is retained within the cells, and only small amounts are shed slowly into the medium.

Let us consider the idealized curves shown in Figs. 1 and 2. In these, concentrations of virus are shown on a logarithmic scale and the concentrations in the cells and the medium are both referred to the same volume. In Fig. 1 it can be seen that antigen was first detected in the cells between four and six hours after infection but that a definite

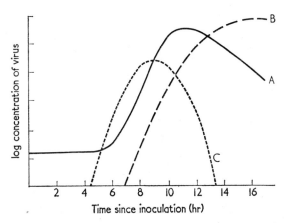

FIG. 1. Graphical presentation of the results of a hypothetical experiment on the growth of a virus in cells in an *in vitro* system.
A, Virus concentration in cells; B, Virus concentration in medium; C, Antigen concentration in cells.

increase in the concentration of infectious virus was first detected after six hours. The antigen behaved like a virus precursor in that it declined in concentration as the concentration of infectious virus reached a peak and was not released into the medium. In some systems it is possible to assay also the infectious RNA formed prior to its incorporation into intact virus particles. In our example infectious virus was present in the cell fraction from the start of the experiment at a "base line" level in spite of the fact that the cells were thoroughly washed after exposure to infection; this is due to virus which is irreversibly adsorbed on the cell surface but fails to penetrate into the cell (see Chapter 4). Its presence unfortunately prevents detection of very small amounts of newly produced virus, so that one cannot say that no virus production at all occurred before six hours. However, no virus was detected in the medium during the latent period, and so one can be sure of the time of its first appearance in this situation. It is theoretically possible to estimate the time taken by a virus particle to escape from the cell as the interval between the appearance of the first

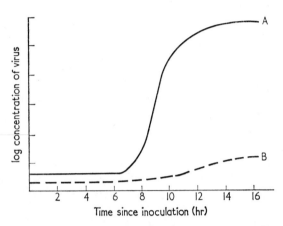

FIG. 2. Idealized growth curve of a virus which is retained in the cells.
A, Virus concentration in cells; B, Virus concentration in medium.

new virus particle in the cell and the first new particle in the medium, but this estimate can only be an approximation because of the uncertain length of the latent period. Moreover, the speed of release when virus production is fully under way may be greater or less than when the first virus particles are being released.

In this example a little over two hours elapsed between the end of the latent period and detection of free virus in the medium. Virus was then rapidly released into the medium, giving a straight line or "logarithmic" curve, until about 10 hours. The rate of release then slackened, and shortly thereafter the concentration of virus in the cells began to fall. We can conclude, therefore, that the cells shed virus for a period of about four hours from eight to 12 hours after infection.

Comparison of the maximum levels of virus concentration attained in the cells and in the medium gives some indication of the relative rates of virus maturation and virus release. In the examples illustrated by Fig. 1, virus concentration in the cells reaches a level which is nearly as great as the maximum concentration in the medium. This occurs because virus matures faster than it is released, so that newly formed virus accumulates in the cells. Later, virus production is slower than release and the concentration in the cells falls. On the other hand, virus may mature slowly and be released soon after completion. Then the concentration of virus in the cells will remain more or less constant at a relatively low level, while the concentration in the medium steadily rises.

2. Virus readsorption

So far we have assumed that the phenomena observed represent the summation of identical phenomena occurring in a large number of cells. In fact, the cells are inhomogeneous, and this inhomogeneity may make interpretation of the results of growth curve experiments somewhat difficult. For example, it may be impossible to infect every cell initially, and as a result the virus released may be rapidly readsorbed to cells not previously infected and the growth curves distorted. Fortunately, this difficulty is largely surmountable in the case of most myxoviruses. The receptors of cells remaining uninfected after exposure to virus can be destroyed by treatment with neuraminidase (RDE), so that virus readsorption is prevented although the infected cells can still produce virus in normal amounts. With other viruses readsorption may be prevented to a large extent, provided that they can be grown in suspended cell cultures. Simple dilution of the suspension during the latent period reduces to negligible proportions the chances of collisions occurring between released virus particles and fresh susceptible cells.

3. Infectious-centre counts

The number of cells which yield virus may be estimated in tissue-culture systems by infectious-centre counts. The cells of an infected monolayer are dispersed by trypsin, freed from extracellular virus by washing and treatment with antisera, diluted and assayed, usually by a plaque method. In this case each plaque is initiated by a single infected cell rather than by a single virus particle. From the total amount of virus in a culture and the number of cells present which yield virus one can estimate the average number of virus particles produced per infected cell.

4. Measurement of virus release from single cells

Even if all or most of the cells are infected, virus maturation and release are unlikely to occur synchronously and to the same extent in all cells. To be able to describe virus release fully it is necessary, ideally, to measure the time at which each cell begins to shed virus, how fast it releases it in the succeeding days or hours and the total amount of virus released. One method of obtaining such information is as follows. Cell suspensions obtained from infected-cell monolayers are diluted so that a given volume is unlikely to contain more than one cell, and this volume is then inoculated into a number of similar tubes. The amount of infectious virus found in each tube is assayed. This gives a measure of the varied yields of virus which, in sum, produce the sort of growth curve we have described. A more refined technique is to pipette individual cells into tiny drops of medium in oil by using a micro-pipette. The medium in the drop may be removed after a period of incubation and the virus released by individual cells may be deter-mined. With even greater manipulative skill the medium in individual drops may be removed at regular intervals and replaced by fresh medium; in this way the curve of virus release for a single cell may be obtained, and finally the cell itself may be taken and disrupted and its content of virus measured. By such means one may measure both the variations in time of release, total amounts of virus produced and amounts released.

In methods using single infected cells it is often assumed that the cell produces virus in the same way when it is contained in an intact cell sheet or a thick suspension as it does when incubated separately in a large volume of medium or confined within paraffin in the micro-drop. This may not be so. It is therefore desirable to confirm that the summation of curves of virus release from individual cells gives results similar to those obtained with mass cultures. Provided this can be done, there is no doubt that single-cell techniques can give the most complete analysis of the process of virus release in mass culture, and examples of this will be discussed later. However, such experiments are impossible with some viruses; for example, if a high degree of oxygenation is required for virus production it is impossible to use microdrops.

5. Growth curve experiments when little release occurs

In many growth curve experiments the amount of virus released into the medium may be very small relative to the amount produced and retained in the cells. Such a growth curve may be seen in Fig. 2. Some spurious virus release may appear in such experiments if the cells are grown in monolayers, because some of the cells may become detached from the glass surface. It is therefore important to centrifuge the medium at low speed to sediment cells in suspension before assaying for extracellular virus.

When studying viruses which give growth curves of this type it is desirable to establish whether the virus can be transferred from cell to cell by a mechanism in which it never enters the medium. This cell-to-cell transfer can be demonstrated by observing the formation of plaques in cell monolayers in the presence of specific virus-neutralizing anti-bodies. The standard plaque technique depends on an agar overlay to prevent released virus from travelling far from the cell in which it was produced. The agar overlay, however, does not prevent short-distance travel to neighbouring cells, so that infected centres are set up which lead to plaque formation. The addition of antiserum to the overlay results in the neutralization of any virus released into the medium, so that in this case plaques can only develop if the virus is able to pass direct from cell to cell without coming into contact with the antibodies. Indeed, plaques may develop in a cell monolayer without any agar overlay, provided that antiserum is added to the nutrient fluid. Herpes virus is an example of a virus which behaves in this way.

These general growth-curve studies can be fully interpreted only when the results are correlated with information obtained by the cytological methods discussed below. On the other hand, cytological methods can be applied most fruitfully to systems in which the kinetics of virus maturation and release have been fully studied by growth-curve methods. Growth-curve studies thus form the framework into which other observations can often be fitted.

B. FLUORESCENT-ANTIBODY STUDIES

The immunofluorescent methods of Coons and Kaplan (1950) are based on the conjugation of fractionated immune serum with a fluorescent dye. In order to help in the study of virus release, the conjugates are used as a specific stain for virus antigens. Host cells are fixed and stained with a conjugate prepared from an antiviral antiserum and from which all antibodies against normal cells have been absorbed. The uninfected cells are seen dimly by virtue of their autofluorescence, but virus antigens are seen clearly as areas of bright specific fluorescence. It is therefore usually possible to see whether the antigen is in the cytoplasm or in the nucleus. Also, cells can be photographed after fluorescent staining and again under phase contrast or after staining with ordinary stains; if the photographs are now compared the site of the antigen in the cell can be determined exactly (Plate 1, Chapter 5). Nevertheless, the method has limitations. It will give no inkling of the presence of a virus component (nucleic acid, for example) against which there is no antibody in the antiserum used. Moreover, it is impossible to tell from the appearances seen whether, or where, the antigen is incorporated into a virus particle. All the same, the method can show quite clearly where, in the cell, virus components and particles accumulate, and it will also show directly whether cells are infected and, if so, how many are infected. In some cases it is possible to demonstrate that virus synthesis and release have come to an end, because stainable antigen is no longer demonstrable in the cells. Fluorescent-antibody studies can be particularly useful in visualizing the process of direct cell-to-cell transfer of virus referred to in the previous section.

C. HAEMADSORPTION

Certain haemagglutinating viruses (myxoviruses, vaccinia and Arbor viruses) produce the phenomena of haemadsorption; that is to say, red cells adsorb to the surfaces of cells producing virus (Vogel and Shelokov, 1957). This is a useful way of detecting virus at the surface of tissue-culture cells, although it cannot tell us whether the virus has found its way into the medium. It is possible to detect a very few cells in this state in the presence of many cells which are not releasing virus. A modification of this method based on the mixed-cell-agglutination technique of Coombs has also been described (Fagraeus and Espmark, 1961) which can be used for non-haemagglutinating viruses. Tissue cultures are treated with antivirus serum and then with sheep red cells coated with an antibody directed against the species of animal used to produce the antivirus serum. The first antibody is fixed to virus present at the surface of the culture. The red cells are then tied to this antibody by the second antibody directed against the species-specific antigens of the first. The facts that the method of Fagraeus and Espmark does not reveal poliovirus at the surface of cells and that haemagglutinating ECHO viruses do not haemadsorb suggest that when certain viruses are released they do not remain exposed at the surfaces of the host cells.

D. ELECTRON MICROSCOPY

Virus release can be studied with the electron microscope by using the methods developed for the study of cell cytology. Infected tissue is fixed in buffered osmic acid solutions, and ultra-thin sections are cut and examined under the electron microscope. For this purpose it is necessary to use enlarged photographic prints rather than direct observation of the screen. The osmic acid acts as a "stain" by being adsorbed to various cell components. Even more intense "staining" can be obtained by exposing the sections to solutions of salts of other heavy metals such as uranium or lead. Virus particles and other components or products can, at times, be readily recognized in sections of infected cells. However, virus particles take up heavy metals much as do various cell components though perhaps rather less intensely. In addition, many of the particles and vesicular components of cells are of about the same sizes as virus particles and their sub units. Therefore virus particles can usually be recognized only if they appear in large numbers with uniformity of size and outline. Their recognition is considerably easier if they form crystalline arrays. Large numbers of characteristic virus particles may be present in cells and yet not be detected on electron micrography because only a very small fraction of the cell can be seen in one section. Nevertheless, no study of virus release is complete without electron microscopy, for it is the only way we have of visualizing how individual virus particles leave cells or pass through their substance. This point will be illustrated later when we describe the influenza viruses.

Virus particles may be seen by another method, that of "negative contrast" (Brenner and Horne, 1959). If a virus is mixed with sodium phosphotungstate, the latter provides an electron-dense background against which the less dense virus particles can be seen in sharp outline, much as bacteria are visualized in the classical india ink method of film preparation. The virus-surface structures may also be revealed to some extent. The method is of particular value for the study of free virus particles but as yet has found little application in studies of virus release in which the relationship of the virus particle to cell components is of particular interest.

E. VISIBLE LIGHT, PHASE CONTRAST AND DARK-GROUND MICROSCOPY

All the cytological methods so far mentioned can be used only on fixed and non-living material, although it may yet become possible to apply electron microscopy to unfixed virus-infected cells. As a complete virus particle is non-motile, it is necessary to look for cell activities and movements which bring about its extrusion into the medium. Certain of the larger viruses can be seen by light microscopy, but virus particles cannot usually be detected with visible light. Light microscopy is used to give a picture of the morphology and movements of living, unfixed cells in the process of producing virus. It is possible to see by dark-ground microscopy the formation of structures which are probably virus filaments at the surface of cells producing influenza virus. Detailed permanent records may be obtained if time-lapse cinemicrophotography is used, and in the work of Lwoff et al. (1955) such morphological studies of infected cells in microdrops enabled the release of virus into the medium to be correlated with certain characteristic movements of the cell.

F. CELL FRACTIONATION

Cells may be disrupted by grinding and the sub-units then separated by various methods. Centrifugation in sucrose solution or in sucrose density gradients has proved to be particularly useful. If a virus particle develops in one part of the cell and then migrates to another, it may be possible to detect this by breaking up cells at different stages of infection and looking for the virus in various sub-fractions. Conclusions drawn from such attempts must be made with great caution. A centrifugation method which will give a purified fraction of normal cell nuclei may not give a comparable fraction from infected cells. In addition, a special intracellular structure in which virus is developing may sediment together with a normal cell component of the same density, in which case some relationship between the virus and the normal component may be erroneously deduced from the fact that both become concentrated in the same fraction. This is the apparent explanation of the observation that virus infectivity can be found in the mitochondrial fraction of ascites cells infected with encephalo-myocarditis virus—the virus particle in its free state remains suspended during the sedimentation of mitochondria, but prior to release it exists in association with a larger structure (Martin and Work, 1961). Virus may be adsorbed on to a normal cell component during fractionation and again lead to results which mislead the incautious. Kaplan and Melnick (1953) thought on the basis of cell fractionation that poliovirus was associated with nuclear fractions, although it is currently believed that infectious virus develops in the cytoplasm.

III. The Release of Certain Viruses

In this section certain viruses in which the mechanisms of virus release have been studied in some detail are considered. The material presented has been highly selected, and most prominence has been given to research in which co-ordinated studies of virus growth and release have been made, using a variety of techniques. For this reason particular attention will be paid to work on tissue-culture systems, and to studies on the multiplication of myxoviruses in the chorioallantois of the chick embryo. Interesting variations in the mechanism of virus release will be emphasized.

Different viruses are completed at different sites in the cell, so that those which mature almost at the surface have only a little way to go to be released, while those which mature within the nucleus have to pass through cell membranes and long tracts of cytoplasm in order to escape. Now, it is known that many normal cell components and also the sub-units of some viruses travel into the cytoplasm from the nucleus and through cell membranes. Possibly in some cases a mature virus particle also is able to utilize the normal transport mechanism of the cell, but even using our present crude methods it is obvious that a variety of things may happen. Sometimes a virus escapes with little sign of any disturbance to the functioning of the cell, but in other instances it seems to leave the cell only when the latter disintegrates.

In order to classify the data in some way we have grouped the viruses according to the site at which the mature particles seem to appear. This method brings together viruses of similar biological groups and also those which have, so to speak, similar barriers to pass in order to escape into the exterior.

A. VIRUSES DEVELOPING IN THE NUCLEUS

1. Cell disintegration

It is known that the nucleus plays an important part in the growth processes of myxoviruses and that some of the virus sub-units may be synthesized there; however, in this section we shall deal with viruses which are largely completed in the nucleus. The adenoviruses belong to this group, and their growth in monolayer and suspended cell-tissue cultures has been well studied with clear-cut results. The analysis of growth curves shows that for many hours after its first appearance only a small fraction of the infectious virus is released from cells (Kjellén, 1961). In a culture in an advanced stage of degeneration produced by any of the adenovirus types, the titre of the cellular fraction may be a hundredfold to a thousandfold higher than that of the medium, though there are some differences between strains in other aspects of their growth curves (Denny and Ginsberg, 1961). There are gross pathological changes in the nucleus from a fairly early stage of infection; yet the nuclear membrane remains intact even when the whole cell has become rounded up in the way characteristic of adenovirus cytopathic effect. This is consistent with the long retention of virus in the cell demonstrated by growth curves. Fluorescent-antibody studies have been directed mainly to the early stages of virus multiplication; the first antigen is detected in the nucleus before infectious virus appears. Later, an antigen appears in the cytoplasm. Electronmicrographs of thin sections show that inside the nucleus there are characteristic developing and mature virus particles which are often arranged in crystalline arrays (Morgan et al., 1956a; Morgan and Rose, 1959; Pereira, Allison and Balfour, 1959). Few particles are seen in the cytoplasm, and those which do occur there are often found near breaks in the nuclear membrane. From these results it may be suggested that virus particles leave the nucleus only when the nuclear membrane ruptures, and that virus particles are released from cells only when the cell disintegrates completely. In a sense no special virus-release mechanism can be discerned, only the spilling of virus from the broken fragments of a cell into the medium in which it is bathed.

2. Passage through the cell without disintegration of structure

Virus particles may develop in the nucleus and may be found passing into the cytoplasm of a relatively intact cell. Herpes is a virus of this type which has been well studied, and some attention has also been given to the related virus B of monkeys. Analysis of growth curves in rabbit-kidney tissue cultures (Kaplan, 1957) reveals that herpes virus develops in cells after five hours and is shed into the medium after seven hours. The mean virus release time (Rubin, Franklin and Baluda, 1957) was 2·3–3·5 hours (see p. 228). On the other hand, when isolated in microdrops, HeLa cells released virus between 16 and 33 hours after infection (Wildy, Stoker and Ross, 1959). Late in the multiplication cycle there seems to be as much virus inside the cells as outside them (Scott *et al.*, 1953).

The release of this virus can be studied in various cell systems, as it is possible to make accurate measurements of infectious virus by pock counts on the chick chorioallantois or by plaque counts in tissue cultures. However, the use of too many virus strains and cell lines tends to lead to confusion, because there are large and still undefined differences in the way in which various virus–cell combinations behave.

Fluorescent-antibody staining reveals that herpes virus antigens appear first in the nuclei of infected cells and later in the cytoplasm (Lebrun, 1956). Profiles of virus particles can be seen by electron microscopy in the nuclei of both chick embryo and HeLa cells (Morgan *et al.*, 1959b; Stoker, Smith and Ross, 1958). These particles have one membrane surrounding a central nucleoid. In the cytoplasm are found particles possessing a double membrane, and other similar particles are found at the surface of the cell (Plate 3). The virus particles may be found in the cytoplasm inside vacuoles. Those at the cell surface are apparently being released without gross disruption of the structure of the cytoplasm, although it is difficult to be sure that particles seen at the surface of a cell or within its cytoplasm have not been released from an adjacent and more seriously damaged cell and then attached to its neighbour and taken up into the cytoplasm. It is therefore uncertain which of the intracellular particles are really complete and infectious and therefore being "released". Some may still be incomplete structurally and functionally and may have been reabsorbed. Morgan and Rose (1959) consider that the virus particles in the nucleus acquire their second membrane from a folding of the nuclear membrane as they enter the cytoplasm. The second membrane may therefore be derived mainly from the cell and may not be an essential part of the virus particle. They also believe that the virus is released from the intracytoplasmic vacuoles without disintegration of the cells. Gray and Scott (1954) have shown virus infectivity to be associated with the nuclei of fractionated chick-embryo-liver cells in the early stages of virus synthesis, but not in later stages. The virus would not adsorb to the isolated nuclei of normal cells. It could be extracted from infected nuclei with hypertonic NaCl. The authors thought the virus was probably replicating within the nuclei. Ackermann and Kurtz (1952) found the virus in mitochondrial fractions from chick-embryo-liver cells collected at a late stage when gross lesions were present. All such results, as indicated above, have to be viewed with caution but might indicate that in different sets of experiments the virus was caught at different stages of the release process.

3. Cell-to-cell transfer

Working with herpes B virus, Reissig and Melnick (1955) showed that plaque formation occurred in monolayer cultures, whether the overlay medium contained normal serum or immune serum, and concluded from this that the virus could pass from cell to cell without becoming exposed to the surrounding medium (see Section II A 5). Hoggan, Roizman and Roane (1961) shed more light on the details of this process when investigating the behaviour of two variants of herpes simplex virus. These strains were identical antigenically and grew to similar titres in the cell system used. If the medium contained chicken serum, both viruses produced a generalized cytopathic effect. If the medium contained horse serum, which has some virus inhibitory activity, one strain, MP, produced large plaques, while the other, mP, produced small plaques. It was found, by staining with fluorescent antibody, that cells infected with the MP strain contained virus antigen in the cytoplasmic threads joining infected syncytia to adjacent cells, while cells infected with the mP strain manifested similar threads, but these contained no virus antigen. This suggested that the MP strain could form large plaques because it could spread efficiently by the cytoplasmic processes.

Stoker (1958) approached the problem of virus spread differently. He exposed a culture of HeLa cells to herpes simplex virus and then counted the number of infectious centres by planting on sheets of HeLa cells. Similar cells were dispersed in microdrops and incubated, but when these were broken up by freezing and thawing little or no infectious virus could be recovered from them. In addition, when the cells were planted on chorioallantoic membrane instead of sheets of HeLa cells there were apparently few infectious centres. He concluded that the virus could produce a focus of infection by spreading from cell to cell if they were of similar type, but that it could not be extracted from the cells in infective form; it might be analogous to the vegetative form of bacteriophage.

It has been found (Hoggan and Roizman, 1959) that when cells infected with herpes virus are held at a reduced temperature, 30°, virus is still formed but it tends to accumulate in the cells rather than to be released. Poliovirus also accumulates in cells held at a low temperature (Roizman, 1959). It is possible, therefore, that a common release mechanism is inhibited at this temperature. The cell merging process by which the virus spreads in an immune environment seems to be temperature-dependent also, since the virus spreads from cell to cell most rapidly at 37°, although the maximum amount of virus is formed at 34° (Hoggan, Roizman and Turner, 1960). In another system (Maben cells), it has been shown that a "latent" infection, in which only a small proportion of cells actually produces virus, can be induced by reducing the temperature of the culture, but it is not clear whether this is mediated by altering the rate of virus release (see Chapter 8, p. 327).

In the herpes group of viruses it is probable that the particles make use of some cell-transport mechanism to pass from the nucleus to the cell surface while the cytoplasm is still in a relatively normal state. The hypothesis that this is due to passage down the endoplasmic reticulum is interesting but unproved and deserves more study. Phase-contrast cinemicrophotography shows that there is a great deal of movement within the cytoplasm of a normal cell, in which particulate matter may be transferred from the cell nucleus to the surface of the cytoplasm and also in the reverse direction. It would be interesting if a technique were developed which enabled one to follow the movement of virus particles also. Perhaps paralysis of the mechanism would lead to retention of virus in the cell.

The experiments with immune serum seem to show that virus can pass from one cell to the next either without leaving the cytoplasm or by passing through a portion of the extracellular fluid sequestered from the surrounding medium. Alternatively, it may be transferred in a non-antigenic form, perhaps as nucleic acid, although this would probably survive only a short time in medium. Whatever the details of the process may be, direct cell-to-cell transfer may be very important for a virus such as herpes simplex, which survives for long periods and produces lesions in persons with high levels of circulating antibody. It is possible that the virus survives in a latent form in skin cells, the temperature of which is lower than that of deeper tissues and approximate to that which *in vitro* favours the retention of virus in cells.

In summary, it seems that herpes simplex virus in tissue culture is transferred from cell to cell both by release and reabsorption and by direct cell-to-cell transfer. The strain of virus, the type of cell and the conditions of culture determine how much of each occurs in any given system.

Chickenpox-zoster virus also matures in the nucleus and may be related to herpes simplex. Typical cytopathic effects are produced in tissue cultures inoculated with vesicle fluid from a human case. The vesicle fluid apparently contains free virus particles. However, it has been found impossible to transfer infection from one culture to another except by the use of intact cells (Weller, 1953; Taylor-Robinson, 1959). In fact, there is little or no release of infectious virus from infected-tissue-culture cells, which fluorescent-antibody studies show to contain a great deal of virus antigen (Weller and Coons, 1954); as might be expected, foci of degeneration in tissue cultures spread by the infection of successively more and more cells in a centrifugal fashion. There are, therefore, differences between the mechanisms of maturation and release of virus developing in human-skin epithelial cells and in cultured cells. It is possible that cells in culture lack some physiological activity by means of which cells in the skin produce fully infectious particles.

B. Viruses Maturing in the Cytoplasm

1. Pox viruses

The pox viruses appear to be synthesized and to reach maturity in the cytoplasm of the host cell. In the case of vaccinia the evidence for this is that virus antigen, DNA-ase-resistant DNA, and typical virus particles can all be detected in the cytoplasm of infected cells, but not in the nucleus (Loh and Riggs, 1961; Anderson, Armstrong and Niven, 1959).

There is a good deal of evidence to support the view that in cell-culture systems release of the mature virus into the medium depends chiefly upon disintegration of the infected cells. Thus, growth-curve experiments show that there is far more virus in the cells than in the medium until the stage at which the cytopathic effect of the virus is very marked (Furness and Youngner, 1959). Microscopy and electron microscopy (Morgan et al., 1954) indicate that the virus particles develop in foci within the cytoplasm, and little is seen to suggest that they migrate towards the cell surface. It is true that, at a time when the tissue cells as a whole are releasing virus, particles can be seen by electron microscopy at or near the surface of some cells or attached to cell processes, but it is not possible to decide whether these represent virus which is leaving the cells or has just been readsorbed from the medium. That virus spread from cell to cell is not entirely dependent upon its release into the medium is shown by fluorescent-antibody studies in which virus antigen is demonstrable in the long cytoplasmic processes of infected cells (Noyes and Watson, 1955), coupled with the fact that discrete plaques develop in cell monolayer without agar overlay (Postlethwaite, 1960). Thus, both the potentiality of direct cell-to-cell transfer and the mechanism of virus release by cell disintegration are likely to be factors of great importance in the pathogenesis of natural infection.

2. Enteroviruses and related viruses

The enteroviruses, which also seem to mature in the cytoplasm, form a very large family of viruses. Among these the polioviruses have been the subject of most intensive study, but a great deal of what is known about their behaviour may apply to the family as a whole.

Growth-curve experiments with poliovirus have been performed in monolayers prepared from trypsin–dispersed monkey-kidney cells and in cell lines which can be propagated serially either as monolayers or in suspension. The virus infectivity and the infectious RNA can be measured accurately by plaque assay (Dulbecco and Vogt, 1954a; Alexander et al., 1958) and the formation of virus antigen can be detected by complement fixation (Roizman, Höpken and Mayer, 1958). Virus nucleic acid and protein develop virtually simultaneously in the cells, and infectious virus particles appear shortly afterwards (Darnell et al., 1961). The new infectious units are retained in the cells for a short time before their release (Darnell, 1958; Howes, 1959). The amount of virus synthesized per cell seems to depend on the size of the cell (Dunnebacke and Reaume, 1958) and the amount escaping from the cells varies with the type of cell used (Howes and Melnick, 1957; Roizman et al., 1958). Usually much of the virus appears in the medium when a cytopathic effect develops. Virus release is prevented by maintaining cultures at room temperature (26–32°C), and little release occurs at 33°C; as a result, under these conditions virus accumulates inside the cell (Roizman, 1959). Virus release may also be affected by the medium. Takemoto and Habel (1959b) have described a gamma-globulin found in normal horse sera which can inhibit the adsorption and release of certain strains of poliovirus.

We have already referred to the work of Lwoff et al. (1955), in which virus release from single cells immobilized in microdrops was measured. Cinephotomicrography of the cells being studied showed that most of the virus escaped into the medium within half an hour from the time when the cell suddenly began to be rounded up and became granular and vacuoles appeared in the clear peripheral zone. This suggested that the development of the cytopathic effect was intimately associated with the release of infectious particles into the medium. Reissig et al.

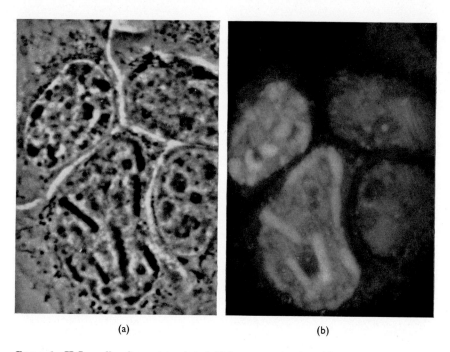

(a)   (b)

PLATE 1. HeLa–cell cultures inoculated 48 hours previously with adenovirus type 5. The same group of cells is shown both on the left (a) and on the right (b). The nucleus at the bottom contains protein crystals visible by phase contrast in (a) and stained with fluorescent antibody in (b). The nucleus above it shows areas of antigen formation, some of which correspond to small inclusions while others do not. The nuclei to the right contain a little antigen and the lower contains two inclusions which fail to stain for antigen. (× 1900). (Reproduced by courtesy of Dr. H. G. Pereira.)

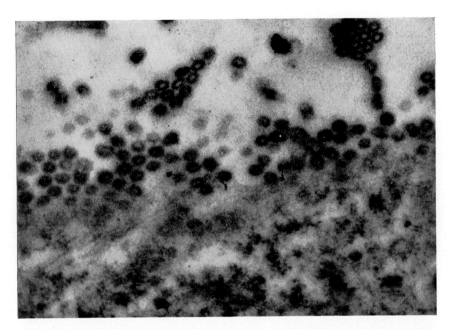

PLATE 2. An electron micrograph of a section of a calf-kidney cell 24 hours after inoculation with influenza A virus (Niven *et al.*, 1962). The rounded profiles at the surface and in the upper part of the picture represent virus particles or filaments forming at the cell surface and entering the culture medium. The lower part of the picture shows cell cytoplasm. (× 65,000).

(Reproduced by courtesy of the Editor of the *Journal of Pathology and Bacteriology*.)

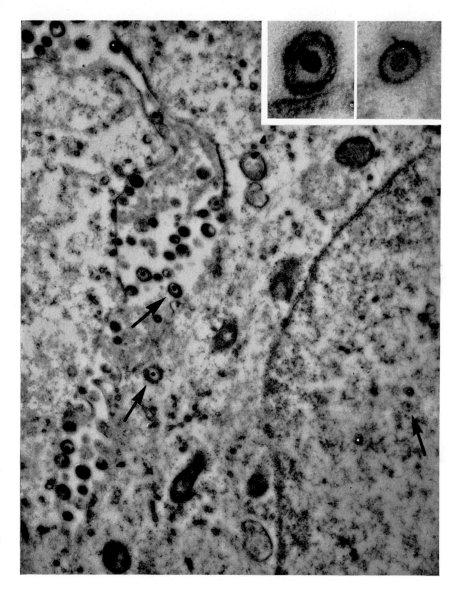

PLATE 3. Electron micrograph of a section of calf-kidney cells inoculated 15 hours previously with the virus of infectious bovine rhinotracheitis, a virus which is closely related to that of *Herpes simplex* (Armstrong, Pereira and Andrewes, 1961). Intranuclear, cytoplasmic and extracellular particles are indicated by arrows ($\times$ 27,000). The inserts ($\times$ 102,000) show higher magnifications of intranuclear (right) and extracellular (left) particles. Note the difference in the virus "membrane".

(Reproduced by courtesy of Dr. J. A. Armstrong and Dr. R. C. Valentine.)

(1956), using stained cells, also showed that the cytopathic effect and virus release occurred almost simultaneously. However, other workers have shown that virus-infected cells treated with fluorophenylalanine, which prevents virus maturation, show a cytopathic effect like that of untreated cells (Ackermann *et al.*, 1954), and cells treated with proflavine degenerate and produce viral antigens but no infectious virus (Ledinko, 1958). There may also be at least one strain of poliovirus which, during its replication, produces a toxic substance capable of inducing morphological changes without cell infection (Ackermann, Rabson and Kurtz, 1958). On the other hand, some attenuated strains of poliovirus multiply in tissue culture without causing obvious cytopathic effects. All this suggests that the maturation of particles, virus release and cytopathic effect may be due to distinct and separable processes, although they normally occur close together in space and time. This view is supported by the findings of Dunnebacke and Mattern (1961) working with amnion cells. They found that virus release and cytopathic effect occurred almost simultaneously in cells infected with poliovirus, but a similar cytopathic effect occurred in cells infected with Coxsackie A10 only hours after virus release was over. Foot-and-mouth-disease virus, which behaves in many ways like enteroviruses is, in one system, released from cells after they have become rounded up (Ribelin, 1958).

Morphological studies show that virus antigen can be detected in the cytoplasm in small areas staining darkly with Giemsa (Buckley, 1956). The failure to detect polio and enteroviruses at the cell surface by haemadsorption methods suggests that the virus is rapidly transferred from below the cell membrane to the medium. By electron microscopy Horne and Nagington (1959) found particles contained in bag-like structures when they disrupted infected cells and stained them by the "negative-contrast" method. Crystalline arrays of virus particles have been detected in the cytoplasm of FL and other cells infected with various enteroviruses, such as Coxsackie B5, ECHO 9 and an unknown ECHO virus (Fogh and Stuart, 1959; Morgan, Howe and Rose, 1959a; Stuart, Fogh and Plager, 1960). Coxsackie 5 virus has also been found in rosettes quite separate from the vesicles of the cytoplasm. It therefore seems certain that viruses of this group mature in the cytoplasm as particles arranged in a variety of ways. Rifkind *et al.* (1961) have evidence that ECHO 9 virus is released through minute breaks in the cell membrane, but particles may also be found in vesicles within the cytoplasm. It has been reported that porcine enterovirus particles may be found within the intracellular canalicular system (Bjorkman and Sibalin, 1960). It may be concluded that, although the exact way by which poliovirus and enteroviruses escape from the cytoplasm is unknown, there is probably a specific mechanism in addition to cell disruption.

The EMC (encephalomyocarditis) group of viruses seems to be related to the enteroviruses and the general pattern of multiplication is very similar. Sanders (1957) and Martin *et al.* (1961) have carried out growth-curve studies of EMC in ascites-tumour cells. These show most of the virus to be released shortly after synthesis, although release times have not been calculated. The virus particles are apparently assembled in the cytoplasm, since haemagglutinin and infectivity are found in the cytoplasmic-cell fractions of ascites-tumour cells producing the virus and virus-like particles can be seen on electron microscopy scattered through the cytoplasm of infected cells. Single-cell studies have not been performed, but the cytopathic effect appears at about the time that virus is released.

Some viruses isolated from common colds in man, and named rhinoviruses (Andrewes *et al.*, 1961) have affinities in their size and general behaviour with the enteroviruses. However, they are fastidious in their requirements, needing for growth a temperature about 33°, a pH close to 7 and a continuously rolled culture (Tyrrell and Parsons, 1960). Even in optimal conditions almost 50% of virus may be found in the cell phase, and the formation of microplaques is only slightly affected by immune serum in the medium. Recent preliminary experiments (Hucker and Tyrrell, 1962) on the growth of strain H.G.P. in tissue culture indicate that although all these requirements are important they each affect different phases of the growth cycle. Thus, virus is formed in the cells rolled at 30°C but is not released into the medium, while little infectious virus is formed in cells rolled at 36°C, though virus is rapidly released into the medium. Adverse pH and stationary conditions do not exert their effects primarily on virus release. It therefore seems that in this system virus release is not complete and is readily inhibited by low temperature, and that cell-to-cell transfer may occur under conditions in which optimal growth occurs in tissue cultures.

3. Arbor viruses

A very large number of Arbor viruses is now known. They fall into several groups and it is by no means certain that they all have the same method of multiplication and release. Their behaviour in tissue cultures varies; in some systems virus may reproduce without any cytopathic effect, while in others rapid and complete destruction occurs. Detailed studies have been performed by Dulbecco and Vogt (1954b) on western equine encephalomyelitis virus (WEE). This Arbor virus belongs to group A, multiplies rapidly in many host species and causes severe cytopathic effects in cultures of chick-embryo tissue. Cell suspensions were made by dispersing monolayers with trypsin. After being infected the cells were washed and resuspended in saline. The suspension was divided into aliquots in test tubes. These aliquots were titrated individually after various periods of incubation; the method used for virus assay was by the formation of plaques in chick-embryo cells under agar. The results indicated that new infectious virus appeared in the cells after $2\frac{1}{2}$ or $3\frac{1}{2}$ hours, depending on the multiplicity of infection. There was a typical logarithmic incremental phase to the growth curve, which then flattened out. When single cells were studied it was found that there was a large variation in the time at which individual cells started to release virus. The first cells to yield virus did so by three hours, and by seven hours all cells began to produce virus. Each cell apparently released virus over a period of time, rather than in a sudden "burst", as in the case of phage particles being released by lysis of the host bacteria. However, if one compares the periods during which infectious virus particles are formed, the two systems are not as dissimilar as seems at first sight. In the case of the bacteriophage this lasts for several minutes, a fairly large proportion of the total length of the growth cycle, and is suddenly terminated by the complete disruption of the cell and the release of the phage particles. Release of the WEE virus commences shortly after the virus is synthesized, and is a more gradual process which does not lead to the immediate disruption of the host cell and the termination of all synthetic processes. In the case of WEE growing in chick-embryo-tissue cultures, the cell is destroyed, but in the case of other related viruses the cell is preserved intact and virus synthesis and release can continue for much longer.

Detailed fluorescent-antibody studies have not been made with these viruses, but antigen is demonstrable in the cytoplasm. If appropriate cells and buffers are used, haemadsorption can be detected with culture cells infected with several Arbor viruses (Buckley, 1959). This implies that the virus haemagglutinin is present at the surface of the cell. As some Arbor virus haemagglutinins are definitely associated with virus particles (Cheng, 1961), we can conclude that virus particles probably spend some time at the surface of the cell during the process of release. Recently, very interesting electron micrographs of cells producing WEE have been published (Morgan, Howe and Rose, 1961). These show groups of virus profiles 22 mμ in diameter around vesicular spaces in the cytoplasm. Larger mature particles are present within the spaces and it is possible that these are in process of passing down the canaliculi to the cell surface. Earlier photomicrographs had failed to detect virus particles inside the cell but did show numbers of virus particles just outside the surface of disintegrating cells. It is therefore probable that this virus can escape across an apparently intact cell surface and also through the disintegration of the cell.

C. Viruses Maturing at the Cell Surface

1. The influenza-virus group

Influenza viruses were the first animal viruses in which the replication processes were studied in detail, and the mechanism of release of viruses in this group is better understood than is that of any other group. Growth curves of influenza viruses have been fully reviewed elsewhere (Henle, 1953), but a few relevant points should be reiterated.
(a) *Growth-curve studies*. The growth curves of influenza A and B in the chick-embryo allantois are affected significantly by the doses of virus inoculated. With small doses most or all of the virus particles formed are infectious, but with large doses incomplete virus may also be produced which is non-infectious though haemagglutinating. Both complete and incomplete virus are released from the cells and can be found in the medium. When "unsuitable" cells are used, such as L or HeLa cells, a non-infectious virus is formed which is not released. Also, if non-neurotropic strains of virus are inoculated into mouse brain, spread of virus from the cells primarily infected does not occur, probably because newly formed virus is not released.

When diluted normal or "standard passage" virus is inoculated into the allantoic cavity of the embryonated egg, soluble (S) complement-fixing antigen is the first virus component to be detected. This antigen is viral ribonucleoprotein. Shortly after this, virus haemagglutinin appears and also new infectious virus. It may be difficult to determine exactly when the first haemagglutinin is formed, because both cells and allantoic fluid contain non-specific inhibitors of haemagglutination, which are probably mainly mucoproteins. These inhibitors, however, are destroyed by the enzyme neuraminidase, so in order to detect haemagglutinin production as early as possible it is usual to treat cell extracts and allantoic fluids with bacterial neuraminidase (or receptor-destroying enzyme) before testing with red cells. The haemagglutination test itself is relatively insensitive; one haemagglutinating unit corresponds to about 10^7 morphological particles of virus. Because of these factors it is difficult when evaluating growth curves to decide whether haemagglutinin, S antigen and infectivity are being formed and released in comparable amounts.

The concentrations of HA and of infectivity rise rapidly and almost concurrently in the cells and in the medium. Shortly after virus release has commenced, the amount of virus outside the cell is much greater than it is in the cell. The release time has been estimated by Cairns and Mason (1953). They titrated the concentration of haemagglutinating virus in membranes, some of which were treated with RDE to remove loosely adsorbed virus; they also measured the amount of virus released into the fluid in each half-hour period. From their results they concluded that virus normally spent about an hour at the surface of cells before being released but that if the cells were treated with RDE the time was reduced to minutes. This implied that in the presence of RDE a virus particle was released from the cell almost as soon as it was completed. About 10% of the virus produced remained in the cells and could not be released by RDE.

Rubin et al. (1957) studied the growth of another myxovirus, Newcastle-disease virus (NDV) in chick-embryo-tissue cultures. They measured the concentration of virus in the cells and in the fluid as in a normal growth curve. For several hours the concentration of intracellular and extracellular virus gave parallel straight lines when plotted logarithmically, and over this period it was possible to determine the mean time between the formation and release of a virus particle. In their system the time was some hours.

(b) *The composition of influenza-virus particles.* Influenza virus can be highly purified by techniques of adsorption and elution, using either red cells or columns of materials such as calcium phosphate. In such purified virus which has been grown in embryonated eggs, much of the protein is very similar to the membrane protein of the chick-embryo cells (Hoyle and Davies, 1961). Similarly, the lipid composition of virus produced in chick cells or in calf cells closely resembles the lipid of the cells in which it was grown (Frommhagen, Freeman and Knight, 1958, Kates et al., 1961). Furthermore, by complement-fixation tests it appears that purified virus contains antigens, probably of the Forssman type, similar to those found in the host cells (Smith, Belyavin and Sheffield, 1955).

Negative-contrast electron micrographs of the virus surface show that it contains a membrane, much like the normal cell membrane, through which project "spikes", which have been interpreted as representing the viral haemagglutinin (Hoyle, Horne and Waterson, 1961). It is therefore necessary that any description of the release of the virus include an explanation of how a substantial part of the virus particle comes to be formed of cell protein and lipid.

(c) *Cytological studies.* Cells infected with myxoviruses may or may not become degenerate after infection, depending on the strain of virus and the cells used. Examination of chorioallantoic membranes and tissue cultures in the fresh and stained state indicate that cells can produce virus and remain grossly normal (Negroni and Tyrrell, 1959).

Studies in chick-embryo-tissue cultures infected with fowl plague (Breitenfeld and Schäfer, 1957) and in the mouse lung infected with swine influenza virus (Hers *et al.*, 1962) have shown that the V antigen (haemagglutinin) is detected first in the central cytoplasm and later is found nearer the cell surface. The S antigen can be detected first in the nucleus before V antigen appears; it later enters the cytoplasm. The haemagglutinin demonstrable in cytoplasmic fractions seems to be associated with ribosomes (Schäfer, 1959). Hoyle (1954) observed filamentous structures being released from infected cells, although something rather similar could also be seen in uninfected cells in the system he used. He thought some of these structures broke up into spheres. In electron micrographs of thin sections virus particles can be detected only at the very surface of the cytoplasm (Morgan, Rose and Moore, 1956). There they are seen in two main forms, both originating as projections of the surface of the cell and distinct from the normal microvilli found there. The virus protusion may become "pinched off" into short spherical objects or as larger rod-like segments which are found in infected allantoic fluid as filaments. Recently, faint outlines of small objects about the size of a virus particle have been seen in the cytoplasm under the surface at which virus release is taking place, and these outlines may represent the assembly of virus precursors or components (Niven *et al.*, 1962). (Plate 2).

By combining haemadsorption and electron microscopy, Hotchin *et al.* (1958) have shown that the red cells are closely applied to the surfaces of cells which do not show the appearance of virus particles in the process of formation. Although this appearance might be due to the red cell being "tied down" to the cell at points where particles are being formed out of the plane of section, the authors conclude that the appearances are best explained by a transformation of the surface of the cells into virus haemagglutinin.

All these facts, combined with the evidence given above on the structure and composition of the particles, lead to the conclusion that when influenza-virus particles are maturing haemagglutinin becomes embedded in the cell membrane and this modified membrane then forms the outer coat of the fresh virus particle. Now, virus neuraminidase is closely associated with haemagglutinin and it is therefore probable that the virus enzyme is concerned in dissolving the last connections between the haemagglutinin and the mucoprotein receptors coating the surface of the cell.

(*d*) *Single-cell studies.* Isolated-cell studies with influenza virus have not been made, but attempts to discover how single cells behave have been reported. By using fluorescent-antibody staining, or by haemadsorption, the cells of a culture can be seen to produce antigen and to yield virus at different times; it is, therefore, probably true that during the incremental phase of the multiplication and release of this virus there is, in most systems, asynchrony of the infectious process. With fluorescent antibody it can be shown that chick-embryo fibroblasts can be infected simultaneously by using a large inoculum of fowl-plague virus (Breitenfeld and Schäfer, 1957). Another approach has been to sample repeatedly eggs infected with a single infectious dose in order to get an idea of the time course of the initial phase of the yield of a single cell. The incremental phase commenced at very different times in different eggs, but Cairns (1957) concluded that this was due to differences in the times at which effective unions of cell and virus occurred rather than to different rates of the replication process subsequent to cell infection.

In the case of virus release from a system such as this, it is interesting to conjecture what stops virus being released. It cannot be, as in the case of, say, poliovirus, that no more cells remain to yield virus, for there may be little or no cytopathic effect. If there were a block in the release mechanism this would lead to accumulation of virus in the cells while the concentration outside the cells remained static, and this is not found. Instead it seems that the synthesis of virus is inhibited, probably by the formation of an interfering substance, such as interferon.

(e) *An attempt to interpret the data.* It is now possible to bring together the available data in order to build a hypothesis about the details of the release of the myxoviruses from the cell. The inner helical RNA component of the virus is completed in the nucleus of the cell, migrates to the cytoplasm and passes towards the cell surface. At about this time the haemagglutinin, which seems to be synthesized in association with the microsomal elements, is transported towards the cell surface. There it is incorporated into the surface of the cytoplasm, which forms the cell membrane. These processes modify the behaviour of the cell surface, perhaps by altering the enzyme activity of the underlying cytoplasm, or the charge density or structure of the surface. The underlying viral RNA may be carried into the protrusions passively or may in fact control the "nipping off" by which the protrusions are converted into filaments or spheres. The particles naturally tend to attach themselves to adjacent unmodified cell surface or overlying mucoprotein but can release themselves from these by the activity of the neuraminidase enzyme groups, protruding, with the haemagglutinin, from the outside of the particles. Although speculative, this hypothesis does suggest a function for the viral neuraminidase.

It was mentioned earlier that "incomplete" virus or non-infectious haemagglutinin is not released from "unsuitable" cells, such as L cells, in which it develops, although incomplete virus produced by overdose of chick-embryo cells is released. This difference probably shows that the processes of virus maturation and release are more severely disorganized in the first case than in the second. Incomplete virus produced by the use of undiluted passage virus is deficient in S antigen and pleomorphic when released from the cell. However, when fowl plague virus is inoculated into L cells the S antigen remains within the nucleus (Franklin and Breitenfeld, 1959) and virus haemagglutinin is found associated with small particles, possibly microsomes. It is possible that in this case the RNA has failed to perform some important organizing function in the cytoplasm, or that the haemagglutinin is not transported to or incorporated in the cell membrane.

Certain myxoviruses, for instance NDV and fowl plague, are very cytopathic, and although virus release may begin by a mechanism such as that described above it is probable that when cells disintegrate viral components will be released directly from deeper parts of the cytoplasm. Without single-cell studies it is not possible to be sure whether virus release can continue after the occurrence of a marked cytopathic effect. The general impression obtained by examining mass cultures is that virus release is declining when cytopathic effects are developing. Morgan et al. (1961) have seen appearances which suggest that influenza-virus filaments and particles form at the membrane lining vacuoles in the cytoplasm. These might well be infectious but, apart from them, virus shed from the cytoplasm directly as a result of cell disintegration is likely to be imperfect and non-infectious.

2. Parainfluenza viruses

It has been found recently that a number of myxoviruses, such as mumps and parainfluenza virus, types 1, 2 and 3, produce giant cells or syncytia in tissue cultures. Types 1 and 3 do this in continuous cell lines but not in primary cultures of kidney cells, and type 2 does so in all cells. The phenomena found with parainfluenza 3 virus growing in KB and FL cells have been studied in some detail by cytological and other methods (Lépine et al., 1959; Deibel and Hotchin, 1961). It seems that infected cells engulf the adjacent normal cells. The infected cell may start to fuse with other cells, although it is not showing haemadsorption and may not contain new infectious virus. Later on, haemadsorption may be detected and infectious virus appears. The adjacent cell seems to play a passive role even when it is infected with another virus. It is believed therefore that the virus can induce some change in the way the cell surface reacts with surrounding cells. It is interesting that a change in cell surface reactions is also believed to play a fundamental part in the conversion of a normal cell to a malignant cell, and this might be a mechanism by which certain viruses induce a malignant transformation. This engulfing process leads to the infection of more and more cells without true virus release. As the process is initiated before virus is completed it has been suggested that it may be due to a substance, other than virus, called syncytin (Chany and Cook, 1960); the evidence for the existence of such a substance is not strong. In studies on similar syncytia induced in other cells by certain strains of Sendai virus, other workers (Bukrinskaya and Zhdanov, 1961) have suggested that the effect is due to a virus enzyme, possibly related to the haemolysin. In certain of the systems in which giant-cell formation occurs, virus is not freely released into the medium (Marston and Vaughan, 1960; Deibel and Hotchin, 1961), although older syncytia haemadsorb. Possibly virus particles are not formed properly—after all, in cells of this type influenza virus fails to form particles at all. The reported data are difficult to evaluate, and we need a really exhaustive study of the growth and release of one virus both in circumstances in which syncytia are formed and when they are not.

Parainfluenza 3 virus may persist in carrier cultures of KB for a long time without obvious cytopathic effect. It may not be eliminated by the action of antibody, and this suggests that the virus can reach an infectious form and be transferred to other cells without entering the medium or alternatively that virus may survive inside an intact cell for some weeks. There is still a great deal to be learned about this system, and a thorough electron-microscopic study of infected cultures of various sorts would be of great interest. When the parainfluenza viruses grow in monkey-kidney cells, virus is shed freely into the medium in a way reminiscent of the production of influenza virus in the chick embryo.

D. CERTAIN TUMOUR VIRUSES

Tumour viruses are probably released according to a variety of patterns and mechanisms—just as are the viruses of acute infectious diseases which we have considered so far, but only a few of them have been studied in isolated systems such as tissue cultures. Further, it is probable that in tissue cultures they reproduce in a manner which is different in many important respects from that in which they reproduce in the intact host, either within tumour cells or in the stages prior to frank tumour formation. Nevertheless, the precision of the results obtained in isolated systems makes them worth close attention.

1. Rous-sarcoma virus (RSV)

Temin and Rubin have recently made a series of studies of the Rous-sarcoma virus in which they have developed plaque techniques for assaying virus and infective centres, and have also used fluorescent antibody to study the morphological aspects of virus release. The virus produces foci of hyperplastic cells in chick-embryo cell cultures. It seems from these results that, shortly after inoculation, virus is released from cells into the medium at the rate of about one PFU per cell every 5–10 hours over a long period of time. In the absence of an overlay such virus can infect further cells. However, infected cells are also formed by another mechanism, that is by the continued division of cells (Temin and Rubin, 1959). With fluorescent-antibody staining, the virus antigen is seen in the superficial layers of the cytoplasm shortly after infection. These layers seem to become detached but antigen is later found in the deeper parts of the cell. Since antibody forms in some tumour-bearing birds it is probable that virus release also occurs in the intact animal, but it is not known whether it is by the shedding of superficial layers of cytoplasm or by the disintegration of transformed and sarcomatous cells. No electron micrographs have yet been published which show any details of the process of release of virus from the surface of tissue-culture cells, but it is unlikely that it falls outside the range of phenomena which have been observed among the viruses mentioned above.

2. Avian myeloblastosis

Another neoplasm of poultry, avian myeloblastosis, is also caused by a virus which resembles Rous-sarcoma virus in some respects. The properties of the virus have been thoroughly studied by Beard and co-workers. They found large amounts of virus in the blood plasma of infected birds. Recently they have studied tissue cultures of infected monocytes and have shown that the virus particles (and the characteristic ATP-ase enzyme associated with them) are released in large numbers by cells which remain intact and morphologically unchanged (Beaudreau et al., 1958). One thousand five hundred particles per cell may be shed into the medium every 48 hours for periods as long as six months. It is probable that a similar process is occurring in the intact animal. It is, however, difficult to find virus particles in, or on the surface of, cells; they do not seem to accumulate within the cell and there is no clear indication of how they leave the cells (Parsons et al., 1958). They may leave the cells by a "budding" process resembling that of influenza. There is, however, quite enough evidence to indicate that in this system at any rate the process of virus release is quite different from that observed in the tumour virus mentioned below.

3. Polyoma

The polyoma virus causes marked cytopathic effects in mouse-embryo-tissue cultures (Stewart, Eddy and Borghesse, 1958). Antigen and virus particles are found in the nucleus and also in the cytoplasm. The disintegration of cells might explain how the virus gets into the medium; really detailed studies, designed to show whether virus can be released from intact cells would be interesting but have not yet been reported. Virus particles, with an extra membrane like those seen in Herpes virus, are found in the cytoplasm of cells from infected-tissue cultures and may represent virus in transit to the cell surface; such particles were not, however, found in the cells of cultures which were treated with antiserum after virus infection had been initiated. It is possible, therefore, that they represent a readsorption of virus from the medium, rather than newly formed virus in transit to the cell surface (Dourmashkin and Negroni, 1960).

IV. Some Aspects of Virus Release

A. The Relation between Cytopathic Effect and Virus Release

It is very tempting to conclude, on observing marked morphological changes in a cell culture, that the virus which caused them is being released by this means; from what has been said already, it is clear that this is not always the case. Viruses such as parainfluenza 1 growing in monkey-kidney cells may be released from cells which are in no way degenerate, and so also may Arbor viruses, avian myeloblastosis, and others. During the multiplication of adenoviruses the degeneration of the cell follows the gross disorganization of the nucleus as this is replaced with masses of virus particles and antigen; virus release then ensues. In between these two extremes it seems often to be the case that cell degeneration is a separate or co-incidental phenomenon. It may be the consequence of changes in the enzyme activity of the cell cytoplasm, or a disturbance of the cell membrane as the virus passes through it. In other cases it may be due to a non-particulate toxin produced by the virus, or to an incomplete cycle of virus multiplication in which no virus is completed or shed. These cytopathic mechanisms do not necessarily contribute to virus release. Klemperer (1960) has recently found that contact of a red cell with mumps virus leads to a rapid loss of potassium with swelling of the cell and loss of haemoglobin and intracellular proteins. Such a phenomenon might occur in cultures or tissue cells infected with this virus, but it might be due to virus adsorbing onto the cells rather than being released from within them.

B. The Transport of Virus Components and Particles

1. Passage through intact cell surfaces

The sum of evidence suggests, as we have mentioned above, that enteroviruses and WEE may be formed in the cytoplasm and be released before any obvious cell damage occurs and without any evidence of the formation of villous projections. There is also suggestive evidence that such viruses, and also others such as herpes simplex, appear in the lumen of the endoplasmic reticulum of the cytoplasm. This reticulum is widely believed to be a canalicular system and elements contained within it near the cell surface may, from time to time, be connected with or become continuous with the cell surface. This might be either a normal cell process or an abnormality induced by the presence of a foreign particle in the cell. In either case one can envisage the virus being brought to the surface and pushed out as the surface of the cell swells and churns and folds.

It has now been shown that, in systems in which there is no gross cytopathic effect, the cell may nevertheless be abnormally permeable during the time when virus release occurs. For example, chick allantoic cells which are producing PR8 virus release lactic dehydrogenase into the medium (Kelly and Grieff, 1961). To some extent the barrier between the cell and medium has broken down, although the membrane seems to be little affected morphologically. Physiological and chemical studies of such phenomena might help us to understand better how some viruses leak into the surrounding medium, as well as how cells degenerate.

2. Intracellular transport

The matter of the transport of virus particles across cell membranes is really a part of a larger problem. How do the virus constituents or the completed particles move about the cell? Cinemicrophotography shows that cell constituents are normally in constant and extensive motion. Adenovirus particles are formed in the nucleus and remain there; yet herpes virus particles which are largely formed in the same area seem to travel across the cell. Are they, because of their structure, able to utilize some cell mechanism intended for a normal component? Are they being treated as though they were a cell secretion? Because they can be recognized morphologically and in other ways, virus particles may be valuable in helping to unravel some of these problems closely related to normal cell behaviour, just as the study of the genetic mechanisms of normal bacterial cells has been helped by studying those of cells invaded by viruses. For the moment, however, the most profitable approach may be to correlate what is known of the mechanisms of secretion and phagocytosis in order to see how they may be involved in the transport of a parasite such as a virus. There is suggestive evidence that cells at different phases of the mitotic cycle handle herpes virus in different ways (Roizman, 1961), and this probably reflects changes in the physiology of the cytoplasm or nucleus.

C. The Mechanism of Cell-to-cell Transfer of Virus

Much work remains to be done on the spread of infection directly from cell to cell either with or without the formation of the syncytia which are often seen in such cases. In some tissue cultures cell bridges exist, so that the cytoplasm of adjacent cells is really continuous. Therefore virus particles might move from one cell to another without really crossing a membrane or entering the surrounding media. By phase-contrast microscopy Falk and Richter (1961) have demonstrated particles crossing intercellular bridges in cultures in which herpes giant cells develop. However, in many cases the cell boundaries seem to dissolve or disappear so that some profound change must have taken place in the properties of the membrane. In the case of myxoviruses this could be due to the action of an enzyme associated with the insertion of viral elements into the structure of the cell surface; alternatively there may be interference within the nucleus with the direction or control of cytoplasmic activity.

We do not know in what form virus passes from cell to cell. Virus protein may be detected as specific antigen in both receptor and donor cells, but it is possible that infectivity is transferred as viral nucleic acid without the protein coat which it would need to survive outside the cell. Cell-to-cell transfer, possibly by infectious nucleic acid, could account for the survival of virus in chronically infected cultures and also for the fact that such cultures cannot be "cured" by treatment with antibody even though the virus is thought, under other circumstances, to mature at the cell surface.

D. Mechanisms of Virus Release and Virus Classification

A proper basis for virus classification is the structure and composition of the virus particles. The types of tissue in which viruses grow and the sort of diseases which they cause are very unsatisfactory for this purpose. On the other hand, the essential mechanisms by which viruses reproduce and release themselves from the cells may be more closely related to their fundamental make-up than their host ranges and therefore may be of value in understanding the family relationship between viruses. It has been suggested that all viruses which are ether-sensitive are also released continuously from the cell surface. The lipid component is probably of cellular origin, possibly derived from a membrane. This suggestion seems reasonable, but it would be helpful if we knew more of the details of the release of a variety of ether-sensitive Arbor viruses and whether this is really basically different from the mechanism used by, say, enteroviruses.

It has been noted that adenoviruses are scarcely released at all prior to complete cell disintegration, that chickenpox and herpes viruses tend to spread by direct cell-to-cell transfer, that poliovirus and the EMC viruses seem to be released in the same sort of way, and that the influenza viruses all seem to be completed and rapidly released at the cell surface. These similarities and dissimilarities are in agreement with current views on virus classification. However, the fact that there are inconsistencies within the groups should also be kept in mind; for example there are sublines of herpes simplex virus which do, or do not, transfer infection from cell to cell under an overlay containing antibody. Because most of the relevant information has been obtained by growing the viruses in cells quite different from those in which they grow in nature, it is possible that some of these apparent inconsistencies have been forced on them by a strange environment.

E. Cellular Release and Phenomena seen in the Whole Animal

The mechanisms of cell release must have a good deal to do with the behaviour of a virus in the intact animal and the pathogenesis of any disease which it may cause. For instance, the process of cell-to-cell transfer may enable a virus to spread in the presence of antibody and perhaps to persist in the body for many years after an acute infection. This might be the case with herpes simplex and zoster. If a virus tends to be retained within a cell it may persist in the body and be shed in infectious form, in spite of circulating antibody, because it is "wrapped up" in a necrotic cell; this may apply to the adenoviruses, particularly types 1, 2 and 5. A virus which matures at the cell surface will always be accessible to antibody in its mature form and might therefore be completely eliminated from the body when antibody appears, and this seems to be the usual story in the case of non-fatal infections with myxoviruses. Perhaps in some cases a cell containing virus shed from diseased tissue is the true infectious unit by which the virus is transferred from host to host in nature.

We understand too little of the pathogenesis of virus-induced tumours to be able to speculate very profitably about them, but it is clear that in some cases large amounts of virus are shed into the circulation without much cell destruction and in others virus seems to be locked up inside the malignant cells. If virus is released from a cell in such a way that it is completely enfolded in host-cell components then it will be relatively non-antigenic and also insusceptible to neutralization by any antibodies which may have been formed—and these are features of infection with some tumour viruses. In any case the elucidation of the mechanism of virus release is an essential step in acquiring a proper understanding of the disease.

CHAPTER 7

Virus Pathogenicity

J. C. N. WESTWOOD

*Microbiological Research Establishment Experimental Station,
Porton, Wiltshire, England*

I. Introduction

The pathogenicity of a virus is its ability to produce disease. The term in its widest sense must therefore cover all aspects of the host–virus relationship, but the particular facet which will be considered in this chapter is the mechanism by which virus replication produces disease in the host. Other aspects will be touched on only in so far as they clarify the disease picture. It is clear that pathogenicity must be considered at two different levels since, though the host for a virus disease is the intact animal, the host for the virus itself is the individual animal cell, and the disease process is the summation of the cellular effects brought about by virus multiplication and by the action of any toxic products which may be incidentally produced.

In practice this has tended to develop a wide gulf between the work of the virus biologist, who is concerned with the virus as a biological entity, and that of the medical or veterinary virologist, who is concerned with it as a disease-producing entity. To the former the animal host, with its chemical, immunological and physiological responses to infection, is a source of confusion which must be eliminated as far as possible, while to the latter it is the centre of the problem. This dichotomy of interest is an inevitable step in the investigation of virus disease and will necessarily continue until academic biochemical studies at the cellular level have advanced to the stage where the biochemical lesion which results in the injury or death of the infected cell can be stated in clear terms. This stage is still very far off. When it is reached, however, the two branches of virological study should again converge and lead to an understanding of virus disease of the host animal in terms of cellular as well as gross pathology. Until that time the only substantial links between the two lines of study are likely to remain in the strictly practical fields, such as the development of new diagnostic procedures, the production of vaccines and the study of chemo-therapeutic agents.

It is the purpose of this chapter to examine the disease process both at the cellular level and at the level of the intact animal, and to try to trace a connection between the two. It may be thought that the task is doomed to failure from the outset, and, indeed, Cohen (1959b) has stated that "until the biochemical behaviour of the infected animal cell, the unit of viral disease, is clarified it does not appear fruitful to consider in detail the problem of the biochemical pathogenesis of viral disease in an intact multicellular organism. Indeed questions relating to this problem have not yet been posed in suitable forms". One could go further and assert that the biochemical behaviour of the infected cell cannot be clarified until that of the normal cell is understood. Nevertheless, there are some indications that this despondent attitude may not be altogether justified. It is at least possible that examination of the problem might serve to indicate lines of investigation which could be followed even with the knowledge and techniques now available.

When virus infections are viewed as a whole it is evident that the disease picture is a blend of two different factors, the first of which is attributable to the focal effects of the virus and the second to its general or constitutional effects. The signs and symptoms due to focal effects are the direct result of the destruction of particular types of cell or of virus attack on particular tissues or organs in the body. The pre-eminent example is provided by poliomyelitis, in which constitutional symptoms are trivial by comparison with the results of destruction of motor neurones, but in other diseases also the focal effects may be conspicuous or even dominant. Apart from such diseases as trachoma and lymphogranuloma inguinale in which local disease is produced as a result of the very limited distribution of the virus, these diseases are almost exclusively infections of the central nervous system—rabies and the virus encephalitides. But among the severe non-neutotropic infections yellow fever presents a picture which may be dominated by the focal effects of massive necrosis of liver tissue, and likewise the cyanosis and cardiac failure of fulminant influenzal pneumonia may be ascribed to the gross pulmonary oedema characteristic of this condition. In most virus diseases, however, the clinical picture is dominated by the constitutional disturbance, and death, when this occurs, is not attributable to the effects of virus multiplication in, or destruction of, any particular cell type or tissue.

Thus, there are two separate problems to be discussed, and it is fortunate that diseases representing the two types of effect in almost pure form have been investigated in some detail. For the first aspect, poliomyelitis selects itself as the infection on which most work has been carried out both on the disease itself and on the virus as a biological entity. For the second, the choice is perhaps wider, but it is proposed to examine the pathogenesis of the pox group of infections, since this has been the subject of much recent work.

Although no discussion of pathogenesis in virus infections could be considered complete without some reference to virus-induced neoplasia and synergism, it is not proposed to include these aspects of the subject, since the basis for their discussion in the terms proposed for this chapter is still lacking. In the case of neoplasia the critical change, genetic or cytoplasmic, which confers the property of free multiplication on the cells of a metazoan host is not understood and without this understanding it is not possible to suggest mechanisms by which it might be brought about by virus infection. Similarly, the problem of synergism has not been investigated from the point of view of the mechanism by which a combined infection induces disease differing from those of the individual pathogens involved. Indeed, such an investigation would hardly be possible until the mechanisms of the individual infections are understood.

II. Pathogenesis Dominated by Focal Effects—Poliomyelitis

Poliomyelitis is of much intrinsic interest in relation to the problems of pathogenicity since, although the virus responsible for the disease is one of the most consistently cytopathogenic agents to be cultivated *in vitro*, it is one of the least damaging to the cells of the infected animal host. For a full understanding of this anomaly it is necessary to consider the disease process as a whole, and the present state of knowledge with regard to this process will first be summarized.

A. INFECTION AND INVASION OF THE HOST

Although there is still disagreement as to the route by which the central nervous system is invaded by the virus of poliomyelitis, its sites of multiplication in the body and their sequence of invasion have now been very thoroughly worked out, largely as a result of the studies of Sabin and Bodian and their associates using chimpanzees as the experimental host. The pathogenesis and clinical development of the disease in these animals differs but little from that in man, so the detailed investigations which have been carried out on the progress of virus through their tissues may with some confidence be applied to the human disease.

There are two primary sites of lodgment of the virus following feeding, the oropharynx and the ileum; and of these the ileum is thought to be the more susceptible, since small doses of the virus tend to cause primary ileal infection without infection of the oropharynx. Bodian is of the opinion that the tissue of lodgment in which the first multiplication occurs is the lymphoid tissue in close apposition to the gut lumen—the Peyer's patches of the ileum and the tonsillar and associated lymphoid tissue of the oropharynx. He has demonstrated virus in the Peyer's patches in high titre when virus was not detectable in the gut wall after removal of these structures. Sabin, on the other hand, produces evidence that strains of virus which are incapable of multiplication in lymphoid tissue will still become established in the ileum and that secondary invasion of the oropharynx may occur and progress even after the appearance of neutralizing antibody which is known to prevent multiplication in lymphoid tissue. He considers that virus establishment and multiplication take place in the superficial mucosa lining these two regions of the gut and that the finding of virus in the regional lymph nodes, which occurs even with strains incapable of multiplying in lymphoid tissue, is due to drainage of virus from the gut mucosa. Despite this dispute as to the ability of virus to multiply in the lymphatic tissue, both workers are agreed that virus passes from the gut to the regional lymph nodes and thereafter rapidly invades the blood-stream. Viraemic spread is responsible for the invasion of the secondary sites of virus multiplication in the systemic lymph nodes and the suprasternal, axillary and paravertebral depots of brown fat. In these the virus may reach concentrations of 10^4–10^5 monkey infectious doses per gram of tissue, the tissues forming a dangerous source of virus, maintaining the viraemia and increasing the danger of invasion of the central nervous system. Of the extraneural tissues, the lymphoid tissue and brown fat constitute the principal sites of virus multiplication and are probably involved to a greater or lesser extent in all cases of infection. The third site, namely the central nervous system, is involved only in a minority of cases.

The route by which the central nervous system is invaded is again the subject of controversy. Bodian and his associates consider the blood-stream to be the usual route, while Sabin, Faber and others produce evidence that the virus reaches the brain or cord by neural spread via the regional ganglia. The alternative views and the reasons for them are clearly set out in Sabin (1956) and Bodian (1955, 1959), but recent work (Nathanson and Bodian, 1961) suggests that both routes may be operative, depending on the strain of virus. Once the central nervous system is invaded, however, rapid multiplication of the virus again takes place, peak titres being reached in about three days after its first detection. Although the virus concentration then falls rapidly, low concentrations may persist in surviving animals for several weeks.

B. Cytopathology *IN VIVO*

1. Systemic phase

Although poliomyelitis must be regarded as a primarily systemic extraneural infection with the principal sites of virus multiplication in the gut, lymphoid tissue and brown fat, no histological lesions directly attributable to virus multiplication have ever been reported to occur in these tissues. An immense amount of work on human post-mortem material has been carried out by Faber (1955) and, although he has reported hypertrophic changes in lymph nodes and occasional degenerative lesions elsewhere, he considers these to be secondary in nature and not due to virus replication. Yet the virus titres attained—10^4–10^5 monkey infective doses per gram of tissue— are such that lesions should be detectable, if only in the form of an inflammatory reaction, were virus multiplication accompanied by cell destruction. Taken at face value, therefore, the evidence suggests that the infection is non-cytopathogenic. Yet this stage of the disease is accompanied by sore throat, nausea, headache and fever in most patients. Nonspecific constitutional symptoms of this kind are charac- teristic of the early stages of most systemic infections, be they viral or bacterial, but their causation is unknown. In the case of bacterial infections they are vaguely ascribed to bacterial "toxins" or to reaction to foreign protein, and in viral disease to reaction to tissue breakdown products. In the total absence of cytopathology, however, they are not easy to explain even in such evasive terms.

2. Central-nervous-system involvement

With involvement of the central nervous system the vagueness of both symptomatology and cytopathology vanish. There is no question that the critical cytopathology lies in the destruction of the motor neurones of the anterior horn and bulbar regions of the spinal cord.

The motor neurone is a large pyramidal cell with the motor axon originating from its apex and dendritic processes from its body. It usually possesses a single, round, centrally placed nucleus containing a single strongly basophilic nucleolus surrounded by a fine-mesh chromatin. The cytoplasm contains Golgi apparatus, mitochondria and granular inclusions similar to those of other cells, but it also contains two structures—neurofibrils and Nissl granules—peculiar to cells of the central nervous system. The neurofibrils are fine threads which form an interlacing skein of bundles of parallel fibres throughout the cell body. The fibres pass into the axon and dendrites and extend to the synaptic junctions, at which point they terminate. These fibrils are visible in the living cell and are not, therefore, fixation artefacts. The Nissl granules are the most striking feature of neurones stained with appropriate dyes and may also be seen with phase-contrast microscopy in living cells. They are large, strongly basophilic bodies, of irregular size and shape, distributed throughout the cytoplasm with the exception of the region termed the axon hill, from which the axon itself originates. These granules have been shown to contain ribonucleic acid and protein and are seen by electron microscopy to contain dense concentrations of ribosomal particles. Profound changes may occur in them under various physiological and pathological conditions including poliomyelitis.

It is not known to what extent the various anatomical features of the neurone contribute to its primary function of conducting nervous impulses. The Nissl granules are not thought to be of importance in this respect for a variety of reasons, including their absence from certain neurones, and it is unlikely that the Golgi apparatus, mitochondria and ribosomes play a specialized part. They are probably concerned, as in other cells, with the metabolic activity of the cytoplasm. The one structure known to be directly concerned in the passage of the nervous impulse is the cell membrane, polarization of which provides the basis for the electrical discharge which constitutes the nervous impulse. Whether this discharge also implicates the deeper structures, notably the neurofibrils, is not certain.

It is the neurones which exhibit the first pathological changes following invasion of the cord by poliovirus. Concomitant with the onset of virus multiplication in the spinal cord, a process of dissolution and fragmentation of the Nissl substance sets in. This process of "chromatolysis" continues until the deeply basophilic granules are completely eliminated from the cell and the cytoplasm takes on the appearance of a structureless acidophilic mass. This is the stage described as acidophilic necrosis, and almost certainly represents cell death. In certain cells acidophilic necrosis does not occur, the process of chromatolysis ending instead in a condition of diffuse basophilia affecting both the cytoplasm and the nucleus. Cells undergoing acido-philic necrosis tend to be destroyed by lysis, while those undergoing the basophilic changes become shrunken and deformed and are even-tually removed by phagocytes. At the same time as or shortly after the onset of chromatolysis, changes are seen in the nuclei of affected cells. The fine chromatin network of the nucleus becomes aggregated, the nucleus shrinks, deforms and becomes displaced towards the side of the cell. In some cells eosinophilic intranuclear inclusions develop. The nucleolus does not appear to be affected by the degenerative process and remains clearly distinguishable. The nuclear changes progress further in the cells which become basophilic and do not undergo lysis. Mitochondria and neurofibrils persist apparently unchanged until very late in the chromatolytic process but both ultimately disappear at the stage of acidophilic necrosis. Death of the cell is followed by degenera-tion of the axon in a manner and time sequence similar to that of Wallerian degeneration following nerve section.

The changes taking place in the neurones may be completely unac-companied by any inflammatory changes whatever, and cells in the final stages of acidophilic necrosis may be surrounded by apparently normal tissue. The inflammatory response which is such a conspicuous feature of the later stages of the pathological process follows at an uncertain interval after the onset of neuronal changes and must be considered as a secondary process.

3. Relation of neuronal changes to virus multiplication

Bodian (1948) carried out an extensive analysis of the relationship of the neuronal changes to virus multiplication and to the onset and severity of paralysis. His results show, first, that virus multiplication in the central nervous system coincides accurately with the onset and progress of chromatolysis at a time when this may be the only change detectable in the spinal cord. It may therefore be assumed that the virus in fact multiplies in the neurones and that chromatolysis and cell degeneration are the direct results of virus multiplication. At the same time it must also be accepted that this is an assumption. There is as yet no direct evidence either that the virus does multiply in these cells or that they are exclusively involved. Secondly, statistical analysis showed that function is lost from the cells at the stage of "severe" chromatolysis shortly before they pass into acidophilic necrosis or diffuse basophilia. This stage represents the almost complete destruc-tion of the Nissl substance. Thus, the onset of paralysis depends on two factors: whether a sufficiently large number of neurones is affected to produce clinically observable weakness, and whether the changes in these neurones progress to the critical stage of chromatolysis at which function is lost. Even when this stage is reached the changes are still reversible, and cells which do not then progress to the final stages of degeneration are capable of both functional and morphological recovery. The latter results from the regeneration of Nissl substance in apposition to both the nuclear and cytoplasmic membranes to give rise to the bizarre appearances classed as "central chromatolysis". Morphological recovery is a slower process than functional recovery and takes months to complete.

Two features of outstanding interest in the processes described are, first, the fact that the function of the motor neurone is not lost until a late stage in the pathological changes affecting the cell, and second, that cells in which the virus is presumed to be multiplying are capable of recovery. The evidence on these points is necessarily indirect, and is built up from an extensive series of correlations and the assumption that the virus does in fact multiply in the neurones. Nevertheless, it is strong. The motor neurones alone consistently show pathological changes at the time when the virus is multiplying in the cord. Therefore, either the virus multiplies in these cells or it is non-cytopathogenic even in the central nervous system, in which case the neuronal changes must themselves be a secondary phenomenon due to some toxic reaction to products of cells in which the virus is multiplying without producing demonstrable damage. While this latter possibility cannot be ruled out on the evidence, it seems far less likely than the direct interpretation. The evidence as regards recovery is based on a combination of clinical and pathological observations which are set out in detail in Bodian (1948). Suffice it to say here that Bodian states that in animals infected with "mild" strains of virus and showing minimal limb weakness, over 90% of the motor neurones of the affected segments may show chromatolytic changes and the titres of recoverable virus may be as high as in the cords of severely paralysed animals. These mildly affected animals will show complete clinical recovery, and their cords, examined at various time intervals during convalescence, show neurones first in the stages of central chromatolysis and eventually morphologically normal.

It seems likely, therefore, that *in vivo* the virus is capable of multiplying in neurones without destroying them.

C. CYTOPATHOLOGY IN TISSUE CULTURE

The lack of demonstrable cytopathogenicity of poliovirus for extraneural tissues *in vivo* and the apparent capacity for recovery of infected neurones are in sharp contrast to its uniformly destructive character for those cells in which it will multiply in tissue culture. In fact, cell

destruction *in vitro* is not averted even when full replication is inter-
fered with by virus inhibitors, (Ackermann, Rabson and Kurtz, 1954;
Ledinko, 1958).

From the many detailed studies which have been carried out on the
cytopathological effects of poliovirus in tissue culture it is possible to
construct a reasonably clear picture of the changes brought about in a
variety of cell systems. The course of infection with several strains of
all three types of the virus has been followed in monkey-kidney,
human-adult and human-foetal cells and in serially cultivated cell lines
of human origin. It is agreed by all workers that the course of events is
the same whatever the strain or type of virus used and there is also
little to choose between cell types as regards their response to infection.
The single exception in this respect is the response of cells from the
human amnion as described by Dunnebacke (1956b). In all other cell
types closely similar changes seem to occur and even human-amnion
cells in the hands of Bernkopf and Rosin (1957) gave very similar
results. The following synthesis is derived from the observations of
various workers using both fixed and stained material and also phase-
contrast microscopy of living infected cells.

1. Nuclear changes

Reissig, Howes and Melnick (1956) and Shaver, Barron and Karzon
(1958), using Zenker fixed material stained by a modification of the
haematoxylin and eosin technique, reported that the first detectable
changes in poliovirus-infected cells occurred in the nucleus at four
hours. Reissig *et al.* reported loss of staining of the central nuclear
chromatin as the first change, progressing to complete loss of chromatin
from the central region and its aggregation at the nuclear margin. At
the same time eosinophilic intranuclear inclusions appeared and increased in size as the infection progressed. Shaver *et al.* did not see the
early changes in nuclear chromatin and found that eosinophilic granules
were a feature of the nuclei of normal cells. These granules were,
however, small—less than 1 μ in diameter—and stained palely. Few
normal cells contained granules larger than 1 μ in diameter. The first
change following infection was an increase in the number of cells
containing large intranuclear eosinophilic granules. The increase was
first detectable at four hours and the number of cells showing such
granules increased progressively up to eight hours, at which time
60% were affected. Thereafter the number declined again.

Following these early changes shrinkage of the nucleus, first detectable as a wrinkling of the nuclear membrane (Dunnebacke, 1956a;
Bernkopf and Rosin, 1957), sets in, the nucleus at the same time becoming progressively displaced towards the side of the cell. Shrinkage

of the nucleus continues ultimately to the stage of complete pyknosis and fragmentation.

More recently Mayor (1961), using acridine-orange staining, has reported changes in the distribution of nuclear DNA and increased brilliance of the nucleolar RNA staining as early as three hours after infection and before any other evidence of cytopathology could be detected.

2. Cytoplasmic changes

The most consistent change occurring in the cytoplasm of infected cells is the development of a juxtanuclear cytoplasmic mass which increases progressively in size, displacing and indenting the nucleus and leading ultimately to the division of the cytoplasm into a granular eosinophilic central region surrounded by a clear, basophilic peripheral zone. This cytoplasmic mass was first reported by Barski, Endo and Monaci (1953) in fixed and stained preparations, and its development was later followed by time-lapse cinematography in living cells (Barski, Robinaux and Endo, 1955). These studies were carried out in human tonsillar fibroblasts in which the evolution of the lesion was slowed down by incubation at 30–31°C. Under these conditions the first development of the mass is detectable at 20–24 hours and consists of a cytoplasmic condensation, with reduced Brownian movement, at a point in close relation to the nuclear membrane.

With increase in size of the mass the nucleus becomes indented and displaced towards the side of the cell, while stiffening of the material of the mass itself leads to a complete cessation of Brownian movement. As the mass increases in size the nucleus becomes difficult to discern, so that nuclear changes are not as easily seen as in fixed and stained material. The formation of the division between the centrally placed cytoplasmic mass and the clear peripheral zone is well demonstrated, however, and is accompanied by retraction of cell processes and rounding of the cell. At this stage, vacuolation of the peripheral zone is of frequent occurrence and is followed by "bubbling" of the cytoplasm in a manner similar to that occurring in the final stages of cell division. Lwoff et al. (1955) also found this bubbling to be a regular feature in their studies of living infected cells isolated in individual droplets, bubbling being followed rapidly by shredding of the outer layers of cytoplasm and, eventually, by cell disintegration. The final dynamic events do not form a part of the descriptions based on fixed and stained material, though cytoplasmic protrusions clearly related to the bubbling phenomenon have been described (Dunnebacke, 1956b).

The occurrence of strongly basophilic cytoplasmic granules lying outside the central mass was described by Barski et al. (1953) and later by Ackermann *et al.* (1954) in HeLa cells. They were very conspicuous in the studies of Buckley (1956, 1957). Reissig *et al.* (1956) noted their presence in a small minority of cells, and Shaver *et al.* (1958) estimated that they were present in only about 1·6% of the infected cell population.

As has been stated, the changes appear to be uniform regardless of the virus strain or cell type investigated, with the single exception of the findings of Dunnebacke (1956b) relative to infection of cultures of human-amnion cells. Dunnebacke describes a strikingly different course of events. The development of poliovirus in her cultures was slower than in monkey-kidney cells, and the first observable change in the cell population was a loss of staining ability by the nucleoli and nuclear chromatin. Not until the nucleoli of a cell had completely disappeared did cytoplasmic changes become evident. These observations emphasize the very early involvement of the nucleus in the cytopathology of poliovirus infection, but it is not certain where they stand in relation to the changes observed by others as well as those reported by Dunnebacke herself (1956a) for other cell types. Bernkopf and Rosin (1957) did not observe this very early nucleolar involvement in amnion cells but did confirm the absence of a clearly defined cytoplasmic mass as reported by Dunnebacke (1956b). Its place was occupied by a somewhat ill-defined eosinophilic area not sharply demarcated from the peripheral basophilic zone. Their description suggests a quantitative rather than a qualitative difference in response, and they suggest that differences in cultural technique might underlie the discrepancies reported.

The time relationships of the cytopathic changes to virus production are fairly clear despite some variation in the reported sequence of events, and are of particular interest in relation to the site of virus replication discussed below. The earliest detectable changes occur in the nucleus, three or four hours after infection, at a time which corresponds closely with the end of the eclipse phase and the first emergence of new infective virus within the cells. According to Reissig *et al.* (1956) the nuclear changes may just precede the first detectable increase in infective virus, and Mayor's results also suggest that this is so (Mayor, 1961). Release of virus from the cell has been clearly correlated by Lwoff *et al.* (1955) with the stage of cytoplasmic shredding which immediately follows cell bubbling. It would appear, therefore, that almost the whole sequence of cytopathic change up to the time of cellular disintegration occurs during the time when virus is being assembled and released. The period of the eclipse phase, during which the major part of the synthesis of virus material occurs, is not associated with any changes in the morphology and behaviour of the cells except possibly some ambiguous changes in the nuclear DNA.

3. Location of virus synthesis

Schwerdt and Pardee (1952) found that four fifths of the virus present in the central nervous system of infected cotton rats was located in the microsomal fraction of the disrupted cells, and Kaplan and Melnick (1953) found virus earlier in the "cytoplasmic" than in the "nuclear" fraction of infected mouse brains. They were able, however, to release as high concentrations from the washed "nuclear" fraction as from the "cytoplasmic" fraction during the later stages of infection. Mass fractionation procedures applied to infected brain tissue in which the majority of the cells are in any case not infected might be expected to yield somewhat inconclusive results, but it is surprising that even the large volume of work performed in tissue culture has not greatly improved our knowledge of the intracellular localization of poliovirus synthetic activity. Although there is a wealth of information on the intracellular localization of many other viruses, reports on poliovirus are extremely few.

The earlier histochemical studies are almost uniformly negative in this context. The eosinophilic intranuclear inclusions appearing in infected cells *in vivo* and *in vitro* naturally aroused interest, but the presence of similarly staining granules in normal cells, and the facts that they have been consistently found to be Feulgen-negative and that Shaver *et al.* (1958) also found them to be negative for RNA glycogen and lipid have left both their nature and significance a mystery. Since, however, the peak in the frequency of their incidence lies at eight hours after infection, when virus replication is complete, they are unlikely to be directly associated with the virus and are probably a secondary response of the nucleus to infection.

The nature of the cytoplasmic mass has also been somewhat inconclusively investigated. It is Feulgen-negative and contains a variable amount of glycogen and fat. Harding *et al.* (1956), using decreased basophilia after ribonuclease treatment as their criterion, reported that, though the mass itself might contain a little RNA, there was a marked increase in RNA in the surrounding clear basophilic zone. This finding suggests that the virus may be peripherally situated and is therefore in line with observations on the release of virus by shredding of the outer cytoplasmic zone and with the observations of Buckley (1957) that this zone was more strongly fluorescent than the cytoplasmic mass following fluorescent-antibody treatment. Mayor (1961) showed that at the time of virus release the cytoplasm was heavily loaded with both RNA and virus antigen and that cell bubbling was associated with the release of fragments of antigenic material into the medium surrounding the cells. In addition these findings would seem to accord well with the presence of basophilic cytoplasmic granules, which have usually been reported to be confined to the outer cytoplasmic zone, though Buckley (1957) also reported their presence in, or overlying, the nucleus. Moreover, these basophilic bodies occur at a time when virus might be expected to be aggregated near the cell surface.

Although at first sight these various observations seem to hang well together, a closer examination introduces considerable doubt as to their true significance. In the first place, the cytoplasmic granules have been shown by Shaver et al. (1958), using methyl green pyronin staining in combination with ribonuclease treatment, to be devoid of RNA. According to these workers, moreover, they occur in under 2% of infected cells. These granules, therefore, cannot be accepted as virus aggregates. Secondly, as will be discussed later, the amount of specific viral RNA in an infected cell is probably very small in comparison with the amount of normal or abnormal cellular RNA, and consequently localization of RNA by histochemical methods cannot be accepted as indicating the localization of virus. Even the extreme sensitivity claimed for the acridine-orange technique (Mayor and Diwan, 1961) would not permit the viral increment to be detected against the background fluctuations in cellular nucleic acid. This situation could be changed only if, as Mayor suggests, a technique could be developed for the selective degradation of cellular RNA, but no such technique is as yet available.

Although the fluorescent-antibody studies are not open to the same criticism of non-specificity, they indicate only the distribution of virus antigen, not of formed particles. Since it is known from the work of Lwoff et al. (1955) that virus is released during the shredding of the peripheral cytoplasm, it is not in itself surprising that antigen is also released at this stage. More surprising is the amount of antigen that is left associated with the substance of the disintegrated cells. Under normal conditions very little virus remains associated with the debris from poliovirus-infected cells and ultrasonic treatment of the latter fails to release a significant increment. It seems likely therefore that the antigen demonstrable in cell debris is not associated with formed virus particles, and hence the evidence for virus localization obtained by this technique must be accepted with caution. Nevertheless, Buckley (1956), Lebrun (1957) and Mayor (1961) are all in agreement that the first indication of specific fluorescence occurs in the cytoplasm and not in the nucleus. Lebrun detected an increase in the cytoplasmic fluorescence of some cells as early as one hour after infection. On the other hand, spread of fluorescence to the nucleus occurs late, at a time when cellular integrity is breaking down, and is almost certainly due to spread of antigen from the cytoplasm.

Using the electron microscope, Ruska, Stuart and Winsser (1956) reported the presence of intranuclear particles in infected cells, a finding which might suggest a nuclear origin for the virus, or at least nuclear participation in its formation, but this report has not been confirmed. Kallman *et al.* (1958) were unable to locate developing virus by electron microscopy and considered it unlikely, for mathematical reasons, that the virus could in fact be detected by this technique; however, Stuart and Fogh (1959) demonstrated crystalline arrays of particles of the appropriate size in the cytoplasm but not in the nuclei of infected cells of the FL line of human amnion.

On balance, therefore, the evidence suggests a cytoplasmic rather than a nuclear origin for the virus and certainly points to a cytoplasmic origin for the virus antigen. It does not, however, indicate the origin of the viral RNA. The findings of Ruska *et al.* (1956), the early nuclear changes in the cytopathology of infection, the nucleolar changes observed by Dunnebacke in human-amnion cells and the changes in the distribution of the nuclear DNA reported by Mayor all point to the involvement of the nucleus in the very early stages of virus replication, so the possibility of a nuclear origin for the viral RNA cannot be ruled out. Not only is there precedent in the replication of the myxoviruses for such a division of virus synthetic activity, but Bellett and Burness (1960), examining the site of replication of the infective RNA of the much more closely related mouse-encephalomyecarditis virus, found that this made its first appearance in the nucleus as little as 30 minutes after infection.

D. Metabolic Studies

It is clear from the cytopathology which has so far been discussed that there is a certain lack of precise definition in the picture which has emerged. In certain virus infections, for example those due to herpes and adenovirus, the cytopathology points clearly to the nucleus as the region of the cell which is likely to be implicated in the basic biochemical changes. By contrast, in the case of the pox viruses, the primary pathology as well as the primary biochemical disturbance affects the cytoplasm. In the case of poliovirus, however, the cytopathological picture is vague and "non-specific". The whole cell is clearly affected but no one part more than another, and consequently the pathology has given no clear guidance to the biochemist in his search for the disturbances which lead to cell death. Biochemical studies have therefore been devoted largely to an examination of the general changes affecting the major facets of cell metabolism.

Prior to the advent of tissue-culture techniques for the study of the metabolism of poliovirus-infected cells, results on whole tissues were so imprecise and uninformative that they will not be considered here. Even the more precise results obtained in tissue culture are contradictory, though certain facts may be taken as well established.

The poliovirus consists of a ribonucleic-acid core surrounded by a protein shell, both RNA and protein being specific for the virus and the latter carrying the specific antigenic activity. The materials needed for the synthesis of both virus components are derived from the cellular pools of precursors (Darnell and Levintow, 1960; Salzman and Sebring, 1961), and Zwartouw, Taylor-Robinson and Westwood (1960) showed that cultured cells contain an adequacy of all the components necessary for the elaboration of complete infective virus, including a sufficient energy reserve. Provided that adequate oxygenation is ensured, cells in suspension at a concentration of 10^7/ml are capable of synthesizing a full yield of infective virus in the complete absence of all added nutrients including glucose. Under anaerobic conditions, however, the addition of glucose becomes necessary, suggesting that the intracellular reserves of energy-producing carbohydrate are adequate only if oxidative pathways of utilization are employed by the cell. At lower cell concentrations of 10^6/ml Darnell and Eagle (1958) have shown that glutamine and glucose are needed to produce full yields of virus, while at still lower cell concentrations progressively more added nutrients become necessary (Darnell, Eagle and Sawyer, 1959). It would seem that progressive dilution of the cell suspension leads to progressive leakage of essential constituents which must be made good from the suspending medium if full yields of virus are to be produced. Since the cell concentration *in vivo* is higher than could be obtained even with the most concentrated suspension in tissue culture, it may be assumed that the reserves of the cell are sufficient to supply all the materials and energy required for the replication of virus in infected animals.

The replication of poliovirus requires the synthesis of RNA and protein, and the effects of infection on the synthetic activities of the cell for these components has been the subject of intensive studies yielding highly contradictory results. Ackermann's group, using HeLa cells infected in a maintenance medium which did not support cell multiplication, studied separately the nuclear and cytoplasmic components during the first seven hours after infection, (Maassab, Loh and Ackermann, 1957; Ackermann, Loh and Payne, 1959). They observed an immediate increase in synthetic activity leading to a net increase in cytoplasmic RNA to 250% of the control value and in protein to an extent representing a doubling of the cell mass in six hours. There was also an increase in the nuclear RNA and DNA and an increase of up to 150% in the rate of ^{32}P incorporation into nuclear DNA. The cytoplasmic RNA yielded base ratios which indicated it to be cellular and not viral in type, and only that fraction of the RNA which deposited along with the microsomal fraction of the disrupted cells gave base ratios tending towards those of poliovirus. These results were interpreted as indicating that infection with poliovirus triggers a tremendous increase in cell-synthetic activity, resulting in the production of a large amount of cellular RNA and protein in addition to the relatively small amount of viral material.

The findings of Salzman are wholly contradictory to those of Ackermann's group. These workers studied HeLa cells in the log phase of growth in suspension in a fully nutrient medium and did not separate the nuclear and cytoplasmic components. They found an early inhibition of the synthesis of RNA, DNA and protein such that no measurable increase in these components occurred during the first six hours following infection. According to the published figures (Salzman, Lockart and Sebring, 1959), the inhibition only became detectable at six hours, the figure at three hours being, in fact, slightly higher than in the control. Between six and 12 hours 60% of the cellular RNA and 30% of the protein were lost into the medium, but there was no loss of DNA. These losses coincided with the period of virus release from the cells. These two series of studies are the most informative yet published on the effects of poliovirus on cellular metabolism and it is not yet possible to reconcile the contradictory findings. Partly for this reason, and partly because they are concerned only with the overall effects on major metabolic systems, they give no direct indication as to the detailed biochemical lesion underlying the changes studied.

Recently a more detailed approach has been made to the problem using the mouse-encephalomyocarditis virus—an RNA virus of very similar structure to poliovirus. Work, Martin and their associates analysed the changes in synthetic activity occurring in various fractions of infected Krebs II ascites-tumour cells, (Martin *et al.*, 1961; Martin and Work, 1961). They found that there was a progressive inhibition of RNA turnover in the nucleus following infection and also some loss of nuclear RNA. On the other hand, there was a progressive increase in RNA in the mitochondrial fraction of the cytoplasm, the increase being equivalent to the amount lost from the nucleus. The turnover of "mitochondrial" RNA increased enormously at a time corresponding with the production of infective virus, and reached the impressive figure of 320% of the control value. There were similar but smaller changes in the microsomal RNA. It was calculated that only 5–8% of the newly formed RNA could be incorporated into mature virus. The general pattern of these changes, which, despite the fact that no overall changes in the cellular content of RNA or protein were found, are reminiscent of those of Ackermann's group, is supported by the findings of Baltimore and Franklin (1962) on the closely similar if not identical Mengo virus in L cells. Using autoradiographic techniques and also estimations of DNA-dependent RNA polymerase activity in cell nuclei, these workers also reported immediate and progressive depression of nuclear RNA synthetic activity, such that only about 10% of the activity remained after two hours. At this time there began an increase in the rate of RNA synthesis in the cytoplasm.

The investigation by Work and his associates represents the first major attempt to break down the problem of infected-cell metabolism into its component parts by cell-fractionation procedures, and it is no criticism of the work that the results are not easy to interpret in the light of present knowledge. The investigation has shown very clearly the increased precision which can be achieved by this approach. The depression of nuclear RNA synthesis is confirmed by the findings of Baltimore and Franklin (1962), who also noted the increase of RNA synthesis in the cytoplasm, though with rather different time relationships. These workers interpreted their findings simply in terms of direct disruption of cellular RNA synthesis by the virus followed by cytoplasmic synthesis of viral RNA. However, the time of increase in the RNA synthesis in the microsomal fraction in the studies of Martin *et al.* (1961a,b) coincides with the appearance of infective virus relatively late in the replication cycle, while Bellett and Burness (1960) found that the first appearance of infective RNA was in the nucleus as early as 30 minutes after infection, with peak titres being reached at four hours. Only after this time did infective RNA appear in the cytoplasm of infected cells. Martin and Work therefore suggest that the fall in nuclear RNA synthesis is due to the direct damage inflicted by the virus, and the fall in net nuclear RNA to drainage of infective viral RNA to the cytoplasm after its synthesis in the nucleus. The net increase in cytoplasmic RNA, which corresponds in amount to that lost from the nucleus, would then represent mainly infective RNA of nuclear origin. This interpretation, however, leaves the formidable increase of 320% in RNA synthesis in the mitochondrial fraction unexplained, as is also the fact that this increased synthetic activity is not accompanied by any net increase in the RNA of this fraction over and above that derived from the nucleus. Infective virus appeared in the mitochondrial fraction and increased in amount in conformity with the increase in RNA synthesis by this fraction, but the implied geographical relationship may not be as close as would at first sight appear. The fractionation procedures used by Martin *et al.* (1961) did not separate the so-called "fluffy layer" from the underlying layer containing the majority of the mitochondria in the deposit obtained at 10,000 g. This "fluffy layer" contains the enzymic activity attributed to lysozomes and is also rich in RNA derived from fragments of endoplasmic reticulum bearing ribosomal material (de Duve, 1959; Novikoff, 1957). The significance of the term "mitochondrial RNA" is therefore doubtful. Nor does the simultaneous deposition of virus and mitochondria from the debris of disrupted cells necessarily imply any special relationship between the two other than those of size and density of the deposited particles. To be deposited with the mitochondria the virus must be present in aggregated rather than free form, possibly in the manner suggested by Horne and Nagington (1959) for developing poliovirus, but geographical relationships within the cell are not indicated. It is to be hoped that with continuing development of cell-fractionation procedures many of the questions raised by this work will be answered soon, but in the meantime certain general inferences may be drawn.

Since the protein and nucleic-acid requirements of the infecting virus must be met, it is clear that the RNA and protein metabolism of the infected cell must continue at least until a late stage in the cycle of virus replication, and the experimental evidence shows this to be the case. While there is a sharp difference of opinion as to whether there is a net increase or decrease in RNA and protein synthesis, there is no divergence of opinion as to the continuation of these activities. Precursors of both continue to be incorporated into both cellular and viral components. Interference with either of these metabolic systems results in depression of virus production and is the basis of much work on the possible chemotherapy of virus infections (Tamm, 1958; Staehelin, 1959). Similarly, as the synthesis of both RNA and protein requires energy, it may be expected that the energy metabolism of the cell should also continue, and this too is found to be the case. Provided that an internal or external energy source is available, either oxidative or glycolytic, aerobic or anaerobic pathways of metabolism may be utilized, indicating further that the versatility of the system is not impaired, (Eagle and Habel, 1956; Gifford and Syverton, 1957; Zwartouw et al., 1960; Taylor-Robinson, Zwartouw and Westwood, 1961). Again, as with the other two systems, interference with energy metabolism results in depression of virus synthesis.

On the subject of DNA synthesis there is less evidence available, but, since active synthesis of DNA is a function only of cells which are growing and multiplying, it is unlikely to be intimately concerned in the replication of poliovirus, at least *in vivo*. One can assert with confidence, therefore, that the major metabolic activities which are most closely associated with the synthesis of poliovirus continue to function in the infected cell. Why, then, should the cell suffer injury which ultimately causes its death and disintegration?

E. CELL DEATH

King *et al.* (1959) investigated the changes associated with cell death in Erlich-ascites-tumour cells subjected to three different forms of injury: exposure to a non-nutrient Krebs–Ringer phosphate solution, X-irradiation and poisoning with salyrgan (a mercurial poison acting on all –SH enzymes, including those of the respiratory and glycolytic pathways). Their results showed that a uniform series of events preceded the death of the cell, irrespective of the type of injury. Four stages were described, but only the first of these is likely to be relevant to the present discussion, since the second stage was ushered in by metabolic failure, and subsequent changes, such as the disruption of the ionic balance of the cell and its eventual structural breakdown, were presumably consequent upon this. The onset of metabolic failure, however, followed upon a first stage during which all the aspects of metabolism studied remained apparently normal, and no cytopathological changes could be detected. Nevertheless, during this stage there was a decrease in the DNA content of the nuclei and protein was lost to the medium. Unfortunately, changes in the cellular content of RNA were not followed. There is to some extent a parallel between these events and those occurring in poliovirus-infected cells in that no damage is evident in either case during the initial period when the critical injury is probably being inflicted. The loss of protein to the medium is interesting in view of Salzman's observation of the loss of both RNA and protein from infected cells, but it is not possible to relate these findings closely, since the timing of the event in the two cases is widely different. In King's studies the loss of protein was immediate and continuous while, in those of Salzman, RNA and protein were lost late, coinciding with disintegration of the cytoplasm at the time of virus release.

It is clear that the observations of King *et al.* (1959) cannot be pressed too far in relation to poliovirus-infected cells, since the pattern of events leading up to the final death of the cell must be related to the type of injury inflicted—this is clearly shown by the differences in cytopathology seen following infection with different viruses. In the experiments of King *et al.* the cells, on removal from the mouse, were suspended in a non-nutrient salt solution devoid even of amino acids, and at the cell concentrations used the leakage of amino acids from the intracellular pool would rapidly halt protein synthesis. Both X-irradiation and salyrgan treatment were superimposed on this basic injury, to which the infected cells in Salzman's experiments were not exposed.

The main interest in this work from the virological point of view lies in the fact that it was deliberately concerned with the process of cell death. Although the results as they stand do not throw direct light on the type of injury inflicted by viruses, they could do so if extended to the vital questions of how far metabolic injury may be pressed without causing irreversible damage, and the nature of the metabolic changes associated with partial cycles of virus replication.

F. POSSIBLE MECHANISMS OF CELLULAR INJURY

1. Relation of viral to cellular metabolism

The cytopathological and biochemical evidence seems to show that no detectable damage is suffered by the infected cell until towards the end of the eclipse phase of virus replication. Despite the recent surprising report of Darnell et al. (1961) on the lateness of synthesis of poliovirus RNA, the weight of evidence, with this and other viruses, indicates that the synthesis of the greater part of the viral material occurs during the eclipse phase and is therefore completed before cellular damage becomes evident. The earliest abnormality detectable is the alteration in the distribution of nuclear chromatin, which may just precede the appearance of new infective virus. Not only is there no evidence of cellular damage prior to this change, but there is considerable direct evidence that the normal metabolic activities of the cell continue and may even be enhanced. Following this 3–4 hour period, however, progressive changes occur which culminate, in a further 2–3 hours, in the complete disintegration of the cell.

Gottschalk (1957c) has reviewed the arguments for supposing that the enzymes responsible for virus synthesis are derived from the host cell and not contributed by the infecting virus. These arguments are based partly upon the complete failure of many workers to demonstrate the presence, in virus particles, of any metabolic enzymes, other than those which may be acquired through superficial adsorption from the host tissues, and partly on the more positive evidence derived from bacteriophage studies. It is also unlikely that the very small amount of protein present in the smaller viruses would permit the carriage of a sufficient variety of enzymes for their synthetic requirements. While arguments based on the absence of metabolic enzymes in the infective form of the virus leave out of account the possibility that the information for their elaboration may be present in the viral nucleic acid, the duplication of enzymes already present in the cell would seem to be unlikely. Arguments based on evidence derived from bacteriophage studies are more suspect. For instance, in the case of the T-even phages there is an immediate cessation of the normal bacterial-DNA synthesis upon infection of the cell. This is followed after a short interval by a recommencement of synthesis of DNA, but this time of the phage type. The synthesis of the phage DNA starts and continues at a high steady rate which is independent of the concentration of phage material. It is argued that this can only be explained as a diversion of the preformed bacterial-enzyme system into a new channel under the direction of the infecting phage DNA. All the biochemical evidence discussed above is entirely at odds with such a dramatic switch of cellular metabolism occurring following infection with poliovirus, nor is there evidence that it does so with any other animal-virus infection. In the case of the bacteriophage, the final yield of which may account for as much as 70% of the dry weight of the infected bacterial cell, diversion of cellular synthetic activity to the production of virus might be quite enough to account for the death of the cell, but in the case of the animal viruses the situation is different. Poliovirus draws directly on the amino-acid and nucleotide pools of the cell for its basic materials. This has been shown by direct experiment by Salzman and Sebring (1961), using radioactive tracers. They showed, moreover, that these materials came directly from the respective pools and were not derived from breakdown of preformed host protein and nucleic acid. It must be accepted, too, that the virus draws on the host energy metabolism and on the enzyme systems responsible for RNA and protein metabolism. However, the total amount of virus formed has been calculated to represent not more than 5% of the dry weight of the infected cell (Schwerdt and Fogh, 1957), and the results of Ackermann et al. (1959), supported by those of Tenenbaum (1957), Mayor (1961) and, in part, Martin and Work (1961), indicate that the infected cell is capable of more than doubling its output of RNA and protein. The drain on the cell's metabolic resources represented by the virus moiety must, therefore, be trivial and could not in itself possibly cause the death of the cell.

This situation is very different from that obtaining with a bacteriophage representing 70% of the dry weight of an infected cell, but the difference could be only quantitative. The question arises, therefore, whether in the polio-infected cell there is in fact a very much greater diversion of cell metabolism into virus channels than is represented by the total dry weight of formed virus. Gottschalk (1957c) suggested that the infecting RNA acts, not by pre-empting and redirecting the host nucleic-acid-synthetic mechanisms, but by direct competition with a host-RNA counterpart at the enzyme level. By acting as a competitive coenzyme in the nucleic-acid-synthetic or protein-synthetic cycles it could divert a proportion of the synthetic activity into virus-specific channels. The degree of competition would depend, by the normal physico-chemical laws governing competitive equilibria, on the relative concentrations of virus RNA or its active derivatives present in the cell, and would increase as these increased. This suggestion is an interesting anticipation of some of the recent theories that virus RNA acts as a "messenger RNA" within the cell and might therefore act in direct competition with a cellular messenger (Tsugita *et al.*, 1962).

If the mechanism of competition envisaged by Gottschalk were in fact operative, it seems possible that it could give rise not merely to a cumulative but to a progressively accelerating diversion of metabolic activity. Moreover, if the competitive viral system escaped whatever controlling mechanisms govern the normal synthetic activity of the cell, the accumulation of virus-specific products would mount at an ever-increasing rate and the limit would be imposed only by the final breakdown of cellular metabolism. A toxic mechanism of this type would depend on the production of a large excess of virus material over and above that built into virus particles, and in several virus infections this is known to occur. The soluble antigens of the pox viruses and myxoviruses and the intranuclear protein crystals produced by some adenoviruses are examples. The estimate of the amount of viral material present in polioinfected cells was based on total particle counts which would not take into account soluble material (Schwerdt and Fogh, 1957). Hence the total amount of viral RNA and protein and their precursors might be considerably greater than this estimate indicates. That antigens at least are produced in excess is suggested by the fact that antigenic material remains associated with the cell debris after release of the virus.

Gottschalk's hypothesis implies a basic antagonism between virus and cellular metabolism. The hypothesis presented above for the toxic action of virus on the cells in which it is multiplying endeavours to show how this basic antagonism might build up into a factor sufficiently large to cause metabolic disruption and cell death. It implies that cell damage depends not on the amount of virus, active or inactive, which is produced, but on the total amount of virus-specific material synthesized and acting in competition with the cellular metabolic intermediates. Since formed particles are likely to be much less efficient competitors than unorganized material, besides being present in relatively small amounts, it is the latter which is likely to be the more damaging factor.

In the context of poliovirus there is a clear objection to this idea in that Ackermann, *et al.* (1959) found the excess RNA formed during infection of the cell to be cellular and not viral in type. Several points must, however, be remembered in relation to this finding. Firstly, the characterization of the RNA rested solely on the base ratios obtained on hydrolysis and these would give no indication as to whether this excess material was functionally normal or abnormal. Secondly, poliovirus contains single-stranded RNA and there is as yet no definite evidence as to whether complementary strands are formed in the cell and accumulate there. Such strands would not give the base ratios of poliovirus RNA. Thirdly, competitive disruption of metabolism might well be highly selective and affect only a specialized part of the relevant systems. About 70% of the cytoplasmic RNA of a normal cell is located in the ribosomes and, as far as is known at present, forms only a structural basis for active synthetic activity. The proportion of RNA, such as the transfer RNA, which is directly involved in synthesis is relatively small. Viral competition, therefore, might be effectively toxic at concentrations which are still small by comparison with the total RNA content of the cell.

2. Virus release

It is not possible to state the point at which a cell can be considered to die, nor can one say at present at what stage the damage suffered is irreversible. However, Barski *et al.* (1955) noted that poliovirus-infected cells continued to show active movements right up to the time of cytoplasmic bubbling but were completely inactive after this had ceased. Since this stage represents the release of virus from the cell, it raises the point as to whether the cell is in fact killed as a result of the rupture of its surface membrane. Nothing is as yet known of the mechanism by which cytoplasmic shredding is brought about, nor is it possible to say whether, if shredding and virus release could be prevented, infected cells could recover. Roizman (1959) showed that virus release from poliovirus-infected cells was prevented if incubation was carried out at room temperature. Mayor (1961) used incubation at 30°C for experiments with acridine-orange staining. She found that release did not occur at this temperature and the cells remained intact, but raising the temperature to 37°C was quickly followed by release of virus with cell destruction. Coleman and Jawetz (1961) have succeeded in establishing persistent infection with herpes virus by incubation of infected cultures at 31°C. The cells showed some evidence of cytopathic effect but continued to multiply slowly and could be sub-cultured. Virus in low titre was continuously released into the medium over a period of many months. Transfer of the cultures to 34°C caused the rapid liberation of large amounts of virus to a peak titre of 10^9 infective units per millilitre with prompt destruction of the cells. Additional information is required before the mechanism underlying these findings is clear, since the virus content of the cells when incubated at the lower temperature was not reported. The rapid production of virus on transfer of the cultures to the higher temperature could have been due either to the sudden release of preformed virus, in which case the death of the cell might be directly due to the process of virus release, or to enhanced virus replication with death of the cell occurring through metabolic interference. The authors in their preliminary communication mention but do not discuss the alternative explanations. Whichever mechanism is operative, the system suggests a method of controlling the degree of cellular damage which might prove useful in investigating the mechanisms by which viruses damage cells.

G. The Anterior-horn Cell

The discussion so far has related solely to the problem of how virus multiplication could cause damage to the infected cell, and all the relevant information has been derived from *in vitro* observations. As has been pointed out, however, the critical lesion in poliomyelitis is loss of function of the anterior horn cell, so the central point of the present argument must lie in the question of how far the possibilities discussed can contribute to an understanding of this loss of function.

1. Cytopathology

A comparison of the *in vivo* changes leading to acidophilic necrosis and the cytopathic changes in various cell types *in vitro* suggests that they are on the whole compatible. The *in vivo* picture is dominated by the presence of Nissl substance in the motor neurone, and the dramatic picture of chromatolysis tends to mask the other cellular changes, but underlying similarities may nevertheless be distinguished. Both *in vivo* and *in vitro* nuclear changes affecting the distribution of the nuclear chromatin occur early and are accompanied by the frequent formation of intranuclear eosinophilic inclusions. Shrinkage of the nucleus with wrinkling of the nuclear membrane is followed in both cases by its progressive distortion and displacement towards the periphery of the cell. *In vitro* the distortion and displacement have been traced directly to the development of the cytoplasmic mass and, though the latter has not been described *in vivo*, the similarity of the nuclear changes suggests that a similar cause may well operate. The final stages of acidophilic necrosis *in vivo* are accompanied by swelling of the cell and are followed by lysis. *In vitro*, where the cells are not bound down by dendritic processes or confined by connective tissue, lysis is preceded by cell rounding and cytoplasmic bubbling. The similarities in the processes occurring under the two sets of conditions are sufficient to give some confidence that metabolic observations *in vitro* are also likely to apply *in vivo*, but their application must be made with reservations for two reasons. First, there is no clear *in vitro* counterpart to the basophilic necrosis suffered by a proportion of anterior-horn cells, though this type of necrosis may well depend on the presence in the latter of the strongly basophilic Nissl substance. Secondly, and much more important, there is the demonstrable fact of one basic difference in the behaviour of poliovirus *in vivo* and *in vitro* relative to cytopathogenicity. *In vivo*, as has already been stressed, the virus appears to be almost non-cytopathogenic. The only cells demonstrably damaged are the anterior-horn cells, and even these are capable of recovery, while *in vitro* all the cells in which the virus multiplies invariably appear to be destroyed. In the few instances in which non-cytopathic multiplication of the virus has been reported (Ledinko, Riordan and Melnick, 1951; Youngner, Ward and Salk, 1952; Sabin, 1954), the virus yield was very low and the lack of observable damage was probably due to there being too few cells affected to be readily detectable in the cultures (Kaplan and Melnick, 1955).

At least two differences in behaviour are entailed in these observations. In the first place, cell types which are fully susceptible to infection *in vitro* may be insusceptible *in vivo*, as was shown by Kaplan in his attempts to infect monkey-kidney cells by direct inoculation *in vivo* (Kaplan, 1955b). No replication occurred in the inoculated kidneys, but when the organs were then removed and cultivated *in vitro* the virus multiplied in, and destroyed, the cells. A similar insusceptibility is apparent in the central nervous system, where only the neurones are affected, despite the demonstration by Hogue *et al.* (1955, 1958) that all the cultivated cells of nervous tissue are fully susceptible *in vitro*. The discovery by Holland and McLaren (1959) of the presence of a receptor substance in susceptible cells, and by Kunin and Jordan (1961) that human-amnion cells before cultivation would not adsorb poliovirus, may furnish a clue to this type of insusceptibility *in vivo*, but there is as yet no clue as to the mechanism of the second difference in behaviour—the ability of neurones to recover when damaged beyond the point of loss of function.

2. Loss of function

There is no true counterpart in cells cultivated *in vitro* by present techniques to the loss of function of the motor neurone—that is, the loss of ability to transmit a nervous impulse—but the observations of Barski *et al.* (1955) on living cells provide the nearest parallel. These workers reported that active cell movements continued in their preparations right up to the time of cytoplasmic bubbling, the point at which shredding of the cytoplasm occurred. "Purposive" movements ceased at this point, and when cell bubbling ceased the cell was dead. *In vivo*, loss of function occurs in the neurone at the stage of severe chromatolysis (Bodian, 1948). The fact that cells may pass this point and still recover would seem to indicate that physiological function is lost at an earlier stage *in vivo* than the ability to perform purposive movements *in vitro*; nevertheless, it is still late in the sequence of cytopathological changes. It would probably correspond therefore to the period between three and five hours in the studies of Salzman *et al.* (1959) before the stage of virus release. These workers' results would suggest that damage to the RNA- and protein-synthetic systems might already be detectable at this time, although it falls within the period of metabolic stimulation as reported by other workers. No loss of protein or RNA to the medium would yet have occurred and no irreparable damage would have been inflicted on the cell. It is clear that this is meagre evidence on which to base detailed speculation as to the possible mechanisms of loss of function, but consideration of the physiology of the motor neurone raises interesting questions which might form a useful guide for investigation of the problem. First, however, it is necessary to discuss the special problem of the Nissl substance and the significance of chromatolysis.

(a) *Nissl substance and chromatolysis.* Although the precise function of the Nissl substance is not known, the granules contain RNA and protein (Hydén, 1943; Gersh and Bodian, 1943) and consist largely of densely packed ribosomes. They are probably, therefore, concerned in the synthetic activities of the cell. The process of chromatolysis, or dissolution of the Nissl substance, occurs in a variety of physiological conditions, such as fatigue, hibernation and axon regeneration, as well as such pathological conditions as anoxia and poliomyelitis. It would appear, therefore, to be a physiological process occurring when the cells are under special stress.

Gersh and Bodian (1943) studied chromatolysis following nerve section in the monkey and demonstrated a reduction of RNA relative to protein as measured by ultra-violet absorption. They suggested depolymerization of RNA as an explanation of their findings. Swelling of the cells with dilution of the cytoplasm accompanied chromatolysis, and the concentrations of both RNA and protein consequently fell, reaching the nadir at six days and thereafter rising again. The authors did not relate the changes in concentration to cell volume and so did not indicate the effect of the changes on total RNA and protein content. However, Brattgård, Edström and Hydén (1956) carried out similar experiments in rabbits and estimated the total RNA and protein content of the affected neurones from ultra-violet absorption measurements and measurements of cell size. They found that the total protein began to increase immediately and doubled in 40 days. This increase in protein was paralleled by an increase in cell size, so that the concentration did not alter. Their findings give no suggestion of the cytoplasmic dilution reported by Gersh and Bodian. RNA decreased for the first 12 days and thereafter increased to reach a level double that of the normal cell in 40 days. From forty to forty-five days represented the time taken for regeneration of the axon, and this was followed by progressive return of the neurone to normal. In the frog (Edström, 1959) there was no initial fall in RNA content, the total RNA and protein increasing together from the start in parallel with the increase in cell size, so that the concentration of neither was altered.

In the study of Gersh and Bodian the increase in cell size was ascribed to uptake of water due to increased internal osmotic pressure following on depolymerization of RNA. Edstrom (1959) suggests that the depolymerization converts the RNA to a more active state connected with the great increase in protein synthesis accompanying chromatolysis and axon regeneration. While the overall picture does suggest a mobilization of reserves, the explanations offered for the observed changes are not entirely satisfying. In the first place, there is no evidence for depolymerization of RNA beyond the morphological dispersion of the Nissl substance. Reduction in the ultra-violet absorptive power of the cell does not constitute such evidence, since depolymerization should lead to an increase rather than a decrease in absorptive power at 2562 Å. Nor is it safe to ascribe cell swelling to the products of depolymerization, even if this can be shown to occur without reference to the ionic balance of the cell. The process of chromatolysis, affecting as it does the RNA metabolism of the cell, can hardly fail to be of interest and importance in understanding the changes which follow infection with an RNA virus, yet, at the moment, the knowledge available throws no light on its significance relative to virus multiplication, cytopathology or functional failure of the cell. It would seem desirable that the phenomenon should be re-investigated using chemical as well as physical techniques of analysis, and linking the investigation to functional changes in the affected neurones. If the highly sophisticated physiological techniques developed for the measuring of membrane potential in single cells could be linked with the techniques of sub-microgram analysis and applied to neurones in tissue culture, much of the relevant information could be obtained.

(b) *Possible mechanisms of interference with neuronal transmission.* Despite its many complexities, the nervous impulse in a motor neurone consists essentially of an electrical discharge of a polarized cell membrane. The discharge is localized but transmissible by contiguity, and travels in all directions to the extremities of the cell. Under physiological conditions the impulse is initiated at the post-synaptic region by a chemically induced discharge which excites the neighbouring electrically excitable membrane of the cell body and so initiates a wave of depolarization which travels, via the axis cylinder, to the motor end-plate, which responds by the secretion of a chemical transmitter, acetylcholine.

The functional integrity of the cell, therefore, depends on the maintenance and repeated re-establishment of membrane potential, processes requiring active transport of Na and K ions against their normal diffusion gradients and also against the potential difference set up by the process itself. Active transport would break down and membrane polarization would collapse on failure of energy metabolism in an infected cell, so consideration of alternative mechanisms of functional failure would remain a purely academic exercise were it not for the evidence, already discussed, that functional failure *in vivo* occurs at a time when energy metabolism is not only not depressed but may actually be stimulated and the cell still be capable of full recovery.

Short of complete metabolic collapse, there are several possibilities with interesting experimental implications. In addition to energy requirements, normal polarization requires the maintenance of the normal ionic balance of the cell and certain definite permeability characteristics of the cell membrane, and these in turn are closely linked with the water balance of the cell. These properties must be closely interdependent and yet are capable of independent variation. For instance, the swiftly rectified alteration in membrane permeability which is entailed in the transmission of the nervous impulse is not accompanied by alteration of the overall ionic or water balance unless pushed to the extreme of fatigue and induction of chromatolysis. Similarly, chromatolysis is accompanied by disturbance of the water balance, as shown by cell swelling and the cytoplasmic dilution claimed by Gersh and Bodian (1943), but not by failure of polarization, since function is maintained until a late stage. Neuronal membrane permeability and membrane potential are, however, extremely sensitive to local environmental influences and may be profoundly altered by, for instance, the local application of various ions (Coombs, Eccles and Fatt, 1955) or amino acids (Curtis and Watkins, 1960). Curtis and Watkins showed an interesting relationship between the activity and chemical structure of the stimulatory amino acids and their decarboxylated counterparts which are inhibitory in like degree. The presence in normal nerve tissues of the strongly inhibitory γ-aminobutyric acid (GABA), the decarboxylated counterpart of the strongly stimulatory glutamic acid, indicates the presence of the appropriate decarboxylase systems in normal nerve cells. These systems are not notably specific in their action and are strongly influenced by pH. Is it possible that a falling pH, accompanying the RNA changes associated with chromatolysis in an infected cell, could cause the accumulation of inhibitory amino acids through over-activity of decarboxylase systems? Alternatively, could alterations in the phospholipid metabolism of the infected cell affect the integrity of the cell membrane and so alter its permeability characteristics that it becomes incapable of maintaining polarization? Consideration of the known facts of neurone physiology suggest a number of such possibilities which must at the moment remain wholly speculative, but the underlying problem must be solved for a full understanding of the relationship of poliovirus to the infected neurone.

H. Conclusions

Poliomyelitis was selected for discussion as the virus infection *par excellence* in which the disease in the intact animal could be related to the cellular damage caused by the virus, and its examination shows that the possibilities for investigation are by no means exhausted. Some of the gaps in our present knowledge are surprising—particularly the lack of definite evidence that the virus multiplies in the affected neurones and the vexed question of the apparent non-cytopathogenicity of the virus in extraneural tissues *in vivo*. Both these problems should be soluble by the use of fluorescent-antibody techniques as applied by Mimms (1959, 1960) to the pox-virus infections. Of still greater importance are problems relating to mechanisms of cellular injury, solution of which depends upon refinements of dynamic analytical techniques. While workers the world over are applying these techniques fruitfully to the study of the metabolism of normal and infected cells, the field of cellular injury and cell death appears to have been almost wholly neglected. Even the fundamental parameters have not yet been established, as, for instance, a working definition of cell death *in vitro* or the definition of changes which might be taken to correspond to loss of function in cultured cells. Sophisticated techniques would not be required for much of the ground-work on this problem, in which virus infection would be a useful tool rather than an end in itself. If the basic principles could be established, however, the benefits to be reaped in the virological field are sufficiently obvious.

III. Pathogenesis Dominated by Constitutional Effects— the Pox-virus Infections

In considering poliomyelitis as the best example of the causation of virus disease by focal damage, it was pointed out that, even here, generalized constitutional effects were not entirely lacking. The mild upper respiratory episode which frequently precedes the onset of nervous involvement is accompanied by the familiar symptoms of malaise, headache, loss of appetite, pains in the limbs and fever, which accompany the onset of most virus infections. There is no generalized virus infection which is not heralded by such vague and non-specific constitutional disturbance, and clinical diagnosis must always await the more definite signs attributable to the specific tropisms of the virus responsible. The investigation of this type of generalized disturbance in non-fatal infections is an almost impossible task. The major evidence lies in subjective symptomatology, and the few objective signs, such as loss of appetite and fever, are too imprecise to be of much use in the investigation of disease in experimental animals. Such investigations, therefore, must be confined for the moment to that extension of constitutional disturbance which leads to death in fatal infections in animals. Among virus infections it is only those caused by the pox viruses that have been studied for the specific purpose of determining the cause of death. For this reason the pox-virus diseases have been selected for discussion in the following pages.

A. PATHOGENESIS

The virus exanthemata were at one time held to illustrate the property of dermotropism in particular viruses, but it has long been recognized that involvement of the skin represents only one aspect of the pantropism of a generalized infection. In smallpox, for example, many tissues have been shown to yield virus, while in the laboratory the generalized nature of pox-virus infections was shown by Fenner's work on the pathogenesis of mouse-pox and by recent work on rabbit-pox. The disease of primary importance to man within this group is, of course, smallpox, but, since no laboratory animal is susceptible to regularly fatal infection with the virus, information regarding the pathogenesis of the disease is extremely meagre. The pathogenesis of smallpox must, therefore, be inferred from the results obtained with the two pox diseases which have been extensively studied in laboratory animals, namely mouse-pox and rabbit-pox.

Fenner's studies with mouse-pox reveal a clear-cut course of events. Mice infected via the foot-pad, thought to be the normal route of infection, develop a local lesion with rapid involvement of the regional lymph nodes. This is followed by a primary viraemia with spread of the virus to the reticuloendothelial system generally and to the liver and spleen in particular. Rapid multiplication occurs in these two organs, and, if a sufficiently high titre of virus is achieved, the mouse will die at this stage of the disease. In animals which do not die a secondary viraemia occurs with further generalization and involvement of the skin. Subsequent work with rabbit-pox has shown a very similar series of events, though the sequential development of the disease is rather less clear-cut. Fenner's work was not directly concerned with the mechanisms by which the observed spread of virus through the tissues brings about damage to the host, so mouse-pox will not be considered in more detail. A summary of his results and references to the original papers will be found in Fenner (1949, 1959).

Rabbit-pox infection in rabbits has been intensively studied by Downie's group in Liverpool and by Westwood's group at Porton. The origin of the virus, like that of vaccinia itself, is obscure, but it was first encountered at the Rockefeller Institute in 1932, when it appeared suddenly in the normal rabbit stock and, in the course of three years, wiped out the larger part of the rabbit colony of the Institute, (Greene, 1934a,b). Later a similar episode occurred at Utrecht (Jansen, 1942). The virus is closely related to vaccinia and is possibly derived from a laboratory neuro-vaccinia strain which acquired the property of epizootic spread. Its laboratory characteristics have been thoroughly worked out by Fenner (1958). The virus, particularly the Utrecht strain, is highly virulent for rabbits by all routes of inoculation. The disease produced has an incubation period of from three to six days which is followed by the onset of pyrexia as the first sign of clinical illness, the rectal temperature rising rapidly to 104°F or higher. From this point the clinical signs of disease become obvious and consist of refusal to eat, reduced intake of food and water, loss of weight, weakness, listlessness and diarrhoea. Profuse purulent discharges develop from the eyes and nose. Within a day or two of the onset of clinical signs a bright erythema develops around the anus, and this is followed by the development of large pock-like lesions in the perianal region and at the muco-cutaneous junctions around the lips and nose. If the skin has been previously shaved, a visible cutaneous rash also develops and the number of lesions continues to increase over the next few days. The severity of the rash is variable, and some rabbits die before any eruption appears. The rash usually appears on the sixth day after infection but may appear as early as the fifth or as late as the eighth day. The individual lesions do not seem to progress clearly through macular, vesicular and pustular stages; they appear first as reddish papules which develop a yellowish centre and superficially resemble pustules. The yellow centre is, however, composed of caseous material rather than true pus. The superficial epithelium over the lesions becomes scaly, but true scab formation involving the deeper layers does not occur, and the lesions ultimately fade away if the animal survives. Death when it occurs usually supervenes between the seventh and twelfth days after infection. There is little variation in the course of the disease following small doses of virus, whether these be administered as an aerosol or by the intracutaneous or intravenous routes.

Following respiratory infection with small doses of virus, dispersed as a cloud of droplet nuclei of less than 1 μ diameter, primary infection occurs via the lung, the primary lesion lying in the alveoli or terminal bronchioles. Replication of the virus first occurs in the bronchiolar or alveolar epithelium with rapid spread to the neighbouring lymphoid tissue and thence to the regional lymph nodes. Virus multiplication may be detected in lung tissue within 24 hours and in the regional lymph nodes within 48 hours. By the fourth day, virus may be detected in most tissues of the body. Whether rabbits are infected by the respiratory or the intravenous routes, the lungs appear to be highly susceptible, peak concentrations of up to 10^8 pock-forming units (PFU) per gram of wet tissue being reached by the fifth to seventh day of disease. High titres of virus are also reached in the spleen, adrenals, gonads and skin, but not in the liver, kidney or brain, where the concentrations are similar to those occurring in the blood. If the levels

TABLE I

Concentrations of vaccinia and rabbit-pox viruses attained in rabbits infected via the lungs.

| | Peak titres attained in: | |
	Vaccinia	Rabbit-pox
Lungs	5·9 – 6·8	7·5 – 8·1
Hilar lymph nodes	2·0 – 3·1	4·4 – 5·4
Spleen	1·4 – 1·9	4·3 – 6·1
Liver	2·3 – 2·6	3·1 – 4·7
Kidney	1·3 – 1·4	2·4 – 3·3
Adrenal	1·00	5·2 – 7·3
Gonad	1·0 – 3·4	6·8 – 7·3
Brain	1·0 – 1·8	1·2 – 2·1
Skin	2·1 – 2·2	5·7 – 6·4

Figures represent virus concentration expressed as $\log_{10}$ pock-forming units per gram. wet weight of tissue.

of virus attained in the various tissues are compared with those attained by the relatively avirulent vaccinia virus (Table I), it is clear that the latter are trivial by comparison. Following respiratory infection, the highest titres of vaccinia virus are reached in the lung, where substantial multiplication occurs, but the concentrations attained even here are still only one tenth of those reached by rabbit-pox.

However, even in those tissues where high concentrations of rabbit-pox virus are attained, the degree of damage revealed histologically does not seem adequate to account for death of the animal through destruction of vital tissue. Even in the adrenal cortex, where high virus concentrations are found and extensive lesions may be evident, not more than about one quarter of the cortical tissue appears to be destroyed.

Comparison of this description with the clinical course of human smallpox reveals a number of differences. In smallpox the incubation period is remarkably constant at 12 days and seldom extends beyond the limits of 10–14 days. This long incubation period constitutes one of the unsolved problems of the natural disease, for it cannot be reproduced in animals either by the exposure of monkeys to variola virus (Westwood *et al.*, 1963) or by the intranasal instillation of rabbit-pox virus in rabbits (Duckworth, 1958). Intranasal infection of rabbits with rabbit-pox virus probably represents the closest approach possible in animals to the conditions of infection in human smallpox, in which the virus is thought to invade by the upper respiratory tract. This probability is supported by the demonstration by Downie's group that, though the virus may be readily isolated during the incubation period from the tracheas of rabbits so infected, the animals do not become infective by contact until clinical disease is evident. It is precisely this phenomenon in human smallpox which makes possible the control of the disease by the "ring vaccination" procedure.

Commensurate with the longer incubation period in smallpox, the evolution of the disease appears to be slower. This fact may well be linked with the slower replication of the virus both in tissue culture and in the embryonated egg. The rash in smallpox tends to be uniform in the sense that all the lesions in any one area are at about the same stage of development, and the individual lesions progress steadily from the papular stage to scabbing. In rabbit-pox the lesions on the shaved skin appear continuously over a few days and the lesions themselves do not undergo the same sequential changes. Of much greater significance is the fact that, though the gross oedema which follows the intradermal inoculation of rabbit-pox virus indicates severe damage to capillaries with marked increase in capillary permeability, haemorrhage is not a feature of the disease. In human smallpox, on the other hand,

V.I.—K*

haemorrhage, varying from the prodromal petechial rashes to the frank haemorrhages from body orifices which characterize haemorrhagic smallpox, is the most dramatic single feature of the disease. From this it would appear that the capillary damage inflicted during the course of a severe variola infection in man is much more drastic than the corresponding damage in rabbit-pox infection in rabbits. Despite this, it must be remembered that, while the case mortality in human variola major is usually only 30–40%, it approaches 100% in rabbit-pox.

There is no satisfactory information about the distribution of virus in the body in smallpox. Viraemia is demonstrable particularly in severe cases (Downie et al., 1953), and virus has been isolated in high titre from the pericardial fluid of an acutely fatal case, (MacCallum, personal communication) but no systematic survey of the distribution of virus in fatal cases has been carried out. Nor is laboratory evidence particularly helpful. The monkey is the only susceptible laboratory host which has been used for studies on the pathogenesis of infection, and since the disease produced is usually mild and rarely fatal the information obtained is probably of little relevance to man. In a series of studies on monkeys infected by the respiratory route, Westwood et al. (1963) found that even massive doses of virus administered as a 1 μ aerosol, the estimated retained dose being about 10^5 egg-infective units, produced a disease which was intermediate in severity between the almost completely avirulent vaccinia and highly virulent rabbit-pox infections in rabbits. The incubation period was normally five days as opposed to 12 days in man. The onset of the disease was signalled by a rise of temperature, and the animal huddled in the corner of its cage and refused food. A rash usually appeared on the seventh or eighth day after infection, but varied from the sixth to the eleventh day. It showed a similar centrifugal distribution to that in man and underwent a similar development, except that the lesions were smaller, more scanty and tended to dry more rapidly. Even the most severe rash seen did not approach confluence. Recovery occurred abruptly at about the ninth day with a sudden return to liveliness and normal appetite.

As was expected from the route of exposure, the primary site of multiplication was in the lung, in which the virus attained titres varying between 10^4–10^7 PFU per gram, peak concentrations being obtained around the seventh to ninth days. Apart from the lung and skin lesions, virus was only occasionally recovered from other tissues and then usually in low concentrations (10^3 PFU per gram). Hilar lymph nodes and spleen were occasionally positive, and, in one animal which yielded virus to a titre of $10^{4\cdot8}$ PFU per gram from the hilar lymph nodes, virus was also present to a similar titre in the gonads. Out of some 60 animals exposed to virus by the respiratory route for various purposes, including passage experiments, only two died from the effects of the disease. One of these died suddenly following the stress of handling, and showed at autopsy a severe haemorrhagic bronchopneumonia with virus recoverable from the lung to a concentration of 10^7 PFU per gram but without virus in other tissues except the skin. The other animal was suffering from Flexner dysentery with diarrhoea and died on the eleventh day after infection. This animal also showed a severe haemorrhagic bronchopneumonia and had an extensive skin rash. Virus was present in all tissues tested to the following titres: lung, $10^{9\cdot4}$; spleen, $10^{7\cdot1}$; liver, $10^{7\cdot6}$; adrenal, 10^6; testis, $10^{6\cdot4}$ PFU per gram. This episode suggests that even in the relatively insusceptible monkey the virus may occasionally break through the physiological barriers which normally prevent its free multiplication and that when this occurs it is capable of multiplying throughout the body.

In spite of the absence of direct information, therefore, it is safe to assume that in smallpox, as in other pox-virus infections, the disease is a generalized one and the tissues of fatal cases, if tested, would yield high concentrations of virus.

B. Cause of Death

In terms of mammalian physiology, death must be taken as the moment at which the heart finally and irrevocably fails. In searching, therefore, for a "cause of death" in a disease process one is in fact looking for damage which is severe enough to cause cardiac failure either directly or through a chain of effects.

Consideration of the disease pictures described in the preceding section does not suggest any one anatomical or physiological lesion which is in itself sufficiently severe to cause cardiac failure. The high virus concentrations found in the lungs in rabbit-pox might suggest an indirect effect through cardiac anoxia, but the degree of damage to lung tissue as judged from histological examination does not support this suggestion. The two monkeys which died of variola infection in the experiments of Westwood et al. (1963) were both suffering from a severe bronchopneumonia with oedema of the lungs and it is not unlikely that cardiac anoxia killed these animals in heart failure, especially since one of them died as a direct sequel to handling. Primary pneumonia is not, however, a usual feature of smallpox in man, although it does sometimes occur. Although bronchopneumonia has frequently been found to be present in fatal cases and has even been incriminated as the cause of death (Councilman, Macgrath and Brinckerhoff, 1904, Sweitzer and Ikeda, 1927), it has been almost certainly bacterial in origin and has been eliminated by the use of antibiotics, (Bras, 1952). In rabbit-pox the only other organ besides the lung which yields consistently high titres of virus is the adrenal, a finding which confirms the observations of Douglas, Smith and Price, (1929) in infections with neurovaccinia. This combined with the sharp fall in temperature which consistently precedes death raises the suspicion of acute adrenocortical failure, and Boulter, Maber and Bowen, (1961) investigated this possibility, using changes in the blood levels of sodium, potassium and glucose as indicators of adrenocortical function. It was found that, although there was a rise in the plasma potassium during the course of the disease, there was no concomitant fall in the level of plasma sodium. On the contrary, both plasma sodium and glucose levels tended to rise. Indirect evidence of this type cannot be regarded as conclusive, and blood cortiscosteroid levels need to be investigated, but it can be said that the changes in the blood chemistry do not suggest adrenocortical failure as the underlying cause of death.

During these experiments a consistent rise in blood urea was also observed but no evidence was obtained for a primary renal failure, the rise in blood urea being paralleled by a fall in urinary output which was consequent on diminished fluid intake. In recovering animals the change was rectified as soon as the fluid intake recovered. That renal function was not impaired was shown by the secretion of a progressively more concentrated urine at the time that the blood urea was rising.

However, two consistent findings emerged which were thought to be of crucial importance. First, the tendency for a rise to occur in the plasma potassium was found to be more than just an indication of metabolic imbalance. Just before death in fatal cases there was a sharp rise in the plasma potassium to very high levels. In Table II, taken from Boulter et al. (1961), the terminal levels and ranges found in 11 animals dying from rabbit-pox in a single experiment are compared with the levels and ranges found by various workers to induce cardiac failure, both in vivo and in vitro, in experimental potassium intoxication. These figures suggest very strongly that the immediate cause of death in fatal rabbit-pox infection is cardiac failure induced by a toxic level of potassium in the blood. The second important finding was that all animals, whether or not they ultimately survived the infection, suffered a fall in blood pressure around the seventh to eighth day after infection. In fatal cases a precipitate fall from normal to unreadably low levels may occur very suddenly with death following in a few hours, or the fall may be more gradual, an initial abrupt drop being followed by a partial restoration of pressure with a final fall to very low levels just before death. The initial fall in pressure is usually, though not invariably, less severe in animals which ultimately survive, and normal pressure is restored within a few hours. In general it appears that the final outcome of the disease is related to the severity and duration of the hypotension.

The conclusion appears inescapable that, though the terminal event may be cardiac failure through potassium intoxication, the critical physiological lesion which precedes this failure is shock. The problem of the cause of death appears, therefore, to centre upon these two events, and their possible causes must be considered.

TABLE II

Plasma potassium in fatal rabbit-pox and potassium poisoning

Animal	Treatment	K^+ in meq./l	
		Mean	Range
Rabbit	Normal	3·3	2·4 — 4·4
Rabbit	Rabbit-pox	15·2	8·3 — 31·4
Rabbit	KCl i.v.	18·5	10·4 — 27·0[1]
Rabbit	Haemorrhage — KCl i.v.	13·4	12·0 — 15·3[1]
Rabbit	KCl i.v.	—	14 — 16[2]
Rabbit	Isolated heart — KCl	12·0	— [3]
Rabbit	Heart (cardiac arrest)	18·0	— [3]
Dog	KCl i.v.	19·7	— [4]

[1] Tabor and Rosenthal (1945).
[2] Winkler, Hoff and Smith (1938).
[3] McLean, Bay and Hastings (1933).
[4] Spurr, Barlow and Lambert (1959).

1. Adrenocortical failure

Boulter *et al.* (1961) concluded that the blood changes in fatal rabbit-pox infection could not be explained on the grounds of simple adreno-cortical failure, since neither the ionic balance nor the blood glucose altered as would be expected. Nevertheless, the onset of hypotension, the fall in body temperature and the rise in plasma potassium are changes to be expected from such failure, and the clinical course closely approximates to the picture of the Waterhouse–Friderichsen syndrome, which is usually, but not exclusively, associated with fulminant meningococcal septicaemia. This syndrome, as originally described, can be diagnosed only at autopsy, since it comprises fatal shock associated with bilateral adrenal haemorrhages, and the fatal collapse has been attributed to the destruction of the adrenal cortex. In view of these facts the possible role of the adrenal cortex in the collapse which precedes death in rabbit-pox merits further attention.

Although in the classical Waterhouse–Friderichsen syndrome there may be complete destruction of the adrenal cortex, the causal relationship between this event and the circulatory collapse has for long been in doubt. It has been pointed out by many workers that the clinical manifestations of the syndrome may occur without a fatal outcome and also that cases which die may show no haemorrhage into the adrenal glands, and may even show little or no adrenal pathology, (Thomas and Leiphart, 1944; Ferguson and Chapman, 1948). Recently Benson and Boyd (1960) have analysed 68 fatal cases of acute meningococcal infection, of whom 41 showed peripheral circulatory collapse. Purpuric rashes occurred in 40 of the latter, massive adrenal haemorrhage in 16, small localized haemorrhage in 9, and microscopic haemorrhage alone in 3. The remaining 13 cases showed no haemorrhage. Tubular degeneration of the adrenal cortex was present in a high proportion of cases whether or not these suffered circulatory collapse. Adrenocortical hormone therapy was used on 17 of the patients with shock without effect, and blood or plasma transfusions on 11 with, at best, transient improvement. Finally, the authors quote a personal communication from Migeon (1959) to the effect that the plasma corticoids may be normal in this clinical syndrome. Their own analysis of cases and their study of the literature led these authors to conclude that shock was not due to adrenocortical insufficiency. The same conclusion is to be drawn from the work of Spink (1960) on endotoxic shock in dogs. Direct measurements of corticosteroids in the blood from the cannulated adrenal vein of dogs, in which shock was induced by the intravenous injection of Brucella endotoxins, not only showed normally high levels of corticosteroids during shock but also indicated that the injection of endotoxin actually stimulated the secretion of these substances. The adrenals, moreover, retained their capacity for normal response to ACTH stimulation even in moribund animals. The circumstances of these experiments are clearly very different from those obtaining in animals in the terminal stages of an acute infection, especially as adrenal damage may be demonstrable in the latter, but the evidence as it stands justifies the tentative acceptance of the conclusions of Boulter et al. (1961) that shock in rabbit-pox is not caused by acute adrenocortical failure. Clearly, more work is required on this crucial point, and the answer can only come from direct estimation of corticosteroids during the course of the disease.

If adrenal failure be eliminated as the cause of shock then some other factor must be sought for the onset of this syndrome and also for the raised plasma potassium.

2. Origin of the raised plasma potassium

It has been demonstrated in rabbit-pox infection that multiplication of the virus to high titre occurs in many organs of the body and this must be accompanied by extensive cell destruction with release of potassium. Release of potassium from injured tissues has frequently been reported (Millican, 1960), and Tabor and Rosenthal (1945a) measured the amount of potassium liberated from the entire injured area following the induction of tourniquet shock in mice. While it is not possible either to measure or estimate the amount which must be released during the course of an acute generalized virus infection, it seems not unlikely that potassium from this source could contribute to the tendency for the plasma potassium to rise during rabbit-pox. A raised plasma potassium level is a recognized feature of the shock syndrome, and a terminal rise to fatal or near-fatal levels has been frequently observed. Zwemer and Scudder (1938) suggested that potassium might be a critically toxic factor in shock, and Tabor and Rosenthal (1945b) demonstrated a terminal rise in tourniquet-shocked mice. It was found by these authors that the plasma levels in animals dying from fatal shock were similar to those in shocked animals killed by the injection of minimal lethal doses of potassium chloride, but lower than those of normal animals killed in the same manner. These experiments show that shocked animals are more sensitive than normal animals to the toxic effect of potassium and that the blood levels attained naturally in the terminal stages of shock approximate to those necessary to cause death. The picture is, in fact, so similar to that in fatal rabbit-pox that the problem in the latter appears to resolve itself into the single issue of the causation of shock.

3. Origin of shock

The causes and origins of shock in its many forms have been the subject of intensive study since the time of World War I, and a large part of the accumulated knowledge on the subject may be found in the reports of two recent symposia (Washington Symposium, 1960; *Biochemical Response to Injury*, 1960).

There is probably no single definition of shock which would be universally acceptable, but the one factor which is common to all forms is a fall in blood pressure. If the fall is of sufficient severity and duration it leads to irreversible damage terminating in death of the organism. Death may occur without recovery of the blood-pressure and is then directly due to heart failure, or it may occur after recovery from shock and is then ultimately due to irreversible damage to some vital organ, usually the kidney, during the period of hypotension. The shock syndrome is progressive. The fall in blood pressure which initiates the process may be brought about directly by controlled haemorrhage, and shock itself is then evident as the persistence of hypotension after restoration of the blood volume. The syndrome which then builds up includes hypothermia, peripheral circulatory collapse, disturbances in the ionic balance of the blood and tissues, and various metabolic disturbances reflected in the blood chemistry. If shock persists beyond a certain maximum period it becomes irreversible. The heart and blood-vessels then fail to respond to stimuli and no form of treatment will restore the blood pressure and avert death.

The greater part of the work which has been undertaken in the investigation of shock has concerned itself with the syndrome itself after shock has been induced by some form of controlled traumatic procedure and consequently is not such as to throw light on the mechanism of its causation by a virus infection. However, the phenomenon of shock resulting from acute infections has long been recognized, and in recent years a number of diseases of widely different origin have been shown to terminate in the common factor of the shock syndrome.

One of the best documented cases is that of anthrax, in which the syndrome has been clearly demonstrated and the toxin responsible isolated (Smith and Keppie, 1955). The syndrome has also been shown to be operative in plague (Hoessly et al., 1955), gas gangrene in man (Macfarlane and MacLennan, 1945), staphylococcal-toxin poisoning in experimental animals (Thal and Egner, 1956), meningococcal septicaemia (Benson and Boyd, 1960), diphtheria (Pappenheimer, 1955), acutely fatal varicella infection (Montgomery and Olafsson, 1960) and experimental intoxication with rickettsial toxins (Wattenberg et al., 1955). Rabbit-pox infection in rabbits, therefore, joins an array of diseases of diverse aetiology in which the common physiological lesion leading to death has been shown to be shock.

In the case of the bacterial diseases mentioned toxins, either endo- or exo-toxins, are demonstrably associated with the causation of the shock syndrome, although the chemical basis for their action is not known. The problem has been discussed by Smith (1960). The toxins vary in their chemical nature and therefore presumably in their mode of action, but it is likely that they all act on the peripheral vessels, though some, such as diphtheria toxin, may also act directly on the heart. There would appear to be two possible mechanisms by which a peripheral action could initiate the fall in blood pressure which precipitates shock: direct damage to the capillary bed might cause a sufficient increase in capillary permeability to result in a diminished blood volume severe enough to impair the circulation, or dilatation of the capillary bed might produce the same result without actual loss of fluid from the blood. In the case of anthrax the former mechanism undoubtedly predominates, since oedema is a conspicuous feature of the disease and haemoconcentration with a diminished blood volume has been experimentally demonstrated (Smith and Keppie, 1955). Oedema and haemorrhage are also characteristic of plague, and the toxin extractable from *Pasteurella pestis* by ultrasonic disintegration produces oedema on inoculation into the skins of both guinea-pigs and rats (Keppie, Smith and Cocking, 1957; Cocking *et al.*, 1960).

In the investigations of Hoessley *et al.* (1955) on plague in monkeys, however, haemoconcentration was not shown to be present and it seemed likely that serious oligaemia resulting from increased capillary permeability did not occur in these animals. Nor was peripheral vascular stagnation detected, and so the origin of shock remained unexplained. In the other diseases in which the shock syndrome has been shown to be operative it is clear that there is not enough evidence as yet on which to assess the relative importance of increased capillary permeability, but it is significant that in all cases the agents responsible are capable of producing capillary damage. In the case of the extractable toxins oedema at the site of intradermal injection is directly demonstrable. In meningococcal septicaemia, haemorrhage and purpura are frequent, and varicella may take a haemorrhagic course. Such a course is characteristic also of severe variola infections. Massive oedema follows the intradermal injection of rabbit-pox virus, and oedema and haemorrhagic orchitis follow its injection into the testis, both these effects being in contrast to those following the similar injection of the avirulent vaccinia virus.

The question of haemoconcentration has not yet been studied either in smallpox or rabbit-pox, and until definite evidence of its occurrence is available it would be rash to assert that shock in these conditions was due to leakage of fluid from damaged capillaries with a resulting oligaemia, but this seems at the present to be the most likely explanation.

There is as yet no evidence that the heart is directly involved in the pathology of rabbit-pox, and such lesions as may be seen histologically are non-specific and do not suggest direct viral attack on the myocardium, though this possibility is a real one and deserves further investigation.

Once shock is established, however, the heart is certain to be involved, if only as the result of cardiac ischaemia, and Guyton and Cromwell (1961) have shown that the cardiac reserves are severely depleted when shock is established, so that a relatively small additional stress may lead to failure.

If shock in rabbit-pox infection is due to a toxic action on the peripheral circulation with or without additional central action on the heart itself, then it seems an inescapable corollary that there must be some toxic factor circulating in the blood which is capable of exerting this action. In the case of bacterial diseases extractable toxins fulfil this role, but no toxin other than the virus particle itself has ever been demonstrated in virus infections. On the other hand, many chemical substances have been shown to be released from damaged tissues which are capable of inducing increased capillary permeability and, in the case of histamine at least, of inducing shock. The present state of knowledge in regard to these substances has been reviewed by Spector (1958). The release of these capillary permeability factors may be provoked by degrees of trauma varying from severe burning to the minimal types of trauma which have been utilized by Miles in many of his studies (Miles, 1961).

Since there is, in severe generalized virus infection, an extensive destruction of cells throughout the body, it seems possible that released tissue products capable of acting as capillary permeability factors might play the part of the hypothetical toxin. If this were so it might be expected that the severity of the infection would be closely linked with the degree of tissue destruction, and hence with the degree of virus multiplication in the tissues. Although such a correlation is impossible to prove directly, it is certainly true that in fatal infections such as rabbit-pox, virus multiplies to a higher titre than in infections with an avirulent virus such as vaccinia. Fenner (1949) found that early deaths in mouse-pox were associated with high concentrations of ectromelia virus in the liver and spleen of infected mice. In smallpox it is likely that the degree of viraemia reflects the degree of virus multiplication in the tissues, and Downie et al. (1953) showed that the prognosis of the disease in human patients was linked to the titre of virus in the blood during the first few days of the disease. Again, in the adaptation of influenza virus to the lungs of hamsters and mice deaths do not begin to occur until the virus is capable of multiplying to high titre in these organs and producing severe tissue damage. It is true that Hirst (1947a) observed some dissociation between the ability to multiply to high titre and the ability to cause death during the adaptation of influenza virus to mouse lung, suggesting that some other factor may also be involved, but this does not invalidate the generalization.

The simplest logical sequence of events, therefore, in virus diseases of this type would be: virus multiplication – tissue damage – release of permeability factors – generalized increase in capillary permeability – loss of fluid from the blood – shock. Two important considerations, however, militate against too ready an acceptance of this scheme. In the first place, the multiplication of virus in tissues has never been shown to give rise to any toxic product other than the virus itself. This is not, of course, an insuperable difficulty, since the demonstration of toxic products might be technically difficult—it was only after many years of fruitless experimentation that the toxin of anthrax was eventually demonstrated. Moreover, any factors produced might be present in low concentration and exert their effects by cumulative action over an extended period. Nevertheless, any hypothesis depending on the release of toxic products arising from the destruction of cells by virus multiplication must be supported by the demonstration that such products in fact exist. Secondly, even in the case of traumatic shock and inflammation, in which the release of permeability factors has been demonstrated and investigated, it appears that the action of these factors is strictly local. While they increase permeability in the immediate vicinity of the damaged tissue, they do not cause any generalized increase. Tabor, Rosenthal and Millican (1951), for instance, showed that fluid accumulation in the injured hind limbs of tourniquet-shocked mice was accompanied by a *decrease* in water content of the uninjured tissues. It would seem, therefore, that when shock follows tissue injury it results from local fluid loss into the injured tissue and not from generalized increase in capillary permeability mediated by factors released into the general circulation. Such a generalized increase would only appear to arise when the injury is itself generalized as in the case of haemorrhage.

Nevertheless, preparations of viruses and rickettsiae have for long been known to be toxic, and some of these have been shown to operate through the production of shock in experimental animals, so the phenomenon of virus toxicity and its possible relevance must be examined.

4. Virus toxicity

The term "virus toxicity" was coined to cover the production, in the absence of virus multiplication, of lesions or death following the inoculation of virus preparations into experimental animals. Burnet (1942) first demonstrated this property when he showed that the inoculation of Newcastle-disease virus (NDV) into the lungs of mice, in which the virus was incapable of multiplying, was followed by the production of lesions indistinguishable from those of influenza virus fully adapted to multiplication in this organ. Since the initial demonstration of this phenomenon it has been extensively studied, particularly with reference to the myxoviruses and rickettsiae, and the work has been reviewed by Cooke (1961). During the course of this work the characteristics of virus "toxins" have been largely clarified, but at the same time the originally clear-cut picture of the phenomenon has become blurred, owing partly to the application of the term to cytopathic changes in tissue culture under particular conditions, and partly to the recognition of partial cycles of virus multiplication which may be accompanied by "toxic" effects both *in vitro* and *in vivo*.

While there are some differences in detail in the behaviour of viral and rickettsial "toxins", as, for instance, the ability of the latter to recover lost toxicity on incubation with glutamate, the important characteristics of the toxicity of both are the same and the description which follows applies equally to both.

The toxicity of a virus preparation is inseparably associated with the virus particles themselves. The only substance exerting an effect on tissue cells which has been successfully separated from the virus is the cell-rounding factor of Pereira and Kelly (1957) which is produced by adenovirus type 5. This factor, which is a protein antigen produced during the course of virus multiplication *in vitro*, causes the rounding and clumping of cells in tissue culture, but does not appear to damage them permanently, since they remain capable of multiplication. Although, therefore, it cannot technically be classed as a toxin, its existence is important, for it represents a pharmacologically active substance separable from the virus particle and may indicate that other less bland products of virus multiplication await discovery.

Toxicity segregates with the virus particles in fractionation experiments, can be destroyed by all physical and chemical treatments which destroy infectivity and is specifically neutralized by immune sera capable of neutralizing infectivity. Toxicity is not always, however, as sensitive to destructive agents as is infectivity, and the two properties may be partially dissociated by treatment with heat or ultra-violet irradiation, so that preparations which have lost the greater part of their infectivity still retain the greater part of their toxicity.

The toxic effect of virus preparations in animals can only be demonstrated by the inoculation of massive doses many millionfold greater than those necessary to produce infection in susceptible animals. When such doses are used the result tends, as in the case of influenza and NDV in mouse lung, to be independent of whether or not the virus is capable of multiplication in the host concerned. If the host is susceptible to infection the toxic effect may be recognized by its rapidity of onset at a time when multiplication cannot be demonstrated. This is clearly shown following the intravenous injection of massive doses of mouse-adapted influenza virus into mice. Mice which do not die within 96 hours from the toxic effects of the virus become infected and die of the effects of virus multiplication a week or 10 days later. Alternatively, toxic effects may be elicited by the inoculation of virus into a susceptible animal by a route which does not produce infection. Such is the case with the intracerebral injection of non-neurotropic strains of influenza virus in mice. With toxic doses death occurs in convulsions in a manner not seen when death occurs as the terminal event of an established infection.

In many respects, therefore, there are apparently fundamental differences between virus infectivity and virus toxicity despite the fact that both properties are associated with the virus particle and both are inactivated by the same agents. Thus, it is not surprising, that virus toxicity has been regarded as something of a laboratory freak phenomenon having little relevance to the pathogenesis of disease or even to the processes of virus multiplication, (Burnet, 1955). Recent observations, however, indicate that this impression may be wrong.

(a) *Virus toxicity and multiplication.* Virus toxicity was originally defined as the production of pathological changes in the absence of virus multiplication, or, as expressed by Burnet (1955) ". . . in the absence of multiplication adequate to account for them." The first doubt as to the adequacy of this definition arises from the demonstration by Schlesinger (1950) that non-neurotropic strains of influenza virus undergo a partial cycle of replication when inoculated into the brains of mice, and this *in vivo* observation has since been amplified by numerous studies of partial cycles of replication *in vitro*. The advent of tissue-culture techniques inevitably complicated the concept of toxicity, since cytopathic effects on cells *in vitro* are much easier to observe than toxic effects *in vivo*, and partial cycles of replication may be detected by a variety of techniques. If the concept of toxicity be extended to cover the production of cytopathic effects in the absence of production of new infective virus—and this extension has been widely accepted and applied—then it is evident that toxic effects *in vitro* are normally associated with a partial cycle of virus replication. Evidence for such a partial cycle has been found whenever it has been deliberately sought in relation to toxicity, and much incidental evidence to this effect has come from studies of partial cycles in "insusceptible" cells and studies on inhibitors of virus replication. For instance, Henle, Girardi and Henle (1955) made a full study of the partial cycle of replication which influenza virus undergoes in the HeLa cell and showed that the development of haemagglutinin and complement-fixing antigen was accompanied by cell destruction, although no infective virus was produced.

The toxic effect of NDV in ascites-tumour cells both *in vivo* and *in vitro* has been shown to be associated with a partial cycle (Granoff, 1955; Adams and Prince, 1957; Prince and Ginsberg, 1957). Ackermann *et al.* (1954) showed that, although *p*-fluorophenylalanine would prevent the formation of infective poliovirus, it did not prevent its cytopathic effect. A similar phenomenon was observed by Ledinko (1958) in the presence of proflavine, and in this case fully formed particles of non-infective virus were produced. Many similar examples could be cited.

If the cytopathic effect of virus multiplication is not prevented when the final step in the replication cycle—the production of infective particles—is suppressed, then it follows that the critical biochemical lesion must be inflicted, or at least initiated, during the eclipse phase. The conferring of infectivity on the final product may modify the nature of the damage but is not itself the cause of it. Thus, no valid line can be drawn between cytopathic effects of virus multiplication according to whether or not the final product is infective. If this line of reasoning is correct it should be possible to show that single virus particles, which are capable of initiating infection in susceptible cells, will also initiate "toxic" changes in cells which are insusceptible in the sense that they will not support the production of infective virus but are nevertheless susceptible to its toxic effects. The very elegant experiments of Wilcox (1959) have, in fact, shown this to be the case. Newcastle-disease virus produces a typical cytotoxic effect in L cells and can be shown to undergo a partial cycle of replication with the production of non-infective haemagglutinating particles, which are nevertheless capable of protecting normal cells, by interference, from the toxic effects of complete virus. By comparing the numbers of surviving cells in cultures infected with known doses of infective virus and incubated for 48 hours, with the numbers of cells in control cultures, Wilcox was able to show a 1:1 relationship between the numbers of virus particles inoculated over a series of dilutions and the numbers of cells missing, presumed killed, from the corresponding cultures.

Within the pox group of viruses, studies on the toxicity of vaccinia virus have been carried out both *in vivo* and *in vitro* (Cassel, 1957; Nishmi and Bernkopf, 1958; Bernkopf, Nishmi and Rosin, 1959; Brown, Mayyasi and Officer, 1959). In these studies no evidence was found to suggest that partial cycles of replication were occurring under the test conditions, but Appleyard, Westwood and Zwartouw (1962) have shown that the toxic changes induced by rabbit-pox virus in cultured cells are accompanied by antigen production. If cells infected with the virus are extracted at intervals during the eclipse phase and the extracts tested by the agar double diffusion technique, the sequential development of antigens may be demonstrated. Antigen is first

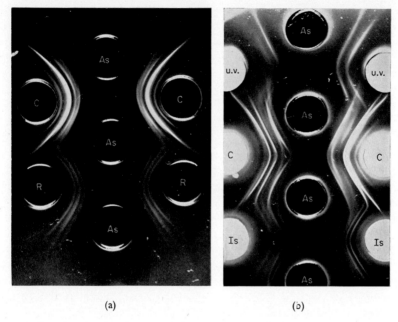

(a)   (b)

PLATE 1. Antigen patterns developed in tissue culture when replication of rabbit-pox virus is inhibited by various treatments. (a) Inhibition by rutilantin A. (b) Inhibition by isatin-B-thiosemicarbazone and by ultra-violet irradiation of seed virus.

In left hand cups of (b), antigens were added 24 hours after antiserum had been placed in central cups, to give better separation of lines. Reagents in all remaining cups were added together.

    As,   Antiserum;
    C,   Control untreated;
    R,   Rutilantin A;
    Is,   Isatin-B-thiosemicarbazone;
    u-v., Ultra-violet.

detectable at about two hours and by three hours three antigen lines may be seen. The pattern becomes complete at about six hours and in fully developed soluble antigen about 15 lines may be detected with the help of chromatographic separation. When the development of infective virus is prevented by prior ultra-violet irradiation of the seed or by the presence of sodium azide, the cells undergo cytotoxic changes indistinguishable from those occurring during the first six hours in normally infected cultures, but only three antigen lines, corresponding to those in the three-hour normal sample, develop. Two further substances are known which will suppress infective virus formation by rabbit-pox and vaccinia viruses without interfering with cytotoxic activity. Isatin-β-thiosemicarbazone (Bauer and Sheffield, 1959; Sheffield, Bauer and Stephenson, 1960) was shown by Easterbrook (1962) to permit apparently normal development of both viral DNA and antigen. The higher resolution of the double-diffusion technique shows that, in fact, antigen production is not complete, two strong lines of the normal antigen being missing from the isatin-inhibited pattern, but the action of the compound is undoubtedly late in the virus replication cycle. Rutilantin A, an antibiotic isolated from cultures of an actinomycete and shown to have anti-phage activity (Asheshov et al., 1954), permits the development of four antigens giving clear-cut lines in the double-diffusion pattern but again does not appear to interfere with viral DNA synthesis (Hume and Westwood, unpublished). The antigen patterns under the various conditions discussed are shown in Plate 1.

These four treatments interrupt virus synthesis by four different mechanisms operative at, at least, three different points in the replication cycle, yet the visible cytotoxic effect produced under all four conditions appears to be the same. This effect does, however, differ from the cytopathology developing in uninhibited cultures in that the final stage of syncytium formation does not occur. It must be presumed that this final change depends on some very late event, possibly associated with the final development of infectivity, which is prevented by all the inhibitors.

(b) *In vivo significance of virus toxicity*. In summary it may be said that there is now strong evidence that cytotoxicity is due to the biochemical disturbance which accompanies the replication of virus material within cells, and the mechanism of damage is closely similar, though not always identical, whether the replication cycle is complete or incomplete. The really important difference lies not in the mechanism of damage but in the transmissibility of the effect, since the ability of the virus to complete the cycle in cells of a particular type or species will determine the susceptibility of the host as a whole, whether this be an animal or a tissue culture, to infection with the virus in question. The implications of this are clear. If the host be susceptible then it is possible for the toxic effect to build up progressively from a small initial infecting dose, while if the host be insusceptible then the factor of transmissibility is absent and a massive dose of virus capable of producing immediate damage in large numbers of cells becomes necessary to produce a demonstrable toxic effect. Moreover, even in a susceptible host, all cells may not be equally capable of supporting virus multiplication; the *in vivo* insusceptibility of monkey-kidney cells to poliovirus (Kaplan, 1955b) is a case in point. If relatively insusceptible cells are capable of supporting even a partial cycle of replication, they too may be destroyed during the course of a virus infection. The amount of infective virus which may be isolated from a particular tissue, or even the nature of demonstrable lesions, may not reflect the degree of cellular damage suffered, particularly in the terminal stages of a fatal infection if high concentrations of circulating virus are present. Under these conditions the cells most open to virus attack would be those of the capillary endothelium, and hence the virus itself could fulfil the role of the hypothetical toxin postulated to account for the circulatory damage which leads to the onset of shock. The myocardium itself would clearly not be immune from similar damage.

This hypothesis for the mechanism of production of shock in virus infection demands that four conditions be satisfied. First, that the virus must be capable of infecting the cells of the capillary endothelium, and possibly the myocardium, and that these cells must be capable of supporting at least a partial cycle of virus replication, being damaged in the process. Second, that capillary damage in fact occurs during the course of the disease. Third, that increased capillary permeability, with or without associated myocardial damage, is capable of initiating shock. Fourth, that sufficient circulating virus is present over the appropriate period to cause the damage in question.

In relation to the pox viruses there is at present no direct evidence as to the susceptibility of the vascular endothelium, but in view of the pantropism of this group of viruses it would be surprising if this tissue were immune from attack. The second condition is, however, satisfied, and the evidence relating to capillary damage has already been discussed at length. The third condition is not virological, but reduction of the effective blood volume as a result of capillary damage is accepted as the basis of shock in a wide variety of circumstances. The final condition is clearly crucial and has not yet been discussed.

By direct inoculation of heparinized blood on to the chorioallantoic membrane of developing hens eggs, Duckworth (1958) has shown that rabbit-pox virus may be present in the blood of infected rabbits from the second day after infection and persists thereafter throughout the course of the disease. Using this technique Boulter and Westwood (unpublished) have followed the virus concentration in the blood of infected rabbits up to the time of death. Some of the results from a single experiment on 18 rabbits are shown in Fig. 1. It was found that three groups of results were obtained. In animals dying before the eighth day from fulminant infection, the concentration of virus in the blood rose logarithmically from the fourth day of disease, the highest

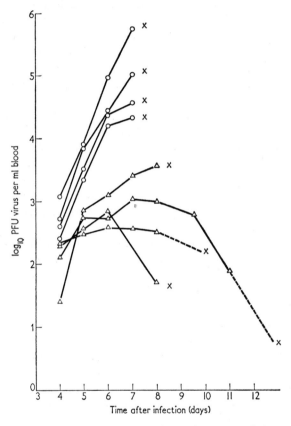

FIG. 1. Viraemia in rabbit-pox. Each curve shows the course of viraemia in a single rabbit. Eight curves have been selected to show the different patterns found in rabbits dying before and after the seventh day after infection.

recovery from the four animals in this group being $10^{5 \cdot 8}$ PFU/ml. In animals dying between the eighth and thirteenth days a mounting viraemia might still be present but the peak concentrations were from one to three logs lower than those in the first group. Finally, in animals which recovered viraemia tended to be irregular, and only in one case did the concentration reach 10^3 PFU/ml. In one animal which died on the eleventh day no virus was recovered from the blood at any time.

The interpretation of these figures is difficult. A considerable viraemia is certainly usual, but it is not possible to set a figure to the "sufficient" amount of virus demanded by the hypothesis, and the death of the animal without demonstrable viraemia is in any case inexplicable. Clearly, many factors require further study before any definite conclusions can be drawn. The sensitivity of the isolation technique is not known nor is the location of the virus. Douglas *et al.* (1929) found that circulating neurovaccinia was located principally in the leucocyes, but this requires reinvestigation in animals dying of rabbit-pox. Intracellular virus could well not be available for infection of endothelial cells; on the other hand, multiplication of virus in leucocytes might constitute a reservoir of virus from which the capillary endothelium could be infected. The virus measured in these investigations was circulating virus and gives no measure of the amount removed from the blood by adsorption to susceptible cells. The animal from which no virus was recovered presents a further problem. Viraemia of some degree must occur in generalized rabbit-pox infection, and complete failure to detect it in repeated samples suggests the intervention of some unknown factor. Finally, the number of rabbits so far examined is too small for the apparent patterns of viraemia to be accepted with confidence. In view of all these uncertainties further investigations are urgently required.

In the case of smallpox Downie *et al.* (1953) found that, if virus was present in the blood to a demonstrable concentration of more than 10^4 infective units per millilitre on the second day of disease, the patient was unlikely to recover. In these cases the viraemia persisted until death, while, in cases which eventually recovered, virus was not present in the blood to a titre higher than 10^2 infective units per millilitre and disappeared after the second day. It is evident, therefore, that both in smallpox and in rabbit-pox a relatively high concentration of virus in the blood is characteristic of the severe case, but it is not possible to decide from the evidence whether the circulating virus is responsible for the terminal events or is merely a reflection of the severity of the infection.

One may conclude, therefore, that in rabbit-pox infection death is due to shock leading to cardiac failure through potassium intoxication of the myocardium; that shock is probably caused by damage to the vascular capillaries, and possibly to the myocardium, by some circulating toxin. While toxic derivatives from virus-damaged tissues could theoretically play the part of the toxin, no such derivatives are demonstrably toxic. The virus particle itself *is* demonstrably toxic and is present in the blood during the course of the disease. In severe cases at least, its concentration in the blood may reach high levels. It is at

least possible, therefore, that the virus particle is itself the toxin.
(c) *Role of virus toxicity in other diseases.* If it is possible that virus
toxicity plays so vital a role in the pox-virus infections, to what extent
could it also account for the clinical manifestations in other virus
infections?

Henle and Henle (1946), as a result of their extensive work on the
toxicity of influenza virus, suggested that this property might be
important in the pathogenesis of human influenza, the generalized
clinical disturbance being, at least in part, the result of virus spill-over
into the blood. Hamre, Appel and Loosli (1956) showed that pulmonary
infection with influenza virus in mice was accompanied by viraemia,
and there are numerous reports in the literature of cardiac and neurological complications in human influenza, (Finland *et al.*, 1945;
Blattner, 1958; Kapila *et al.*, 1958; Sugiara *et al.* 1958; Walsh *et al.*,
1958; Bourne and Wedgewood, 1959; Martin *et al.*, 1959; Oseasohn,
Adelson and Kaji, 1959). These reports are all based on clinical observations, sometimes backed by histological evidence and occasionally virus
isolation from throat washing or autopsy lung. Although the association
of such complications with influenza seems well established in many
cases (see Bourne and Wedgewood, 1959), the role of the virus in
producing them is much less certain. For one thing, they nearly always
follow rather than accompany the influenzal attack, occurring when
the patient is afebrile and to all appearances convalescent. Even if
they are directly caused by the virus, therefore, they can hardly be
ascribed to the immediate toxic effects of circulating virus, though they
might be a late manifestation of toxic damage inflicted during the
acute stage. Again, Hook *et al.* (1962) have shown that the NWS strain
of influenza virus will multiply in the capillary endothelium of infected
chick embryos, and Chang and Kempf (1950) have demonstrated a
direct toxic action of the virus on the myocardium of rats, resulting in
a sudden fall in blood pressure within minutes of the injection of
infected allantoic fluid.

However, haemodynamic collapse is not a feature of influenza, in
which the clinical picture consists rather of subjective symptoms such
as headache, muscle and joint pains, malaise and prostration out of all
proportion to the severity of the disease. While it is entirely possible
that some or all of these symptoms could be caused by the toxic action
of circulating virus, massive viraemia is not observed in influenza, and
in its absence it is not easy to interpret the clinical picture in terms of
the known toxic properties of the virus particle. Experimental investigation of the problem is fraught with the difficulties already mentioned regarding the experimental handling of subjective symptoms.

The possibilities may be better judged in those diseases in which viraemia is known to occur and in which the outcome may be fatal. The group of arthropod-borne virus diseases belongs to this category. In the encephalitides the focal effects of central nervous involvement condition the course of the disease, but in other viraemic diseases such as haemorrhagic fever and yellow fever, constitutional disturbance is the dominant factor. Haemorrhagic fever represents in almost pure form the syndrome of shock and its complications due to direct damage to the capillary endothelium (Oliver and MacDowell, 1957; Smadel, 1959), and should provide an ideal model for the investigation of the syndrome in relation to virus disease when once the aetiological agent can be established in the laboratory. In yellow fever the clinical course can be divided into the stages of congestion and stasis, the latter being dominated by the effects of liver necrosis and renal failure. While death is probably due in most cases to the consequences of failure of these two organs, there is also microscopical evidence of myocardial damage, and bradycardia, hypotension and haemorrhagic diathesis become established during the stage of congestion. This suggests that not only the heart but also the capillary endothelium is directly attacked by the virus and the effects of liver and kidney failure, including the prothrombin deficiency induced by the former, are superimposed upon the direct toxic effects of the virus. Moreover, since viral toxicity is independent of whether or not the virus replication cycle is completed, the liver damage itself may be regarded as due to toxic action.

In rickettsial infections the evidence for the direct contribution of rickettsial toxicity is clear-cut and supported by histological evidence of multiplication of the organism in the capillary endothelium. The skin rashes are due to the direct damage caused in this way and, in severe cases, may be frankly haemorrhagic. Haemoconcentration and hypotension are constant features and death frequently occurs in shock. In laboratory studies on rickettsial toxicity the rapid induction of shock in rats and mice has been demonstrated. Clarke and Fox (1948) and Neva and Snyder (1955) demonstrated rickettsia-induced shock to be accompanied by haemoconcentration which was shown to occur without increase in the specific gravity of the plasma and so was probably due to whole plasma leakage. The latter was, in fact, directly demonstrated by Wattenberg et al. (1955). Greissman and Wisseman (1958) suggested that, since the reactivity of the vessels to epinephrine was unaltered, the action was probably on the capillary endothelium itself and might be confined to that tissue.

The similarity between these findings and the clinical manifestations of severe rickettsial disease in man is too close to be fortuitous. It seems certain that similar damage must be inflicted in both cases. In

the natural infection this damage must build up gradually and progressively as the organisms multiply in the capillary bed throughout
the body, while in the laboratory it may be inflicted at a single stroke
by the injection of a massive dose of organisms which may be incapable of completing the replication cycle.

C. SUMMARY

In summary, therefore, one may conclude that in acute virus infections
the only demonstrable manner in which the virus can inflict damage on
the host is by its direct destructive effect on individual cells and that
this results from the occurrence in those cells of a complete or incomplete cycle of replication. Where this damage affects cells which are
individually important, as in the central nervous system, clinical
manifestations may be directly attributable to cell destruction. Even
in those generalized virus infections in which severe clinical manifestations and death are due to general, rather than focal, physiological
disturbances, selective cell destruction may be so extensive as to
cause the functional failure of a vital organ to such a degree that this
dominates the clinical course of the disease and determines the outcome. Such is the case with the hepatic failure of yellow fever and
infective hepatitis. This, however, is exceptional. In most diseases the
failure of no single organ can be implicated as the underlying cause of
the clinical picture or, ultimately, of death.

There is increasing evidence that the shock syndrome is the common
end-channel in a large number of severe diseases of both viral and
bacterial origin, and that shock is induced in these by direct toxic
damage to the cardiovascular system. In virus diseases it is possible
that the virus particles themselves are the toxic factor and inflict the
critical damage through partial or complete cycles of replication in the
cells of the capillary endothelium. In the rickettsial diseases there is
ample direct evidence that this is the case.

However, even if this hypothesis should prove to be generally true,
it would still leave unexplained those milder and largely subjective
manifestations of constitutional disturbance such as the symptoms of
influenza and the common cold. It is as difficult to imagine that these
could be due to the toxic action of circulating virus as it is to believe
that the extensive tissue destruction of the more severe diseases should
fail to give rise to toxic products which could cause physiological
disturbance.

CHAPTER 8

Virus Adaptability and Host Resistance

G. BELYAVIN

Department of Bacteriology,
University College Hospital Medical School,
London, England

I. Introduction

Viruses are obligatory intracellular parasites and are thus wholly dependant upon the integrity of the cellular systems they parasitize for their survival in an active state. It is something of a paradox, therefore, that many viruses such as the bacteriophages, and the mammalian cytocidal viruses, ultimately destroy the cells they are living in.

Taking the "virus-eye view", the ideal situation would appear to be the one in which the virus replicates in cells without in any way disturbing their normal metabolism. This has been suggested as the ideal biological situation towards which all viruses are slowly evolving; at the same time it must be noted that an almost completely benign equilibrium of this kind between parasitic virus and cellular host can be found as a temporary phase of virus existence. The "latency" of human herpetic infections, and the lysogenic form of bacteriophage are two classical examples of such an equilibrium. It is not by any means certain, however, that normal virus replication proceeds under such conditions of latency. This situation is both biologically intriguing and relevant to the problem of virus adaptation, and will be considered in more detail later.

It is worth noting that if a virus were to attain a state of wholly benign equilibrium with its host cell, it is unlikely that its presence would be readily detected, or that it would be necessarily recognized as a "virus". It is logical to suggest therefore that such a state of affairs could be comparatively common in nature; indeed there are "entities" which can in some cases be just recognized as being transmissible, and yet can only be accepted as "viruses" in the contemporary sense of the word with certain reservations. The factor responsible for the Scrapie disease of sheep may be one such, as it is clearly transmissible not only from sheep to sheep, but also from sheep to goats, a species never affected in nature. Yet the entity concerned, unlike the majority of viruses, is remarkably thermostable, with-standing prolonged boiling, and disease develops only very slowly in experimental animals after an incubation period of several months. This may perhaps be a state of incipient virus–host equilibrium. As a possible example of complete equilibrium one may quote the chroma-toid body found in species of *Entamoeba*. Ultra-thin sections of enta-moebal cells examined under the electron microscope reveal that the chromatoid body is a crystalline array of uniformly spherical particles about 200 Å in diameter and strikingly similar to known intracellular virus aggregates (Plate 1) (Deutsch and Zaman, 1959). If, and it is obviously a very large if indeed, these particles do represent the homologue of a "virus", then this must represent almost complete integration between host and parasite. The stage immediately before this, and closely analogous to the lysogenic state of phage, is perhaps the K substance of paramecium.

If we subscribe to the view that such situations represent the evolu-tionary end-point of virus adaptation, then by making certain addi-tional assumptions, the circumstances of host–parasite adaptation observed in the paramecium and *Entamoeba* are wholly predictable, for what can be regarded as among the most primitive biological forms participate in the most advanced stages of virus adaptation. It should be added, however, that other speculators have suggested that such completely integrated states are really the beginning of virus develop-ment and that the fully "cytocidal" and individual "virus" is a later stage, asserting that the first evolutionary step is the random ap-pearance perhaps of an aberrant cytoplasmic gene. Such a suggestion has already been put forward by Darlington (1944). Obviously these are highly speculative views, but whatever the evolutionary significance of some of these observations may be, the phenomena of cell patho-genicity and intracellular latency are present facts of virus behaviour, and their biological significance must be considered in the light of their possible importance to continued virus survival and propagation.

As was emphasized in the first paragraph, a virus is wholly depend-ent, as far as we know, upon the cell it lives in for replication and continued survival. Clearly, if the cell dies or is destroyed as a result

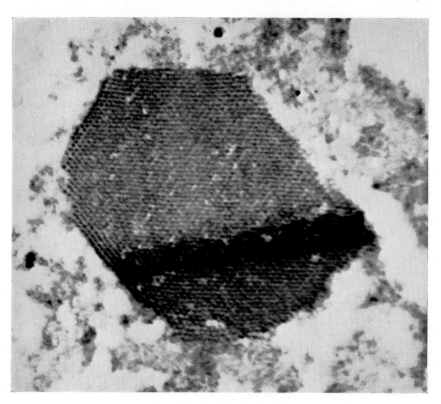

PLATE 1. Electron micrograph of chromatoid body of *Entamoeba Invadens* (Rodhain). (× 33,000).

(Photograph kindly supplied by Dr. V. Zaman.)

of agencies other than virus infection, the virus will cease to replicate, and may become simply a complex, though inert, macromolecule. This will be certain, unless the virus has means of subsequently entering and parasitizing other cells. Such means are undoubtedly possessed not only by actively "cytocidal" viruses but others as well, and the complex mechanisms for doing this which are highly developed among certain viruses, have been discussed in detail in other chapters. It is noteworthy, that a wholly benign virus, completely integrated with the functions of its host cell, and multiplying in step with the divisions of its host's cytoplasm, is trading heavily upon the potential immortality of such protoplasmic clones for its survival. Metazoon hosts are of course highly integrated and complex communities of cells. Virus parasitizing some of these cells may not only destroy a few of them by its cytocidal activity, but may also thereby encompass the death of the whole host, and thus place its own survival in jeopardy. By analogy with the single-cell situation, some means of spread from metazoon host to metazoon host clearly confers advantages in overcoming this difficulty.

These observations may be summarized by the following propositions:

(1) That the biological survival of a virus in a metazoon host is dependent upon the existence of cell-to-cell or intra-host pathways of spread.

(2) That cell-to-cell spread of virus may continue until (a) no more susceptible cells are left; (b) virus is rendered non-functional by neutralizing substances (e.g. antibodies); (c) the host dies as a whole; (d) in the case of a wholly intracytoplasmic "benign" virus, the cells involved are no longer able to replicate and the cell community begins to die—i.e. the normal life span of the metazoon host is achieved.

(3) That these "difficulties" are overcome by adaptation of the virus to methods of transference from one cell community to another— viz. inter-host pathways of spread.

While the transfer of virus along the inter-host pathways from one host to another involves no more in the final analysis than a simple cell-to-cell transfer, it must involve in addition the negotiation of many structural and functional barriers peculiar to the organization of a metazoon host. In addition, therefore, to the adaptive mechanisms acquired by a virus to enable it to pass from one cell to another initiating fresh infection, it must be adapted for negotiating the barriers which lie between the susceptible cells of one host and those of another. The ability of any one virus to negotiate both intra-host and inter-host pathways with a reasonable probability of success is a measure of its "adaptation".

The sum total of host barriers to be overcome are a measure of the resistance of the host system.

II. Inter-host Pathways

The modes of inter-host virus transfer observable in nature seem to be of two kinds: direct and indirect. In the case of direct transfer, virus apparently passes directly from one individual host to another, either by direct contact, or by exhalation and inhalation of, for instance, infected droplets of respiratory secretion. This mode of transfer is probably confined to mammalian viruses. Transfer may also occur by means of contaminated food and drink.

Indirect transfer involves some other host species which intervenes between the two host individuals, and is an active agent of transfer. Arthropod species are commonly found to act in this role, and either mosquitos, ticks, mites, or similar organisms may be involved. Taking the class of viruses as a whole, it is probably true that indirect transfer through some intermediary host species is by far the commoner form of the inter-host pathway, for not only is it involved in the transfer of many animal viruses, but it is also the principal mode of transfer for plant viruses, either aphids or leaf-hoppers being the main intermediary groups involved.

A. DIRECT MODES OF TRANSFER

The simplest version of a direct transfer pathway is where virus is carried directly from the susceptible cells in one host to correspondingly susceptible cells in another. This will be achieved where infection involves superficial layers of cells. Transfer could be brought about by direct contact between infected and uninfected cell layers, but, in fact, rarely occurs in nature in as direct a form as this. There is ample evidence, however, that where virus parasitization involves the respiratory epithelium of a mammal or bird, transfer of virus from the respiratory system of one host to that of another may occur by means of aerosol-formation. Under these conditions, there is no direct contact between infected and uninfected cells, but transfer of virus is nevertheless from cell to cell and is immediate in the sense that no replication of virus occurs or is necessary while passing from original host to new host.

The main problem concerning the virus in this very simple transfer pathway is that it must be able to survive long enough in the aerosol droplet to reach the cells of the new host in a viable form; that is, a reasonable proportion of the virus particles reaching susceptible cells of the host must be able to initiate successfully the stages of cell attachment, penetration and replication. It may be mentioned in passing that, in addition to the problem of virus survival, the host must be in a position to generate an aerosol from the respiratory tract. This is clearly true of most mammals and probably most birds.

Whatever the circumstances of formation of the aerosol may be, it is obvious that only a small fraction of all the virus expelled in the droplets will reach the respiratory epithelium of another host unless conditions of transfer are quite exceptional. This is a simple statistical fact. In theory, it should be necessary for only one viable virus particle to reach another host in order that infection should be established. Virologists, however, are by no means certain that this is so. The question as to whether a given virus particle, when placed in a suitable environment of susceptible cells, will prove to be "infective" (in the sense that it will induce the formation of more virus particles), can be answered in a number of ways. One can imagine witnessing a virus elementary body in an aerosol droplet impinging on the respiratory epithelium of a human being, and the virus particle being brought thereby in direct contact with an epithelial cell. The particle may rapidly penetrate the cell and initiate the replication process—we claim therefore that this particle was infective. Alternatively, we observe that nothing happens; the virus particle remains passively on the epithelial surface until removed by a passing phagocytic cell. Such a particle could be classed as "non-infective". Generally this classification of virus elementary bodies on the basis of a hypothetical observational experiment such as has just been described treats the property of "infectivity" as being an intrinsic property of the particle, and the property, in this sense, is analogous to the simple ideas of "dead" and "living" as we apply them to human beings or other animals. In the "real" world of virus particles we cannot carry out experiments of this kind. We can only place a number of virus particles in the midst of a population of susceptible cells, and see what happens to the cell population *as a whole*. One can estimate for instance the probable proportion of cells which were infected by the given number of particles. Alternatively, one may estimate what is the least number of particles of a given virus preparation which will initiate a self-sustaining infective process in the cell population which will ultimately infect and destroy most of the cells. Theoretically this should potentially be only one particle, but experimentally this hardly ever seems to be so with respect to the sorts of cellular population used in the laboratory.

Tissue-culture monolayers have been used in experiments of this kind. If a sheet of cells growing in a glass bottle is infected with discrete virus particles, then where a given particle initiates a process of cellular infection, sustained from cell to cell, an increasing area of cell destruction will form, provided the virus is cytocidal in the cell system concerned. Provided the virus particles are initially seeded on the cell sheet in a sufficiently well-dispersed distribution, so that the distances between neighbouring particles are very large with respect to the dimensions of the cells, and provided that steps are taken to limit the spread of cell-to-cell infection, the original position of each "infective" particle will be marked by a discrete zone of cell destruction, or "plaque". It is usual to limit the rate of cell-to-cell spread by "overlaying" the cell sheet with agar. By counting the number of plaques formed and comparing the result with the number of particles originally seeded, some estimate of the proportion of infective particles may be obtained. The estimate of the number of actual morphological particles being inoculated is usually obtained by direct counting of samples of the virus preparation under the electron microscope. In every case it is found that more than one particle, on the average, must be introduced into the host system, in order to induce one plaque. Thus, for Mahoney type 1 poliovirus, using monolayers of either human-amnion or monkey-kidney cells, it was found that anything from 20 to 90 particles of purified tissue-culture-grown virus were required to induce one plaque (Dulbecco and Vogt, 1954; Schwerdt and Fogh, 1957). A comparable system is the chorioallantoic membrane of the embryonated hen egg. Many viruses, including those of smallpox and vaccinia will multiply on the membrane with the formation of discrete, heaped up, foci of cells ("pocks") presumably induced by single-particle infections of the chorionic epithelial cells, by analogy with the "plaque" system. Here also, values of between 10 and 20 inoculated particles of purified vaccinia virus have been reported as being equivalent to one observed "pock" lesion (Dumbell, Downie and Valentine, 1957; Kaplan and Valentine, 1959). The exact interpretation of these results is still by no means clear. It is convenient to assume that, in every case, *one* particle of virus *should* be sufficient to initiate a plaque or pock. Supposing this were true, it would appear that even then *one* particle is not enough to produce such unequivocal signs of infection in the host systems studied. It would be too much of a digression to discuss all the implications of these experiments, and all the arguments that surround their interpretation. The immediate point is that we must answer our original question by saying that in all probability a single virus particle is not likely to be enough to induce self-sustaining infection in a natural host. Consideration of the conditions under which epidemic virus infections are propagated, particularly the respiratory infections which we have been discussing as hypothetical models, suggests that only a few particles of virus can be transmitted at each natural transfer of infection. There is very little published experimental data available to suggest just what this number may be. It is obvious, however, that the smaller the number of particles on the average required to infect, the more likely is the virus to establish itself in a fresh contact host; in other words, the greater will be the proportion of hosts successfully infected in any one exposure. This is a very important biological attribute for a virus to possess and it is clearly distinct from its capacity to survive in aerosol droplets. One may term this property the "transmissibility" of a virus. Perhaps the most striking aspect of this virus attribute is the fact that we know very little about it. Nevertheless, it is certain that "transmissibility" in the sense in which it has been defined above facilitates the adaptation of a virus to pathways of direct transfer.

The respiratory system of animals and birds is not the only portal of entry for the direct transmission of a virus. The epithelium lining the gastro-intestinal tract forms a closely analagous system, although the virus no longer travels from epithelial surface to epithelial surface in an aerosol, but simply in those materials which come in contact with the alimentary epithelium, i.e. food, drink and faeces. It is easy to understand how the pathway of transmission is maintained here simply by the contamination of food and drink by faecal matter. The situation is somewhat more complicated for the mammalian and bird viruses concerned in this version of the direct pathway, by the need to negotiate the relatively highly acid conditions of the stomach, and the presence of bile salts in the upper intestine. There is no doubt, however, that man (and probably most apes and monkeys) has become host to a wide range of viruses which parasitize his alimentary tract epithelium and are passed from individual to individual by some such simple chain of transmission as has been implied above. Many of these viruses are benign, in the sense that they do not give rise to any clinically apparent disease, although they are cytocidal in tissue culture, and must be presumed to produce some cellular damage *in vivo*, albeit limited exclusively to the alimentary tract epithelium, and perhaps small in extent. As the poliovirus is a member of this group of enteroviruses, it is clear that not all the members of this large group are equally benign in their current phase of adaptation to man.

All that has been said already on direct droplet transfer of virus infection has emphasized the essential simplicity of the process. Provided the virus is capable of surviving in an aerosol for a period of time which, under given conditions, may be no longer than the period of survival of the aerosol itself in the form of suspended droplets, then transmission can be effected. It is perhaps wise to qualify the word survival in the case of the virus by using the phrase "maintain its transmissibility", whatever that may mean. Nevertheless, the process is relatively simple when compared with the adaptations required of an enterovirus which has to be swallowed and passed through the varying pH and surface-tension-reducing conditions of the alimentary tract.

Where the susceptible cells are situated in deep tissues of the host, the virus may need to negotiate many epithelial and other barriers before establishing itself. There are a number of human-virus infections in which the virus is transmitted by droplet infection, via the respiratory tract, but in which the virus subsequently invades other body tissues, giving rise to a "systemic" type of infection. Measles and smallpox are two examples of such virus infection. Poliovirus is a corresponding example from among the enteroviruses (see Chapter 3).

Viruses which give rise to "systemic" infections of their metazoon hosts must pass through successive structural regions of the host. Thus it may be necessary to traverse certain external and internal epithelial layers, the blood-stream, the extracellular spaces of the host tissues, etc., before reaching the surface of the cell in which the virus will finally multiply. At each of these stages the virus particle is faced with agencies which can potentially arrest its progress. An epithelium can constitute a simple unbroken physical barrier, and the blood plasma and lymphatic fluid may contain specific substances such as antibodies or other "inhibitors" capable of blocking the effective surface of the virus particle. Not every tissue cell that the virus particle comes in contact with may permit either specific attachment to its surface or subsequent penetration and successful parasitization. These are the detailed elements of the host's resistance to infection. It is clear that viruses responsible for extensive systemic infection of metazoon hosts are exposed to a greater element of host resistance than viruses parasitizing more superficial epithelial layers, even though all are dependent on relatively simple direct inter-host transmission pathways for their propagation in the community of hosts. It is legitimate to enquire whether this difference in adaptation is linked to any other significant differences in biological character. This will be considered in a later section.

B. INDIRECT INTER-HOST PATHWAYS

There are many animal viruses which are dependent upon a more complex inter-host pathway for their propagation within a host community. The essential feature of these pathways is that transfer of infective virus from host A1, to host A2 (both members of species A) takes place via host B1, belonging to species B. The chain of transmission involves a strict species alternation, so that transference of virus will go:

$$A1 \rightarrow B1 \rightarrow A2 \rightarrow B2 \rightarrow A3 \rightarrow B3 \rightarrow \ldots \ldots$$

Such a sequence constitutes the "indirect" type of inter-host pathway, and in such a pathway it is found that species A and species B may differ very profoundly in their taxonomic positions. Thus, it is common to find that whereas species A may be a mammal or bird, species B is very commonly an arthropod.

In spite of variations in the biological details of the various indirect transmission pathways found in nature, a certain overall pattern can be discerned. Thus, virtually all the viruses known to maintain themselves by such pathways are "systemic" in their intra-host distribution. That is to say the virus invades the host tissues and distributes itself widely, so that virus multiplication may take place in a number of cellular sites. Under such circumstances virus is always present in the blood of the host at some stage of its intra-host dissemination, although the ultimate pathology may be predominantly localized to one or two viscera. The transmitting host is thus always a blood-sucking one, and also capable of supporting some virus replication. Under these conditions it is found that the host transmissions A → B, and B → A are always direct, being dependent upon the fact that B preys upon the blood of A; and when virus is present in A's blood, B will become infected as it feeds. Once it is infected, B will then infect A again at its next feed.

This fundamental pattern has undergone varying degrees of elaboration in nature. One of the classical examples is that of yellow fever. This disease was known for some 200 years or more as an acute epidemic disease of man occurring in the tropical and subtropical regions of the Americas and West Africa. At the beginning of this century it was conclusively shown that urban yellow fever, in the form that yearly occurred in Havana, was transmitted from man to man by the bite of the *Aedes aegypti* mosquito, which mosquito was shown to harbour the virus in an active state from initial infection by a blood meal contaminated with virus to the completion of its life span. This was dramatically confirmed in the field by the virtual elimination of yellow fever from Havana, by the elimination of *A. aegypti*.

The control measures which were developed from this experience made possible the ultimate completion of the Panama canal and the apparent virtual eradication of yellow fever from tropical America. The true complexity of the situation, however, became apparent within the next 20 years or so, when outbreaks of yellow fever in rural areas and in regions where *A. aegypti* did not normally breed began to be reported (Soper *et al.*, 1933). Since 1940, something of the transmission pattern of what is known as jungle yellow fever has been elucidated. Suspicion had centred from the earliest investigations on certain species of *Haemagogus* mosquitoes. It was shown experimentally that, for instance, *Haemagogus spegazzini* (Shannon, Whitman and Franca, 1938) could transmit and maintain the yellow-fever virus. Sample trappings, however, suggested that this species was rare in the jungle and in marginal jungle lands; too rare, in fact, to be responsible for effective transmission of yellow fever to occasional human intruders. A chance observation gave the clue to the solution. It was found that *H. spegazzini* is a mosquito species that commonly lives largely in the tree canopy of the rain-forest areas. Here the female relies mainly on various species of monkeys for blood meals, as these mammals are relatively common in the tree-canopy level. During tree felling, for marginal clearance or for timber, large clouds of *Haemagogus* mosquitoes may be released at ground level, and under these conditions the wood cutters are particularly likely to be bitten, with the attendant risk of contracting jungle yellow fever.

It is clear from this that the yellow-fever virus can maintain itself in two mammalian hosts; in certain monkeys, and in man. In each host species, transmission from host to host is effected by means of a specific species of mosquito. Occasional transfer of virus may occur from one pathway to the other; for instance, from the jungle monkey–*Haemagogus*–monkey cycle, to the urban man–*Aedes*–man one.

Although it is known that there are many other viruses which depend upon arthropod vectors for their maintenance in vertebrate host communities, the details of the transmission pathways are not sufficiently well-determined for comparison with the yellow-fever pattern to be made. It is certain that in several cases, such as the western and eastern equine encephalitides found mainly in the U.S.A., more than one species of mosquito is involved in the transmission of the virus. Western equine encephalitis, for instance, is primarily a disease of horses and mules, but human outbreaks also occur from year to year, interspersed with occasional explosive epidemics. The virus has also been isolated from squirrels, deer, pigs and birds. Although there is good evidence to implicate *Culex tarsalis* as the main mosquito involved, it is known that other species belonging to the genera *Aedes*, *Anopheles* and *Arliseta* have been found infected in nature, or shown experimentally to be capable of maintaining and transmitting the virus. No field data are available, however, to suggest that transmission from horse to horse and man to man is effected by different species of mosquito. In fact, it is by no means clear that the main pathway of transfer maintaining the virus in its principal host population runs either through man or the horse. It is considered more likely (Hammon, 1948; Reeves, 1951) that the infection is maintained in wild birds by transmission through appropriate mosquito species, and that transfer to equines or man is incidental, so that these species do not constitute separate stable host populations, in which the virus consistently maintains itself.

C. ARBOR VIRUSES AS A BIOLOGICAL FAMILY

There are many known viruses exhibiting a very similar pattern of indirect transmission in nature. As the host intermediate to the vertebrate one is in every case an arthropod, it is customary to class these viruses together as the group of Arbor (or arthropod-borne) viruses. In defining the group it is usual to emphasize the following points:

(a) Transmission is regarded as being primarily from one vertebrate host to another (usually bird or mammal).
(b) The transmitting agent is an arthropod, either insect, tick or mite.
(c) The virus must be capable of multiplication in the arthropod vector, without, however, producing disease; i.e., the virus is not "pathogenic" to the vector.

Paragraph (c) explicitly excludes those circumstances relevant to certain non-Arbor viruses, where the virus may be passively transferred on the proboscis of a blood-sucking arthropod by chance contamination. Considerable evidence has been accumulated to indicate that this is the principal way in which myxomatosis infection is transferred from rabbit to rabbit in Australia. No multiplication of the myxomatosis virus has been demonstrated in those mosquito species principally implicated (Fenner, Day and Woodroofe, 1952; Day, Fenner and Woodroofe, 1956).

Some 46 Arbor viruses are currently distinguishable on the basis of their antigenic structure and general physical and biological properties (Casals and Reeves, 1959). All but four of these have a particle size lying in the range 15–40 mμ, all are rapidly inactivated by ether or sodium desoxycholate, and all invade the tissues of the vertebrate host with some degree of general systemic involvement. Ten of the viruses in this group localize predominantly in the central nervous system of the host, and constitute all the known primary viral encephalitides of man. It should be emphasized that the poliovirus now generally accepted as a member of the enterovirus group does not typically give rise to clinical encephalitis in man, the virus usually localizing in the motor neurones of the brain stem and spinal cord. It is true that other viruses (such as measles or mumps) will not uncommonly give rise to signs of cerebral and meningeal involvement. Extension of viral infection to the central nervous system in these diseases, however, is usually only incidental to the general widespread involvement of other tissues in the body, and is not a typical feature of the disease.

The uniform ability of the viruses in this group to multiply in other than purely superficial cells of their vertebrate hosts, together with their capacity to parasitize certain arthropod tissue cells, are manifestly essential conditions of their adaptation to an indirect inter-host pathway, using arthropod species as intermediaries.

This adaptation is correlated with a notable degree of neurotropism, but there is nothing to indicate what the biological significance, if any, of this fact may be. The general biological uniformity of the group, such as it is, is perhaps best regarded as a reflection of their adaptation to a common form of inter-host pathway.

III. Virus-host Equilibrium

It has already been emphasized that if a virus is to survive it must achieve some independence from the host cell which it parasitizes so intimately. Furthermore, where the cell is integrated in the cell community of a metazoon host, the virus must be to some extent independent not only of the cell but also of the whole host as well. It is because of this, one presumes, that viruses have become adapted to using pathways of intra-host and inter-host transfer. It has been suggested, indeed, that only the constituent ribo- or deoxyribo-nucleic acid of a virus particle, upon which perhaps its capacity to replicate wholly depends, is the true "virus", the external layers which wrap it around being only adaptative structures upon which the "virus" relies for its successful transference from cell to cell and from host to host. This speculative view serves to emphasize that it is only in the cytoplasm of a suitable cell that a virus reveals itself as a dynamic biological entity endowed with self-replicating properties. Outside this cell it is merely a highly modified "spore", adapted specifically for survival in the extracellular environment and for attack on and penetration into a new host cell.

The orthodox biological view is that viruses have become adapted to specific host species in nature by a process of selection, whereby the resistance factors of the host have selected out variant particles capable of circumventing these factors. The adaptation by selection hypothesis may, of course, be applied also from the host point of view, for the virus may select out those host individuals whose resistance factors are most effective. Where parasitization leads to rapid death of the host in the majority of cases, selection pressure must tend to act against the virus, as it is the most "transmissible" particles which will tend to spread and ultimately be lost from the virus population as a result of the rapid death of the majority of the hosts. At the same time the most susceptible hosts are eliminated. A purely qualitative interpretation of this argument suggests that equilibrium will be reached between host species and virus in terms of a less "susceptible" host and a less "pathogenic" virus. We are brought back again at this point to the original question: did viruses originate as disease-producing entities, which are gradually evolving towards a state of wholly benign integration with the cells of their hosts? Or does the process work the other way round by progression from benignancy to malignancy? After all, transfer of a virus to a laboratory animal not normally susceptible in nature will often lead to enhanced virulence of the virus for that species after a large number of passages. Ignoring for the moment the question of how viruses became intracellular parasites at all, the argument initially deployed above suggests that, whatever state of "pathogenicity" is achieved by a virus with respect to a given host in nature, there will always be a tendency towards some degree of ultimate benign equilibrium. On the other hand, as artificial transmission of a virus under laboratory conditions is undertaken whether the infected host dies or not, strong selection in favour of virus pathogenicity would be expected.

The problem of the probable biological origin and evolution of the viruses, fascinating as it is, is largely speculative and cannot properly concern us here. The reality of virus-host equilibria, however, is a question of some practical importance in the study of virus infections in the human community, and is moreover susceptible to observation and experiment. Evidence for the attainment of host–virus equilibria and the nature of the mechanisms involved must therefore be considered.

A. Host–virus Equilibria Observed in Nature

1. General concepts

The concept of a host–virus equilibrium has already been discussed in a very general manner. Before examining the circumstances of this biological situation more closely, it is perhaps proper that our mental picture of it should be more explicitly defined. Thus: A state of equilibrium is deemed to exist between a virus and its metazoon host when the virus can maintain itself in the host's cells without inducing more than the maximum of cell damage compatible with the normal physiological functions and survival of the host. This definition is specifically formulated with the multicellular host in mind. There is, of course, no difficulty in translating it into the conditions of virus–cell equilibrium, which are already implicit in it to some extent. Equilibrium at the cell level, however, which leads on to a consideration of latent virus infections, will be examined in a later section. For the moment, it is convenient to restrict the discussion to the multicellular host; by this restriction one must leave aside any consideration of one of the most classical and well documented examples of virus–host equilibria—the lysogenic or symbiotic bacteriophage state.

Amongst human virus infections, herpes simplex yields one of the best examples of a human host–virus equilibrium state, as defined above. Human infection with the herpes simplex virus is very commonly contracted either in infancy or early childhood, presumably from another human being. Not infrequently the initial infection is a systemic one, and the characteristic skin lesions appear as a fairly widespread vesicular and papular rash. There may be high fever and signs of central-nervous-system involvement such as coma, tremors, and convulsions. A small proportion of infants may die as the result of such a generalized infection.

After recovery, the virus may persist in the tissues of an otherwise perfectly healthy and normal host. This is evident from the fact that certain physiological stimuli in later life, such as exposure to intense sunlight or fever due to a cold, will precipitate a small outcrop of typical herpetic vesicles, usually around the mouth. These can be shown in most cases, to contain infective herpes virus. The precise nature of the virus–host equilibrium in this infection is not known, but is examined in more detail below in the discussion of the phenomena of latency (Section III A 3). At this stage it is appropriate only to enquire how the virus manages to maintain itself in the community as a whole. It seems reasonable to suppose that dissemination of virus must occur from active clinical cases of herpes simplex, the main source of virus being presumably from the vesicles. Frank clinical disease is, however, relatively rare in any community, and its incidence is much lower than would be inferred from the proportion of individuals having herpes antibodies in their serum. The inference is therefore that many primary infections are sub-clinical, and that these infections form the main infectious reservoir. If so, virus transmission in the absence of overt vesicles must be presumed to be by aerosol droplets from the respiratory tract. This supposition is given some basis by the fact that virus has been isolated on a few occasions from the saliva of recurrent cases. It is at least possible that persons carrying the virus as a latent infection will periodically excrete it in the saliva, without necessarily manifesting the presence of active virus by the appearance of a crop of typical vesicles.

There is also the possibility that a latently infected mother will infect her child either *in utero* or in the immediate post-natal period, when there may be very close contact between mother and infant. Cases of neonatal generalized herpes, occurring sometimes within the first week of life, have been reported, but they are rare and no clear relationship has been established with latent infection in the mother.

These facts illustrate the theoretical difficulties of understanding how a virus may maintain itself in a community once some degree of "benign equilibrium" has been achieved with the host. Where the degree of equilibrium is such that cell breakdown is a rare event, spread by direct transfer to daughter cells as a result of cytoplasmic division probably becomes the primary means of maintaining the virus in the host. For its maintenance in the community of hosts some mechanism of inter-host transfer is needed, other than the ones already mentioned which depend upon free release of virus from cells. A mechanism which would serve the purpose effectively is transfer of virus from parent to offspring through the germinal cells. Although this is not known to occur in the case of the mammalian viruses, its demonstration in future would not be surprising, for it is well established as a mechanism whereby certain rickettsiae pathogenic for man are maintained in benign association with the arthropod vectors of the diseases in question.

2. The epidemiology of myxomatosis

Although the way in which viruses may achieve "host equilibrium" can be suggested, most of the virus–host systems already in equilibrium probably achieved this state many thousands of years ago. The systems now in the process of achieving equilibrium, if such is the general tendency of the virus–host relationship, are probably doing it so slowly that it is difficult to discern what is actually happening. It is not easy, therefore, to obtain direct observational evidence of how a virus can achieve equilibrium with its host in nature. In the last decade, however, the use of myxomatosis as a means of eradicating the rabbit in Australia, and the spread of the disease to Europe, have provided situations which have given some very suggestive clues regarding the general trend of the virus–host relationship.

Myxomatosis as a disease of rabbit stocks was first observed in 1896 as an outbreak in experimental rabbits housed in a laboratory in Montevideo. It was shown that the disease was caused by a virus, and Aragão (1943) ultimately demonstrated that this virus was present as a natural infection in the Brazilian "tapeti", *Sylvilagus braziliensis*, which is a species related to the cottontail rabbit of North America. In this wild species, the infection was benign, giving rise usually to small subcutaneous tumours of a mainly fibromatous nature. The virus was shown to be present in the cells of this tumour, and natural transmission appeared to be effected from rabbit to rabbit by the bite of a mosquito. Transfer of the virus to varieties of the European rabbit, *Orycytolagus cuniculus*, resulted in a severe systemic infection, followed by rapid death in more than 99% of the infected animals. Shope demonstrated that the American cotton-tail rabbit (*Sylvilagus spp.*) was also prone to an infective benign tumour in nature, but transmission of this to European rabbit stocks only resulted in the formation of similar moderately sized fibromatous tumours, which regressed rapidly after 10–12 days (Shope, 1932). European rabbits convalescent from the fibromatous tumour were shown to be resistant to infection with virulent myxomatosis virus, and, conversely, any rabbits which recovered from myxomatosis were shown to be refractory to infection with the Shope fibroma. The causative viruses of the two conditions must therefore be extremely closely related and probably represent mutants from a common progenitor virus. To complete the picture, it was also confirmed that the wild American cotton-tail rabbit is virtually immune to experimentally inoculated myxomatosis (Shope, 1932). There is therefore very suggestive evidence here of the establishment of host–virus equilibrium between the myxomatosis virus and species of the genus *Sylvilagus* in the first instance. In the case of the Shope-fibroma virus, equilibrium seems to have been achieved by a combination of increased resistance of the cotton-tail rabbit host, and diminished pathogenicity of the virus. The situation existing in South America differs in the fact that the "tapeti" host has become resistant to the tissue-invasive properties of the virus, although the latter has retained a very high degree of virulence for the European rabbit.

The deliberate introduction of a highly virulent strain of myxomatosis virus into Australian rabbit populations, and the subsequent introduction of this disease into Europe, have permitted some field observations to be made on the interaction between virus and fully susceptible host.

Strains isolated from different field outbreaks of myxomatosis in Australia and in Europe and the United Kingdom have been compared carefully with respect to their virulence for the fully susceptible European rabbit as bred for laboratory stocks (Fenner and Marshal, 1957). By allocating these strains to five defined grades of virulence and tabulating the number of outbreaks in each year yielding strains of these varying grades, it was possible to show that in Australia some diminution in virulence of the epizootic strains had occurred during the five years elapsing since the original introduction of the virus (Table I).

As there had been several re-introductions of fully virulent virus during this period, the accumulation of relatively less virulent epizootic strains is all the more striking. It was noted by Fenner and his co-workers that although there was fairly rapid attenuation of strain virulence to the level at which there was a mean mortality of about 90% among susceptible stocks, there was little apparent tendency for the virus to attenuate further; if any further diminution of strain

TABLE I

Rabbit myxomatosis. "Virulence grades" of virus strains isolated in successive years.*

Grade of virus virulence	I	II	III	IV	V
Case mortality rate in laboratory stock rabbits	99·5%	99·0%	90%	60–70%	0–30%
Mean survival time (days)	<13	>13<16	28> >16	50> >28	—
Australia					
Year of virus isolations					
1950–51	1	0	0	0	0
1951–52	2	3	1	0	0
1952–53	1	1	8	2	0
1953–54	1	4	5	1	0
1954–55	3	2	7	4	0
Europe and United Kingdom					
1953	3	0	0	0	0
1954	7	0	1	0	0
1955	3	0	0	2	1

* See Fenner and Marshall, *J. Hyg. Camb.*, **55**, 149 (1957).

virulence was occurring, it seemed to be proceeding very much more slowly. Thus, although in the 1952-53 warm season there were eight outbreaks yielding eight Grade III strains and two Grade IV, in the season 1954-55 the comparable yields were still seven Grade III and four Grade IV (see Table I). Fenner and his collaborators have attributed this apparent stabilization of virus virulence at this level to the fact that rabbits infected with strains of rather lower virulence have a longer mean survival time. As mosquitoes do not feed on dead rabbits, the prolongation of the period during which the rabbit will have exposed superficial lesions from which virus may be spread will considerably enhance the dissemination of the virus in the community. One presumes that strains of high virulence, killing the rabbit quickly in under 13 days, must spread more slowly, owing to the smaller chance of transmission. Such strains are presumably "self-quenching" and therefore more readily replaced by the strain with the longer killing time.

It is interesting that it has been found that strains of greater attenuation fail, on the whole, to establish themselves in the rabbit communities. This has been observed not only in Australia but also in Europe and Great Britain. Thus, two strains of low virulence (Nottingham and Sussex) have been isolated in Great Britain producing highly atypical lesions, but these have shown little tendency to spread widely in the rabbit populations. It may be presumed that such strains "quench" themselves by virtue of the fact that too few lesions of a suitable kind are formed, and too many rabbits recover and become immune, for the strains to establish themselves rapidly in the population.

The apparently uniform failure of low-virulence strains to establish themselves as dominant epizootic strains in both Australia and U.K. is suggestive of the fact that the fundamental ecology of the disease is very similar in the two countries. It has been pointed out that whereas myxomatosis has spread in Australia by virtue of simple mechanical transmission of virus by appropriate mosquitoes, this is not the case in U.K., where little evidence of mosquito transmission has been found. Although some experimental data have been published suggesting that the virus is capable of overwintering in hibernating females of *Anopheles atroparvus* (Andrewes, Muirhead-Thomson and Stevenson, 1956; Muirhead-Thomson, 1956), simple mechanical transmission has taken place principally through the bite of the rabbit flea *Spilopsyllus*. If the main vectors play a purely passive role in the transmission of the virus, it is perhaps only to be expected that they will not influence the rate at which the virus undergoes modification of virulence. At the same time, information on spread and field mortalities among rabbits in myxomatosis outbreaks in U.K. is not as detailed as that provided by Fenner and his collaborators for the Australian epizootics, and there may be factors present in the British outbreaks which may have independently influenced the pattern of strain virulence. While it is true that the period of observation is shorter, it is notable that there has been a less rapid shift to intermediate virulence levels among strains isolated from outbreaks in Europe and U.K.

A mean mortality rate of 90%, as evinced by the widely epizootic

Grade III strains, is sufficient to allow some selection of relatively resistant rabbits. Putting it in another way, it would appear that strains of this level of virulence will kill all the rabbits in a community except those which are most resistant, amounting to approximately 10%. It is of course quite likely that some of these survivors of natural field epizootics may survive for reasons other than high innate resistance. Their survival may be due to chance protection from exposure or the reception of too small a dose of virus; however, it is not unreasonable to suppose that some of these survivors are drawn from the most resistant fraction of the population. If this is so, and provided the resistance is genetically transmissible, some increase in overall resistance of the rabbit population to myxomatosis may be expected. Experimental data have been obtained recently suggesting that such an increase in innate species-resistance of the Australian rabbit has already occurred (Marshal and Fenner, 1958). Thus, it does not seem unreasonable to suppose that ultimately the Australian rabbit and the myxomatosis virus can achieve an equilibrium comparable to the cotton-tail-fibroma situation of the North American continent. Whether the virologist and agricultural economist will allow this to take place is, of course, another matter. The whole experiment has revealed in a beautiful manner the delicate interplay between virus virulence, host resistance and virus transmissibility that is probably necessary in order to adapt a virus to a condition of relatively benign equilibrium with its host.

3. The phenomenon of "latent" virus infection

In the ultimate state of integration between virus and host the virus replicates intracellularly without disturbing the physiological integrity of the cell. Such a situation is virtually achieved by the symbiotic (or "lysogenic") bacteriophages, where the bacterial cell continues to metabolize and divide, and the replication of the genetic material of the phage keeps pace with the multiplication of the cell's genome, without apparently interfering with its normal functions. The presence of such non-functional phage material may, however, be readily demonstrated by subjecting the bacterial cell to a physiological shock, such as transient irradiation with ultra-violet light. Under these conditions "normal" bacteriophage synthesis may be restored, and the cell lyses with release of active phage. Also, the addition of a "carrier" bacterial culture to a culture of normal uninfected bacteria will rapidly induce proliferation of phage and lysis in the latter. Hence the use of the term "lysogenic" in connection with the symbiotically infected bacterial strain. This suggests that there must be *some* formation and release of fully biological potent phage in cultures of lysogenic strains, but that for some reason this active phage cannot induce progressive lysis of the culture as a whole. Several workers have proposed such an explanation (Lwoff and Gutmann, 1950; Boyd, 1951) and have also demonstrated that bacterial cells carrying a symbiotic phage are fully capable of adsorbing more phage of the same type, so that immunity to lysis is not brought about by failure of the surface adsorption mechanism. Modern concepts of the factors and mechanisms involved in this immunity are discussed in Chapter 2.

It is difficult not to be struck by the superficial similarities between a symbiotic bacteriophage system and latent human infection with herpes simplex virus. The activation of the clinically dormant herpes virus by certain physiological stimuli constitutes a noteworthy point of resemblance. Detailed study of animal-virus behaviour of this kind, however, can only be achieved in tissue cultures, which offer conditions similar to those existing in bacterial cultures, and much work has now been done in this field (see Symposium on Latency, 1958).

In a multicellular organism it is always possible that active cytocidal virus infection of some tissue cells may occur without any gross effects on the physiology of the whole organism. There is ample evidence to show that parasitization of this kind is very common, and constitutes the "sub-clinical" form of virus infection. At the cellular level, however, there is no reason to suppose that this type of infection necessarily differs in any important respect from the same process as it occurs in an overtly "clinically" infected host, and it is usual to ascribe the difference between "clinical" and "subclinical" or "asymptomatic" infections solely to differences in the extent of cellular involvement. Such an assumption may or may not be correct; one certainly cannot assert unequivocally that this is the only reason, for complex intracellular factors may exist capable of modifying both the degree and form of cellular involvement.

The argument may be clarified by considering three basic virus–cell situations which can occur in infected tissue cultures:

(1) The virus is actively cytocidal. Cells are infected and destroyed, the virus spreading quickly through the cell population, by virtue of its rapid growth.
(2) The virus is cytocidal but virus growth is slow, and spread through the cell population is only gradual.
(3) The virus is not cytocidal, and there is little release from cells, spread through the culture being mainly by division of infected cells.

Situation (1) is comparable to the state of affairs when a multicellular host is infected with a virulent virus which causes acute tissue necrosis, as, for example, in the acute liver atrophy of yellow fever. Situation (2) may result in a condition analogous to the host–virus association of a sub-clinical infection. Situation (3) may conceivably arise as a result of true virus latency at the cellular level. In situation (2) the direct recognition of infection depends upon the proportion of cells undergoing degeneration at any given moment. If, say, in a population of 40,000,000 cells about 1,000,000 are degenerating at any one time, the one degenerate cell in 40 might be impossible to detect by simple microscopical observation. Demonstration of the presence of a virus in the culture might indeed necessitate passage to a more sensitive cell system. This is analogous to the subclinical infections of man which are revealed by virus isolations effected by either serial passages through laboratory animals or cell cultures. In situation (3) the intracellular multiplication of virus often results in observable changes which obviously reflect some disturbance of normality, so that neither sub-clinical infection nor true latency comes into question. For example, HeLa-cell cultures infected with measles virus show syncitial giant-cell formation, and in many other systems intracellular inclusion bodies appear. Theoretically at least, however, the spread of virus solely by division of infected cells, and without observable morphological or physiological changes in the cells, is possible. While there is no conclusive evidence that this does in fact ever occur in tissue-culture systems, and therefore no compelling reason for accepting its occurrence in the multicellular host, the possibility derives some support from circumstantial evidence.

It is unlikely that stable equilibrium would persist for any length of time if the only operative factors were the basic ones of cell multiplication and cell infection leading to cell death with release of more virus. *In vivo*, certain extrinsic factors such as circulating antibodies are readily demonstrable, but even from tissue-culture systems there is accumulating evidence that other intrinsic factors may play an important role. Henle *et al.* (1958) showed that Newcastle-disease virus and mumps virus growing in tissue cultures of mouse fibroblasts (MCN cells) give rise to persistent inapparent infections, in which only a small proportion of the cells (about 1 in 10 to 1 in 40) appear to carry infective virus. As the proportion of infective cells appeared to be of the same order of magnitude in several successive tissue cultures, it is a fair inference that this proportion probably remained substantially constant for long periods of time. Subsequently Henle and his co-workers showed that these tissue-culture systems contain measurable amounts of interferon and suggested that it is the interferon which acts as the stabilizing mechanism (Henle *et al.*, 1959).

It is certainly possible that interferon may act in such a way that collisions of virus particles with uninfected cells, while leading to adsorption of virus and cell penetration, fail to result in infection and thus constitute a "feed-back" mechanism which will stabilize the amount of cellular infection at a low level. The effect of the interferon, however, would probably build up to the required level only slowly in the culture, for the essential factor would be that there should be enough interferon present to render a significantly large proportion of the uninfected cells refractory to infection.

The theory of feed-back mechanisms indicates that a simple feed-back arrangement, in which the feed-back acts slowly or with some delay, does not stabilize but results in oscillation with varying frequency about the equilibrium position. As will be mentioned in a later section, human populations exposed to epidemic infections contain feed-back mechanisms of this type where the accumulation of immune individuals forms the essential feed-back control. Such systems can show well-marked oscillations of disease incidence. There is no evidence to suggest that similar oscillations occur commonly in these infected-tissue cultures. This of course does not constitute a conclusive argument against the possible role of interferon as a stabilizing agent. The mere presence of interferon by itself does not, however, indicate that it is the essential controlling factor; its presence may to some extent be incidental.

Some direct experimental evidence has been published recently suggesting that interferon may play some part in maintaining an "inapparent" infection in a tissue culture. It has been shown that vaccinia virus inoculated into a monolayer culture of mouse-embryo cells (3-B line) will stimulate the production of interferon (Glasgow and Habel, 1962). If the conditions under which the culture is maintained are properly adjusted, viz. if the growth medium is changed sufficiently frequently to prevent the accumulation of too high a level of interferon, a fairly high level of infection can be maintained for up to 30 days or more. Thus, by changing the medium approximately every four days and ensuring that about 10–20% of the spent medium was left *in situ* at every change, the virus concentration in the medium could be maintained at around 10^3 PFU/ml for up to 28 days. If, however, the culture was exposed to trypsin or more frequent changes of media (i.e. every two days), then virus rapidly accumulated in the medium and cytopathogenic effect spread through the culture. This could be correlated with a rapid fall in the interferon concentration. It is notable that even in the moderately stabilized culture the virus concentration fell slowly over most of the experimental period, and on the thirtieth day was only a tenth of what it was on the second day after initial seeding. The authors emphasize the fact that whatever degree of equilibrium was achieved in the experimental cultures was always delicately balanced, and it was not difficult to precipitate the culture into a state of total cell destruction, or conversely to engender almost complete elimination of the virus. One of the experiments published is particularly interesting as it suggests the occurrence of oscillations of virus concentration in the culture before finally the cells were virtually overwhelmed (Fig. 1). The initiation of these states was also dependent upon the virus seeding being not too large (apparently of the order of 0·5 PFU per cell).

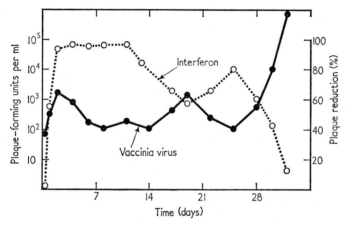

FIG. 1. Levels of vaccinia virus and interferon in tissue cultures maintained for long periods by frequent changing of medium (after Glasgow and Habel (1962). *J. exp. Med.* **115**, 503).

Although these results are of great interest, the suggestion that they constitute good evidence of the role of interferon in maintaining virus–cell equilibria can only be accepted with reservation. Clearly, under the conditions of the experiments frequently changing of the culture medium would wash out not only free interferon but also excess free virus. Furthermore, these conditions could accelerate cell growth to an extent which would surely affect the rate of spread of infection through the cell population quite considerably. Apart from factors of this kind, it is obvious that other selective influences could conceivably be at work, leading to the accumulation of more resistant cells or less cytopathogenic virus in the system.

There is no doubt that a better understanding of the behaviour to be expected in tissue-culture systems under different conditions of virus infection and propagation would be a great help in interpreting the experimental data. A fertile approach would perhaps be the construction of mathematical models utilizing a stochastic approach, particularly as such models would be well adapted to solution by computer.

Although it is not clear whether, in general, animal viruses can adapt to cell populations in such a way as to achieve relatively benign equilibrium, it is now becoming increasingly certain that particular viruses can exist in association with cells in such a way as to lose most of their biological identity as viruses while in the cell. Thus, it has been shown that mouse or hampster cells grown *in vitro* can be infected with polyoma virus, leading to the usual rapid intracellular replication of virus with cell degeneration and release of free virus. A proportion of cells, however, will show a modified response. In these there is a marked morphological transformation, and such cells can be shown to have undergone a neoplastic change, as the derived daughter cells can be propagated as tumours by grafting in appropriate animal hosts. Such cells, however, carry little if any detectable virus, although it is possible that virus elements are still present in the cell, for they are resistant to further infection with polyoma virus (Vogt and Dulbecco, 1960; Dulbecco and Vogt, 1960; Hellström, Hellström and Sjögren, 1962). This perhaps is the closest analogy yet found between the integration of an animal virus with its host cell and the lysogenic phage state. The important difference, however, is the evident physiological modification of the parasitized cell, indicating that the "equilibrium" between parasite and host is not without some grossly disturbing effects on the latter.

The possibility of an intracellular integration by a virus, leading to the formation of a neoplastic growth, is of very considerable interest. From a purely biological point of view, such an outcome can be regarded as being essentially disadvantageous to the virus, for it becomes less transmissible by direct pathways and the metazoon host is likely to die of neoplastic disease. In this sense, it is a form of virus–host adaptation which would have little survival value in nature from the point of view of either virus or host, and in the nature of things would presumably be eliminated by selective forces. It is, of course, remotely possible that "free virus elements" arose initially in neoplasms as a special adaptation to survival, and that the ability of certain viruses to reverse the process is merely the retention of a relatively primitive habit of existence. This highly fanciful speculation has little to support it, except that it suggests the possible origin of viruses as parasites. If, in fact, the tendency of all virus–host interactions is towards a state of relatively benign equilibrium, then it is difficult to see how the initial primitive state could be other than one of active pathogenicity for the host. It is conceivable that this could arise initially by the chance appearance of a spontaneous, transmissible oncolytic agent.

B. ROLE OF ANTIBODY IN ESTABLISHING VIRUS–HOST EQUILIBRIUM

1. General mechanism

Little has been said up to now of the effect of antibody on the establishment of a virus in a host community. Antibody is intrinsically a "host" defence and is a factor which probably contributes largely to the "quenching" of a virus infection in a community. The failure of the least virulent myxomatosis strains to establish themselves in rabbit warrens is presumably due to the relatively large proportion of recovered rabbits with circulating antibody which accumulate in epizootics initiated by such mild strains. Such a factor must be an important contribution to the multifarious biological barriers which a virus must overcome in order to maintain itself in the community of hosts. A virus which is highly virulent seems, on the face of it, to gain the advantage of reducing the accumulation of immunes in the community. At the same time high virulence is not conducive to the preservation of many hosts. Provided, however, a small proportion of hosts survive in a non-immune state, perhaps by virtue of non-exposure, their small numbers and associated high spatial dilution will tend to maintain a slower spread of virus until there is a further influx of susceptibles into the community by immigration, and further breeding.

It is evident from this that it makes little difference whether a virus mainly kills or mainly immunizes its host; the outcome is ultimately the same, in so far as it involves effective reduction of the available susceptibles. It does, however, make a big difference where a virus is capable of surviving in a moderately immune host, in a "latent" form, for this may ensure survival of the virus in the immune community.

It has been suggested that the accumulation of antibody-immune hosts in a community acts as a "feed-back" mechanism which must tend to quench the spread of infection. Such simple direct feed-back mechanisms usually lead to wide oscillations of the system around the point of equilibrium, and it has been shown that this is precisely the mechanism responsible for the periodic epidemicity of measles. In this case, the successive accumulation of immunes and susceptibles ensures the periodic rapid accumulation of cases. Many other virus diseases show an epidemic periodicity, although few as regular a periodicity as that shown by measles.

The accumulation of antibody-immune hosts in a given population could act not only as a suppressive "feed-back" mechanism with respect to virus but also as a selective mechanism. Antigenic variants, if they appear in a population of virus particles as a transmissible variation, must have a selective advantage in such an immune community. Any epidemic periodicity which appears in such a system is more likely to be related to the periodic appearance of antigenic variants than to a "feed-back" mechanism of the kind described above. In relation to these factors, it is interesting to note that viruses seem to fall into two major categories from the point of view of antigenic diversity. There is one group, containing agents responsible for some of the principal epidemic diseases, which are to a large degree antigenically homogeneous. Measles, variola, varicella and yellow fever viruses are all antigenically homogeneous. Poliovirus, though not completely antigenically uniform, has only three known main epidemic types. On the other hand, there are many virus groups such as the ECHO viruses, the adenoviruses, the epidemic influenza viruses, and the Coxsackie viruses, which show considerable antigenic heterogeneity. Viruses of the antigenically homogeneous group show a marked tendency to localize their epidemic spread to certain age groups in the community. In the case of measles, for instance, the disease is principally epidemic amongst children, and its periodicity is dependent upon the accumulation of young susceptibles within this age group. Age-group limitation is not a marked feature of case distribution with infections caused by viruses of the second category. Influenza epidemics sometimes show a surplus of cases in the under-twelve age group; thus, the attack rate in school children between 5 and 15 years old was estimated as being 40–80% during the 1957 epidemics of A2 infection in the United Kingdom. Generally, adolescents and young adults showed lower rates, and the very young and very old the lowest of all. It must be acknowledged, however, that influenzal-attack rates are very difficult to estimate accurately as the disease is not notifiable, and diagnosis is not always clinically certain. It is quite clear, however, that the age distribution of influenzal cases is not as restricted as in the case of measles, for instance.

Patterns of this kind are clearly discernible amongst viruses epidemic in man. Unfortunately, relatively little is known about epizootic viruses with the exception, perhaps, of foot-and-mouth disease, rinderpest, and myxomatosis, so that a full comparative picture cannot be formed. Assuming for the moment that such patterns as we can make out among the human epidemic viruses are likely to have been imposed by host-selective processes as implied in previous paragraphs, it is notable that viruses belonging to the antigenically homogeneous group are those which produce typically a generalized systemic infection. This is not the case with viruses from the second group, which most commonly are localized to either gut or respiratory epithelial cells; systemic invasion amongst this group is a secondary phenomenon, if it occurs at all. The relationship between such relatively superficial cellular parasitism and antigenic heterogeneity is by no means obvious, when antibody immunity in the host is postulated as a potent instrument of antigenic selection.

The possible role of antibody and other factors in host resistance as agents of selection can be inferred from a speculative argument of the following kind. Assuming that with respect to a certain host a virus particle must negotiate a number of different barriers in order to reach the cytoplasm of a susceptible cell, we can postulate that to pass each barrier a particle must possess a specific characteristic. Any particle possessing all the characters will be capable of infecting. It does not, of course, imply that each particle is certain of reaching a susceptible cell, but only that its chances are at a maximum. This follows from the consequence inherent in our initial assumptions, that the loss of any one of these characters will disqualify a particle absolutely from achieving infection. All particles reaching susceptible cells therefore will possess all the characters. Assuming that these characters are not distributed among all the particles in a given virus population, and that their actual distribution both in number and combination is likely to be random, it becomes evident that a process of this kind must be highly selective, and must enforce a high degree of uniformity upon the virus. One must emphasize again the highly speculative nature of this argument; nevertheless, it is interesting that there are particular cases which support it to a remarkable degree. The contrast between mumps virus and the virus of human epidemic influenza is one of these. Both viruses are biologically very similar: they are of about the same size and have a very similar morphology as revealed by the electron microscope, both haemagglutinate human and fowl erythrocytes, and both possess a neuraminidase. Mumps is characteristically a systemic infection, and there is frequent clinical evidence of dissemination of the virus to various deep tissues of the body such as pancreas, ovary, testis, meninges or even thyroid, in addition to the classical involvement of the salivary glands. Influenza is, as mentioned above, typically localized to the respiratory epithelium, and spread even to the lung parenchyma is not common. Antigenically, the mumps virus is homogeneous, influenza quite the reverse. It is obviously an important corollary of this hypothesis that antigenic structure is primarily a reflection of fundamental surface and sub-surface molecular configurations upon which the tissue-invasive and cell-parasitizing powers of the virus depend. In other words, antigenic specificity cannot vary independently *per se*, but only as a result of modifications of particle structure in response to host-selective pressures. Thus, one may conclude that mumps virus is more stringently acted upon by selective agencies (only one of which is antibody) than the influenza virus, in which latter case antibody exerts hardly any selective pressure at all.

The fact that this hypothesis is perhaps more superficially plausible than fundamentally useful is revealed by the observation that there are many aspects of virus behaviour, and influenza-virus behaviour in particular, which it cannot explain.

2. Antigenic variation among influenza viruses

The pattern of antigenic variation found among influenza virus strains is of particular relevance to the ideas briefly discussed above. Taking the epidemic-influenza viruses in particular, the hypothetical mechanism postulated would lead one to expect a number of antigenically dissimilar influenza strains to coexist in human populations. This, in a general way, is the situation amongst the ECHO viruses, and the adenoviruses. In fact, this is not the case where influenza virus is concerned. Although many antigenically distinct sub-types of influenza virus have been isolated, they represent sequential changes in antigenic configuration, one particular sub-type being epidemically dominant at any one period. Furthermore, the antigenic progression is unidirectional, earlier antigenic types showing little tendency to return again to epidemic activity. This phenomenon leads to something of a dilemma: if the progressive change in epidemically prevalent antigens is dependent upon an antibody-selective process, why is there no well-marked restriction to the younger age groups—i.e., why is influenza not a childhood disease? If antibody is not a selective agent in this system, why the *progressive* antigenic change?

The first question can be answered by the possibility that the antibody response to influenzal infection is relatively short-lived, so that a small proportion of adults lose enough antibody to become susceptible. Some further light on this dilemma is thrown by the observation that although antibody does tend to be lost progressively with time, subsequent antigenic stimulus, with whatever influenzal antigen, will induce a recrudescence of antibody orientated to the original inducing antigen—the doctrine of "original antigen sin" (Davenport, Hennessy and Francis, 1953). This means that a recovered individual will have his antibody immunity always directed mainly against the antigens of the influenzal strain which gave him or her the first attack of influenza. Such a situation will clearly militate against the re-establishment of "earlier" antigenic types in a population, and since presumably the virus is not restricted in its surface changes, because of its non-invasive character (see original hypothesis), antigenic variation *per se*, irrespective of other changes in biological characters, is an effective mechanism for ensuring virus survival. It is tempting to deduce from this that antibody immunity will in fact readily select major antigenic changes in influenza viruses. Experimental results are somewhat equivocal in this respect.

Passage of influenza viruses through the allantoic cavity of the embryonated hen egg in the presence of homologous antibody can induce several types of variation, not all of them strictly antigenic in nature. Thus, in some cases the variants re-isolated are basically antibody-insensitive—so-called "Q-phase" variants (van der Veen and Mulder, 1950)—although they appear to be antigenically very similar to if not identical with the parent strain. In other cases a detectable amount of antigenic change has been found (Edney, 1957), although this may also be linked to some inducement of the Q phase. It may be noted that Q-phase variants have been isolated from human cases during epidemics, although it is not absolutely certain that they were not selected out by the isolation process itself.

The degree of antigenic change that has been induced in these egg-passage experiments is comparable with what has been observed in nature. A statement of this kind, however, formulates in seemingly exact words a largely intuitive observation, as there is no absolute, quantitative way of measuring degrees of antigenic relationship. At the same time it must be admitted that major antigenic transitions comparable to those observed in some natural epidemics, such as the Type A → Type A1 transition of 1946–47 and the Type A1 → A2 change of 1957, have not yet been reproduced in experimental systems of this kind. Nor do the "new" antigenic determinants elicited in the experimentally passaged strains resemble any antigenic components which have arisen in subsequent epidemics.

It should not be overlooked that the egg system is highly artificial, as it brings relatively large amounts of virus in direct contact with fairly high concentrations of antibody. This is not presumably the typical situation as it occurs when a previously immunized population is seeded again with a homologous epidemic strain. A more comparable experimental system would seem to be that in which previously immunized mice are inoculated with varying doses of homologous virus, and surviving virus is maintained by continued passage in the immunized mice. However, experiments of this kind yield results substantially similar to the ones obtained in the egg-passage experiments (Gerber, Loosli and Hamre, 1955; Gerber, Hamre and Loosli, 1956; Magill, 1955; Hamre, Loosli and Gerber, 1958 a,b). The interpretation of the data obtained from experimental systems of this kind, however, is complicated by factors inherent in the host used. It seems likely, for instance, that adaptation and passage of influenza virus in the mouse, which is not susceptible to natural infection, can lead to varying degrees of biological modification of the virus independently of the effects of antibody. Thus, marked changes in the haemagglutination inhibitor sensitivity of an Asian strain of influenza virus were observed after prolonged passage in the mouse, even though the haemagglutination inhibitor concerned was not present in either the serum or tissues of the mice (Cohen and Biddle, 1960). These changes could be reversed to a varying extent by transfer back to the egg. Some influence of the intra-host environment must presumably be responsible for modifications of this kind, and the superimposition of such influences upon the selective effects of antibody itself may perhaps be the reason for the somewhat variable effects actually observed in the experiments briefly considered above.

The role of Q-phase variants in the maintenance of epidemic strains of virus in immune populations is by no means clear. While it is common to find strains of this type occurring in a community during an epidemic, as has been mentioned previously, fully antibody-sensitive strains can be readily recovered from the same epidemics at the same time. There is no clear evidence to suggest that previous experience of the same or very similar strain encourages the establishment of a Q variant in a subsequent epidemic.

If, in fact, new antigenic forms are selected in nature by antibody in the human host, it is remarkable that in epidemics associated with a new virus type all the cases from start to finish of the outbreak are, as a rule, caused by the new strain. This would suggest that the selective mechanism acts primarily in the inter-epidemic period, during which time there is usually very little evidence of active virus in the community. Admittedly, sporadic outbreaks of influenza have been described during the summer (inter-epidemic) season (Andrewes, 1950; Isaacs and Andrewes, 1951). But in those cases where virus has been isolated from such outbreaks it has already possessed the antigenic characteristics of the fully epidemic strain emerging some months later. The likeliest possibility would seem to be that antigenic change occurs during the later stages of the previous epidemic, when antibody immunity is building up rapidly in the community affected, and the epidemic is beginning to peter out. No direct evidence of such late antigenic changes has as yet been reported. It is clear from all this that the interactions of virus and the resistance mechanisms of the host are in many cases subtle and complex to a degree.

Bibliography

Ackermann, W. W. (1951). *J. biol. Chem.* **189**, 421.

Ackermann, W. W., Ishida, N. and Maassab, H. F. (1955), *J. exp. Med.* **102**, 545.

Ackermann, W. W. and Kurtz, H. (1952). *J. exp. Med.* **96**, 151.

Ackermann, W. W. and Kurtz, H. (1955). *J. exp. Med.* **102**, 555.

Ackermann, W. W. and Johnson, R. B. (1953). *J. exp. Med.* **97**, 315.

Ackermann, W. W., Loh, P. C. and Payne, F. E. (1959). *Virology* **7**, 170.

Ackermann, W. W. and Loh, P. C. (1960). *Ann. N.Y. Acad. Sci.* **88**, 1298.

Ackermann, W. W. and Maassab, H. F. (1954a). *J. exp. Med.* **99**, 105.

Ackermann, W. W. and Maassab, H. F. (1954b). *J. exp. Med.* **100**, 329.

Ackermann, W. W., Payne, F. E. and Kurtz, H. (1958). *J. Immunol.* **81**, 1.

Ackermann, W. W., Rabson, A. and Kurtz, H. (1954). *J. exp. Med.* **100**, 437.

Ada, G. L. and Anderson, S. G. (1959). *Nature, Lond.* **183**, 799.

Ada, G. L. and French, E. L. (1959). *Nature, Lond.* **183**, 1740.

Ada, G. L. and Perry, B. T. (1956). *J. gen. Microbiol.* **14**, 623.

Ada, G. L. and Stone, J. D. (1950). *Brit. J. exp. Path.* **31**, 263.

Adams, M. H. (1959). Appendix to "Bacteriophages", p. 450. Interscience, New York.

Adams, M. H. and Park, B. (1956). *Virology*, **2**, 719.

Adams, W. R. and Prince, A. M. (1957). *J. exp. Med.* **106**, 617.

Alexander, H. E., Koch, G., Mountain, I. M. and van Damme, O. (1958). *J. exp. Med.* **108**, 493.

Alexander, H. E., Koch, G., Mountain, I. M., Sprunt, K. and van Damme, O. (1958). *Virology* **5**, 172.

Allison, A. C., Pereira, H. G. and Forthing, C. P. (1960). *Virology* **10**, 316.

Allison, A. C. and Perkins, H. R. (1960). *Nature, Lond.* **188**, 796.

Allison, A. C. and Valentine, R. C. (1960). *Biochim. biophys. Acta* **40**, 400.

Ames, B., Dubin, D. T. and Rosenthal, S. M. (1958). *Science* **127**, 819.

Anderson, C. E. (1957). *N.Z. med. J.* **56**, 235.

Anderson, E. S. (1962). *Brit. med. Bull.* **18**, 64.

Anderson, E. S., Armstrong, J. A. and Niven, J. S. F. (1959). In "Virus Growth and Variation", ed. by A. Isaacs and B. W. Lacey, Cambridge University Press, London.

Anderson, E. S. and Felix, A. (1953). *J. gen. Microbiol.* **9**, 65.

Anderson, E. S. and Fraser, A. (1956). *J. gen. Microbiol.* **15**, 225.

Anderson, S. G. (1947). *Aust. J. exp. Biol. med. Sci.* **25**, 163.

Anderson, S. G. (1948a). *Aust. J. exp. Biol. med. Sci.* **26**, 347.

Anderson, S. G. (1949). *J. Immunol.* **62**, 29.

Anderson, S. G., Burnet, F. M., Fazekas de St. Groth, S., McCrea, J. F. and Stone, J. D. (1948). *Aust. J. exp. Biol. med. Sci.* **26**, 403.

Anderson, S. G. and Hamilton, J. (1949). *Med. J. Aust.* **1**, 308.

Anderson, T. F. (1948b). *J. Bacteriol.* **55**, 637.

Anderson, T. F. (1953). *Cold Spr. Harb. Symp. quant. Biol.* **18**, 197.

Anderson, T. F. and Doermann, A. H. (1952). *J. gen. Physiol.* **35**, 657.

Anderson, T. F., Rappaport, C. and Muscatine, N. A. (1953). *Ann. Inst. Pasteur* **84**, 5.

Andrewes, C. H. (1929). *Brit. J. exp. Path.* **10**, 273.

Andrewes, C. H. (1930). *J. Path. Bact.* **33**, 301.

Andrewes, C. H. (1950). *New Engl. J. Med.* **242**, 161.

Andrewes, C. H., Bang, F. B. and Burnet, F. M. (1955). *Virology* **1**, 176.

Andrewes, C. H., Burnet, F. M., Enders, J. F., Gard, S., Hirst, G. K., Kaplan, M. M. and Zhdanov, V. M. (1961). *Virology*, **15**, 52.

Andrewes, C. H. and Allison, A. C. (1961). *J. Hyg., Camb.* **59**, 285.

Andrewes, C. H., Muirhead-Thomson, R. C. and Stevenson, J. P. (1956). *J. Hyg., Camb.* **54**, 478.

Appleyard, G., Westwood, J. C. N. and Zwartouw, H. T. (1962). *Virology* **18**, 159.

Appleyard, R. K. (1954). *Genetics* **39**, 429.

Aragão, H. de B. (1943). *Mem. Inst. Osw. Cruz.* **38**, 93.

Arber, W. and Dussoix, D. (1962). *J. mol Biol.* **5**, 18.

Arber, W., Kellenberger, G. and Weigle, J. J. (1957). *Schweitz. Z. Path.* **20**, 659.

Armstrong, J. A., Pereira, H. G. and Andrewes, C. H. (1961). *Virology* **14**, 276.

Arnoff, H. and Rafelson, M. E. (1959). *Arch. Biochem. Biophys.* **81**, 421.

Asheshov, I. N., Strelitz, F., Hall, E. and Flon, H. (1954). *Antibiot. & Chemother.* **4**, 380.

Avery, O. T., MacLeod, C. M. and McCarty, M. (1944). *J. exp. Med.* **79**, 137.

Aycock, W. L. and Kessel, J. P. (1943). *Amer. J. med. Sci.* **205**, 454.

Bachtold, J. G., Bubel, H. C. and Gebhardt, L. P. (1957). *Virology* **4**, 582.

Baker, E. E., Goebel, W. F. and Perlman, E. (1949). *J. exp. Med.* **89**, 325.

Baltimore, D. and Franklin, R. M. (1962). *Proc. nat. Acad. Sci., Wash.* **48**, 1383.

Barksdale, L. (1959). *Bact. Rev.* **23**, 202.

Barnett, R. J. and Ball, E. G. (1960). *J. biophys. biochem. Cytol.* **8**, 83.

Baron, S., Porterfield, J. S. and Isaacs, A. (1961). *Virology* **14**, 444.

Barricelli, N. A. (1956). *Acta Biotheor., Leiden* **11**, 8.

Barrington, L. F. and Kozloff, L. M. (1954). *Science* **120**, 110.

Barski, G., Endo, M. and Monaci, V. (1953). *Ann. Inst. Pasteur* **85**, 254.

Barski, G., Macdonald, A. and Slizewicz, P. (1954). *Ann. Inst. Pasteur* **86**, 579.

Barski, G., Robinaux, R. and Endo, V. (1955). *Proc. Soc. exp. Biol. N.Y.* **88**, 57.

Bauer, D. J. and Sheffield, F. W. (1959). *Nature, Lond.* **184**, 1496.

Bawden, F. C. (1950). In "Plant Viruses and Virus Diseases", p. 57, Chronica Botanica Co., Waltham, Mass.

Baylis, J. H., Mackintosh, J., Morgan, R. S. and Wright, G. Payling (1952). *J. Path. Bact.* **64**, 33.

Baylor, M. B., Hurst, D. D., Allen, S. L. and Bertani, E. T. (1957). *Genetics* **42**, 104.

Bearcroft, W. G. C. (1962). *J. Path. Bact.* **83**, 383.

Beaudraeu, G. S., Becker, C., Sharp, D. G., Painter, J. C. and Beard, J. W. (1958). *J. nat. Cancer Inst.* **20**, 351.

Bedson, H. S. and Duckworth, M. (1963). *J. Path. Bact.* **85**, 1.

Bedson, H. S. and Dumbell, K. R. (1961). *J. Hyg., Camb.* **59**, 457.

Bedson, S. P. and Gostling, J. V. T. (1954). *Brit. J. exp. Path.* **35**, 299.

Bellett, A. J. D. and Burness, A. T. H. (1960). *Biochem. J.* **77**, 17P.

Bellett, A. J. D. and Burness, A. T. H. (1961). *Nature, Lond.* **190**, 235.

Bennett, S. (1956). *J. biophys. biochem. Cytol.* **2**, Pt. 2., Suppl., 99.

Benson, P. F. and Boyd, M. E. (1960). *Guy's Hosp. Rep.* **109**, 219.

Benzer, S. (1952). *J. Bacteriol.* **63**, 59.

Benzer, S. (1953). *Biochim. biophys. Acta.* **11**, 383.

Benzer, S. (1957). In "The Chemical Basis of Heredity", ed. by W. D. McElroy and H. B. Glass, p. 70. Johns Hopkins Press, Baltimore.

Benzer, S. and Freese, E. (1958). *Proc. nat. Acad. Sci., Wash.* **44**, 112.

Benzer, S. and Jacob, F. (1953). *Ann. Inst. Pasteur* **84**, 186.

Bergold, G. H. (1958). In "Handbuch der Virusforschung", ed. by C. Hallauer and K. F. Meyer, Vol. 4, p. 60. Springer, Wien.

Bernkopf, H., Nishmi, M. and Rosin, A. (1959). *J. Immunol.* **83**, 635.

Bernkopf, H. and Rosin, A. (1957). *Amer. J. Path.* **33**, 1215.

Bernstein, A. (1957). *Virology* **3**, 286.

Berry, G. P. and Dedrick, H. M. (1936). *J. Bacteriol.* **31**, 50.

Bertani, G. (1951). *J. Bacteriol.* **62**, 293.

Bertani, G. (1953). *Cold Spr. Harb. Symp. quant. Biol.* **18**, 65.

Bertani, G. (1956). *Brookhaven Symp. Biol.* **8**, 50.

Bertani, G. (1958). *Advanc. Virus Res.* **5**, 151.

Bertani, L. E. (1957). *Virology* **4**, 53.

Beveridge, W. I. B. and Burnet, F. M. (1946). Spec. Rep. Ser. Med. Res. Coun., Lond., No. 256.

Biddle, F. and Cohen, A. (1962). *Nature, Lond.* **196**, 297.

"Biochemical Response to Injury" (1960). Blackwell, Oxford.

Bjorkman, N. and Sibalin, M. (1960). *Virology* **11**, 513.

Black, F. L. and Melnick, J. L. (1955). *J. Immunol.* **74**, 236.

Black, L. M. (1950). *Nature, Lond.* **166**, 852.

Blake, F. G. and Trask, J. D. Jr. (1921). *J. exp. Med.* **33**, 385.

Blattner, R. J. (1958). *J. Pediat.* **53**, 751.

Blix, G. (1936). *Hoppe-Seyl. Z.* **240**, 43.

Boand, A. V., Kempe, J. E. and Hanson, R. J. (1957). *J. Immunol.* **79**, 416.

Bodian, D. (1948). *Johns Hopk. Hosp. Bull.* **83**, 1.

Bodian, D. (1955). *Science* **122**, 105.

Bodian, D. (1956). *Amer. J. Hyg.* **64**, 181.

Bodian, D. (1959). In "Viral and Rickettsial Diseases of Man", ed. by T. M. Rivers and F. L. Horsfall, 3rd Ed., p. 479. Pitman Medical Publishing Co., London.

Boéye, A. (1959). *Virology* **9**, 691.

Boggs, J. D., Capps, R. B., Weiss, C. F. and McLean, I. W. (1961). *J. Amer. med. Ass.* **177**, 678.

Böhm, P., Ross, J. and Baumeister, L. (1957). *Hoppe-Seyl. Z.* **307**, 284.

Boulter, E. A., Maber, H. B. and Bowen, E. T. W. (1961). *Brit. J. exp. Path.* **42**, 433.

Bourne, G. and Wedgewood, J. (1959). *Lancet* i. 1226.

Boyd, J. S. K. (1951). *J. Path. Bact.* **63**, 445.

Boyd, J. S. K. (1954). *Nature, Lond.* **173**, 1050.

Boyse, E. A., Morgan, R. S., Pearson, J. D. and Wright, G. Payling (1956a). *Brit. J. exp. Path.* **37**, 333.

Boyse, E. A., Klemperer, M., Morgan, R. S. and Wright, G. Payling (1956b). *Brit. J. exp. Path.*. **37**, 461.

Bradley, D. E. and Kay, D. (1960). *J. gen. Microbiol.*. **23**, 553.

Brandt, P. W. (1958). *Exp. Cell Res.* **15**, 300.

Brans, L. M., Herzberger, E. and Binkhorst, J. L. (1953). *Leeuwenhoek ned. Tijdschr.* **19**, 309.

Bras, G. (1952). *Docum. méd. geog. trop., Amst.* **4**, 303.

Brattgård, S.–O., Edström, J.–E. and Hydén, H. (1956). *J. Neurochem.* **1**, 316.

Breitenfeld, P. M. and Schäfer, W. (1957). *Virology* **4**, 328.

Brenner, S. (1957). *Virology* **3**, 560.

Brenner, S. (1959). *Advanc. Virus Res.* **6**, 137.

Brenner, S., Barnett, L., Crick, F. H. C. and Orgel A. (1961b). *J. mol. Biol.* **3**, 121.

Brenner, S., Benzer, S. and Barnett, L. (1958). *Nature, Lond.* **182**, 983.

Brenner, S. and Horne, R. W. (1959). *Biochim. biophys. Acta* **34**, 103.

Brenner, S., Jacob, F. and Meselson, M. (1961a). *Nature, Lond.* **190**, 576.

Brenner, S. and Stent, G. S. (1955). *Biochim. biophys. Acta* **17**, 473.

Brenner, S., Streisinger, G., Horne, R. W., Champe, S. P., Barnett, L., Benzer, S. and Rees, M. W. (1959). *J. mol. Biol.* **1**, 281.

Bresch, C. (1955). *Z. Naturf.* **10b**, 545.

Briody, B. A. (1948). *J. Immunol.* **59**, 115.

Brown, A., Mayyasi, E. A. and Officer, J. E. (1959). *J. infect. Dis.* **104**, 193.

Brown, D. and Kozloff, L. M. (1957). *J. biol. Chem.* **225**, 1.

Brown, F., Cartwright, B. and Stewart, D. L. (1961a). *Biochim. biophys. Acta* **47**, 172.

Brown, F., Planterose, D. N. and Stewart, D. L. (1961b). *Nature, Lond.* **191**, 414.

Brown, F. and Stewart, D. L. (1959). *Virology* **7**, 408.

Brown, F. and Stewart, D. L. (1960). *J. gen. Microbiol.* **23**, 369.

Bruusgaard, E. (1932). *Brit. J. Derm.* **44**, 1.

Buckland, F. E., Bynoe, M. L., Rosen, L. and Tyrrell, D. A. J. (1961). *Brit. med. J.* **i**, 397.

Buckley, S. M. (1956). *Arch. ges. Virusforsch.* **6**, 388.

Buckley, S. M. (1957). *Amer. J. Path.* **33**, 691.

Buckley, S. M. (1959). *Ann. N.Y. Acad. Sci.* **81**, 172.

Buddingh, C. J., Schrum, D. I., Lanier, J. C. and Guidry, D. J. (1953). *Pediatrics* **11**, 595.

Bukrinskaya, A. G. and Zhdanov, V. M. (1961). *Probl. Virol.* **6**, 392.

Burnet, F. M. (1927). *Brit. J. exp. Path.* **8**, 121.

Burnet, F. M. (1929). *Brit. J. exp. Path.* **10**, 109.

Burnet, F. M. (1942). *Aust. J. exp. Biol. Sci.* **20**, 81.

Burnet, F. M. (1946). *Brit. J. exp. Path.* **27**, 244.

Burnet, F. M. (1948). *Aust. J. exp. Biol. med. Sci.* **26**, 371.

Burnet, F. M. (1950). *Aust. J. exp. Biol. med. Sci.* **28**, 299.

Burnet, F. M. (1952). *Aust. J. exp. Biol. med. Sci.* **30**, 119.

Burnet, F. M. (1953). In "The Natural History of Infectious Disease", 2nd Ed., p. 19. Cambridge University Press, London.

Burnet, F. M. (1955). In "Principles of Animal Virology", ed. by F. M. Burnet, p. 190. Academic Press, New York.

Burnet, F. M. (1959). *Brit. med. Bull.* **15**, 177.

Burnet, F. M. (1960. In "Principles of Animal Virology", ed. by F. M. Burnet, 2nd Ed., p. 230. Academic Press, New York.

Burnet, F. M., Beveridge, W. I. B., McEwin, J. and Boake, W. C. (1945). *Aust. J. exp. Biol. med. Sci.* **23**, 177.

Burnet, F. M. and Bull, D. R. (1943). *Aust. J. exp. Biol. med. Sci.* **21**, 55.

Burnet, F. M. and Edney, M. (1952). *Aust. J. exp. Biol. med. Sci.* **30**, 105.

Burnet, F. M. and Fenner, F. (1949). In "The Production of Antibodies", 2nd Ed., p. 102. MacMillan, London.

Burnet, F. M. and Lind, P. (1949). *Aust. J. Sci.* **12**, 109.

Burnet, F. M. and Lind, P. E. (1950). *Aust. J. exp. Biol. med. Sci.* **28**, 129.

Burnet, F. M., McCrea, J. F. and Stone, J. D. (1946). *Brit. J. exp. Path.* **27**, 228.

Burnet, F. M. and McKie, M. (1929). *Austral. J. exp. Biol. med. Sci.* **6**, 277.

Burton, K. (1955). *Biochem. J.* **61**, 473.

Bynoe, M. L., Hobson, D., Horner, J., Kipps, A., Schild, G. C. and Tyrrell, D. A. J. (1961). *Lancet* **i**, 1194.

Cairns, H. J. F. (1951). *Nature, Lond.* **168**, 335.

Cairns, H. J. F. (1957). *Virology* **3**, 1.

Cairns, H. J. F. (1960). *Virology* **11**, 603.

Cairns, H. J. F. and Mason, P. J. (1953). *J. Immunol.* **71**, 38.

Campbell, A. (1957). *Virology* **4**, 366.

Cappell, D. F. and McFarlane, M. N. (1947). *J. Path. Bact.* **59**, 385.

Capps, R. B., Sborov, V., and Scheiffley, C. S. (1948). *J. Amer. med. Ass.* **136**, 819.

Carp, R. I., Kritchevsky, D. and Koprowski, H. (1960). *Virology* **12**, 125.

Casals, J. and Brown, L. V. (1954). *J. exp. Med.* **99**, 429.

Casals, J. and Reeves, W. C. (1959). "Viral and Rickettsial Infections of Man", 3rd Ed., p. 269. J. P. Lippincott & Co.

Cassel, W. A. (1957). *Virology* **3**, 514.

Causey, G. (1948). *J. Anat., Lond.* **82**, 262.

Chamberlain, R. W. (1958). *Ann. N.Y. Acad. Sci.* **70**, 312.

Chamberlain, R. W., Sudia, W. D. and Gillett, J. D. (1959). *Amer. J. Hyg.* **70**, 221.

Chambers, V. C. (1957). *Virology* **3**, 62.

Chang, H. and Kempf, J. (1950). *J. Immunol.* **65**, 75.

Chany, C., and Cook, M. K. (1960). *Ann. Inst. Pasteur* **98**, 920.

Cheatham, W. J. (1953). *Amer. J. Path.* **29**, 401.

Cheatham, W. J., Weller, T. H., Dolan, J. F. and Dower, J. C. (1956). *Amer. J. Path.* **32**, 1015.

Cheng, P. (1961). *Virology* **14**, 132.

Choppin, P. W. and Philipson, L. (1961). *J. exp. Med.* **113**, 713.

Choppin, P. W. and Tamm, I. (1959). *Virology* **8**, 539.

Chu, C. M. (1951). *J. gen. Microbiol.* **5**, 739.

Chu, L. W. and Morgan, H. R. (1950a). *J. exp. Med.* **91**, 393.

Chu, L. W. and Morgan, H. R. (1950b). *J. exp. Med.* **91**, 403.

Clarke, D. H. and Fox, J. P. (1948). *J. exp. Med.* **88**, 25.

Cocking, C. E., Keppie, J., Witt, K., and Smith, H. (1960). *Brit. J. exp. Path.* **41**, 460.

Coffin, D. L. and Liu, C. (1957). *Virology* **3**, 132.

Cohen, A. (1960). *Lancet* **ii**, 791.

Cohen, A. and Belyavin, G. (1959). *Virology* **7**, 59.

Cohen, A. and Belyavin, G. (1961). *Virology* **13**, 58.

Cohen, A. and Biddle, F. (1960). *Virology* **11**, 458.

Cohen, A. and Biddle, F. (1963). *Nature, Lond.* **198**, 508.

Cohen, S. S. (1948). *J. Biol. Chem.* **174**, 295.

Cohen, S. S. (1953). *Cold Spr. Harb. Symp. quant. Biol.* **21**, 221.

Cohen, S. S. (1959a). In "The Viruses", ed. by F. M. Burnet and W. M. Stanley, Vol. 1, p. 15. Academic Press, New York.

Cohen, S. S. (1959b). In "Viral and Rickettsial Diseases of Man", ed. by T. M. Rivers and F. L. Horsfall, 3rd Ed., p. 49. Pitman Medical Publishing Co., London.

Coleman, V. and Jawetz, E. (1961). *Virology* **13**, 375.

Colter, J. S., Bird, H. H. and Brown, R. A. (1957a). *Nature, Lond.* **179**, 859.

Colter, J. S., Bird, H. H., Moyer, A. W. and Brown, R. A. (1957b). *Virology* **4**, 522.

Colter, J. S. and Ellem, K. A. O. (1961). *Ann. Rev. Microbiol.* **15**, 219.

Cook, G. M. W., Heard, D. H. and Seaman, G. V. F. (1961). *Nature, Lond.* **191**, 44.

Cooke, P. M. (1961). *Amer. J. med. Sci.* **241**, 383.

Coombs, J. S., Eccles, J. C. and Fatt, P. (1955). *J. Physiol.* **130**, 291.

Coons, A. H. and Kaplan, M. H. (1950). *J. exp. Med.* **91**, 1.

Cooper, S. and Zinder, N.D. (1962). *Virology.* **18**, 405.

Cordy, D. R. and Gorham, J. R. (1950). *Amer. J. Path..* **26**, 617.

Cornforth, J. W., Daines, M. E. and Gottschalk, A. (1957). *Proc. chem. Soc., Lond.* 25.

Cornforth, J. W., Firth, M. E. and Gottschalk, A. (1958). *Biochem. J.* **68**, 57.

Councilman, W. T., Macgrath, G. B. and Brinckerhoff, W. R. (1904). *J. med. Res.* **11**, 12.

Crick, F. H. C., Barnett, L., Brenner, S. and Watts-Tobin, R. J. (1961). *Nature, Lond,* **192**, 1227.

Crick, F. H. C., Griffiths, J. S. and Orgel, L. E. (1957). *Proc. nat. Acad. Sci., Wash.* **43**, 416.

Crick, F. H. C. and Watson, J. D. (1956). *Nature, Lond.* **177**, 473.

Crowther, D. and Melnick, J. L. (1961). *Virology* **14**, 11.

Curnen, E. C. and Horsfall, F. L. (1946). *J. exp. Med.* **83**, 105.

Curnen, E. C. and Horsfall, F. L. (1947). *J. exp. Med.* **85**, 39.

Curtain, C. C. and Pye, J. (1955). *Aust. J. exp. Biol. med. Sci.* **33**, 315.

Curtain, C. C., French, E. L. and Pye, J. (1953). *Aust. J. exp. Biol. med. Sci.* **31**, 349.

Curtis, D. R. and Watkins, J. C. (1960). *J. Neurochem.* **6**, 117.

Dalmat, H. T. (1958). *J. exp. Med.* **108**, 9.

Darlington, C. D. (1944). *Nature, Lond.* **2**, 164.

Darnell, J. E. Jr. (1958). *J. exp. Med.* **107**, 633.

Darnell, J. E. Jr. and Eagle, H. (1958). *Virology* **6**, 556.

Darnell, J. E. Jr., Eagle, H. and Sawyer, T. K. (1959). *J. exp. Med.* **110**, 445.

Darnell, J. E. Jr. and Levintow, L. (1960). *J. biol. Chem.* **235**, 74.

Darnell, J. E. Jr., Levintow, L., Thorén, M. M. and Hooper, J. L. (1961). *Virology* **13**, 271.

Darnell, J. E. Jr. and Sawyer, T. K. (1960). *Virology* **11**, 665.

Davenport, F. M., Hennessy, A. V. and Francis, T. Jr. (1953). *J. exp. Med.* **98**, 641.

Davenport, F. M. and Horsfall, F. L. (1948). *J. exp. Med.* **88**, 621.

Davies, C. N. (1949). *Brit. J. industr. Med.* **6**, 245.

Davis, E. V. (1961). *Science* **133**, 2059.

Davis, N. C. (1932). *Amer. J. Hyg.* **16**, 163.

Davison, P. F. (1959). *Proc. nat. Acad. Sci., Wash.* **45**, 1560.

Davison, P. F., Freifelder, D., Hede, R. and Levinthal, C. (1961). *Proc. nat. Acad. Sci., Wash.* **47**, 1123.

Day, M. F., Fenner, F., Woodroofe, G. M. and McIntyre, G. A. (1956). *J. Hyg. Camb.* **54**, 258.

de Burgh, P. M., Yu, P. C., Howe, C. and Bovarnick, M. (1948). *J. exp. Med.* **87**, 1.

De Duve, C. (1959). In "Subcellular Particles". Ronald Press Co., New York.

Deibel, R. and Hotchin, J. (1961). *Virology* **14**.

Delbrück, M. (1940a). *J. gen. Physiol.* **23**, 631.

Delbrück, M. (1940b). *J. gen. Physiol..* **23**, 643.

Delbrück, M. (1945a). *J. Bacteriol.* **50**, 131.

Delbrück, M. (1945b). *J. Bacteriol.* **50**, 151.

Delbrück, M. (1948). *J. Bacteriol.* **56**, 1.

Delbrück, M. and Bailey, W. T., Jr. (1946). *Cold Spr. Harb. Symp. quan. Biol.* **11**, 33.

Denny, F. W. Jr. and Ginsberg, H. (1961). *J. Immunol.* **86**, 567.

Denny-Brown, D., Adams, R. D. and Fitzgerald, P. J. (1944). *Arch. Neurol. Psychiat., Chicago* **51**, 216.

de Robertis, E. D. P. and Bennett, H. S. (1954). *Exp. Cell Res.* **6**, 543.

Dettori, R., Maccacaro, G. A. and Piccinin, G. L. (1961). *G. Microbiol,* **9**, 141.

Deutsch, K. and Zaman, V. (1959). *Exp. Cell Res.* **17**, 310.

Di Mayorca, G. A., Eddy, B. E., Stewart, S. E., Hunter, W. D., Friend, C., and Bendick, A. (1959). *Proc. nat. Acad. Sci., Wash.* **45**, 1805.

Dixon, C. W. (1948). *J. Hyg., Camb.* **46**, 351.

Dixon, C. W. (1962). In "Smallpox", p. 23 and p. 37, figure 84. Churchill, London.

Doermann, A. H. (1948). *J. Bacteriol.* **55**, 257.

Doermann, A. H. (1952). *J. gen. Physiol.* **35**, 645.

Doermann, A. H., Chase, M. and Stahl, F. W. (1955). *J. cell comp. Physiol.* **45**, Suppl., 51.

Doermann, A. H. and Hill, M. B. (1953). *Genetics* **38**, 79.

Donald, H. B. and Isaacs, A. (1954). *J. gen. Microbiol.* **11**, 325.

Douglas, S. R., Smith, W. and Price L. B. W. (1929). *J. Path. Bact.* **32**, 99.

Dourmashkin, R. R. and Negroni, G. (1960). Proc. eur. reg. Conf. Electron Microscopy, Delft, 24.

Downie, A. W. (1939). *J. Path. Bact.* **48**, 361.

Downie, A. W. and Dumbell, K. R. (1947). *Lancet* i, 550.

Downie, A. W., McCarthy, K., Macdonald, A., MacCallum, F. O. and Macrae, A. D. (1953). *Lancet,* ii, 164.

Downie, A. W. and McGaughey, C. A. (1935). *J. Path. Bact.* **40**, 147.

Druett, H. A., Henderson, D. W., Packman, L., and Peacock, S. (1953). *J. Hyg., Camb.* **51**, 359.

Druett, H. A., Robinson, J. M., Henderson, D. W., Packman, L. and Peacock, S. (1956a). *J. Hyg. Camb.* **54**, 37.

Druett, H. A., Henderson, D. W. and Peacock, S. (1956b). *J. Hyg., Camb.* **54**, 49.

Duckworth, M. J. (1958). Pathogenesis of Pox Virus Infections M.D. Thesis (unpublished).

Duguid, J. P. (1946). *J. Hyg., Camb.* **44**, 471.

Dulbecco, R. (1949a). *Genetics* **34**, 126.

Dulbecco, R. (1949b). *Nature, Lond.* **163**, 949.

Dulbecco, R. (1950). *J. Bact.* **59**, 329.

Dulbecco, R. (1952). *Proc. nat. Acad. Sci., Wash.* **38**, 747.

Dulbecco, R. (1960). *Cancer Res.* **20**, 751.

Dulbecco, R. (1961). *Cancer Res.* **21**, 975.

Dulbecco, R. and Vogt, M. (1954a). *J. exp. Med.* **99**, 167.

Dulbecco, R. and Vogt, M. (1954b). *J. exp. Med.* **99**, 183.

Dulbecco, R. and Vogt, M. (1960). *Proc. nat. Acad. Sci., Wash.* **46**, 1617.

Dumbell, K., Downie, A. W. and Valentine, R. C. (1957). *Virology* **4**, 467.

Duncan, I. B. R. and Hutchison, J. G. P. (1961). *Lancet* i, 530.

Dunnebacke, T. H. (1956a). *Virology* **2**, 399.

Dunnebacke, T. H. (1956b). *Virology* **2**, 811.

Dunnebacke, T. H. and Mattern, C. F. T. (1961). *J. Immunol.* **86**, 585.

Dunnebacke, T. H. and Reaume, M. B. (1958). *Virology* **6**, 8.

Dussoix, D. and Arber, W. (1962). *J. mol. Biol.* **5**, 37.

Eagle, H. and Habel, K. (1956). *J. exp. Med.* **104**, 271.

Easterbrook, K. B. (1962). *Virology* **17**, 245.

Easton, J. M., Goldberg, B. and Green, H. (1962). *J. exp. Med.* **115**, 275.

Eaton, M. D. (1952). *Arch. ges. Virusforsch.* **5**, 53.

Eaton, M. D., Jewell, M. and Scala, A. R. (1960). *Virology* **10**, 112.

Eddy, B. E., Rowe, W. P., Hartley, J. W., Stewart, S. E. and Huebner, R. J. (1958). *Virology* **6**, 290.

Edney, M. (1957). *J. gen. Microbiol.* **17**, 25.

Edström, J.-E. (1959). *J. Neurochem.* **5**, 43.

Ehrlich, R. M., Turner, J. A. P. and Clarke, M. (1958). *J. Pediat.* **53**, 139.

Eichenwald, H. F., Ababio, A., Arky, A. M. and Hartman, A. P. (1958). *J. Amer. med. Ass.* **166**, 1563.

Elford, W. F. (1931). *J. Path. Bact.* **34**, 505.

Ellis, E. L. and Delbrück, M. (1939). *J. gen. Physiol.* **22**, 365.

Evans, C. A., Byatt, P. H., Chambers, V. C. and Smith, W. M. (1954). *J. Immunol.* **72**, 348–352.

Everett, S. F. and Ginsberg, H. S. (1958). *Virology* **6**, 770.

Faber, H. K. (1955). In "The Pathogenesis of Poliomyelitis". Charles C. Thomas and Co., Springfield, Ill.

Faber, H. K., McNaught, R. C., Silverberg, R. J. and Dong, L. (1951). *Proc. Soc. exp. Biol., N.Y.* **77**, 532

Faber, H. K. and Silverberg, R. J. (1946). *J. exp. Med.* **83**, 329.

Faber, H. K., Silverberg, R. J. and Dong, L. (1948). *J. exp. Med.* **88**, 65.

Fagraeus, A. and Espmark, A. (1961). *Nature, Lond.* **190**, 370.

Faillard, H. (1957). *Hoppe-Seyl. Z.* **307**, 62–86.

Falk, D. and Richter, I. E. (1961). *Arch ges. Virusforsch.* **11**, 73.

Farber, S. and Wolbach, S. B. (1932). *Amer. J. Path.* **8**, 128.

Farquhar, M. G. and Palade, G. E. (1960). *J. biophys. biochem. Cytol.* **7**, 297.

Fazekas de St. Groth, S. (1948a). *Aust. J. exp. Biol. med. Sci.* **26**, 29.

Fazekas de St. Groth, S. (1948b). *Aust. J. exp. Biol. med. Sci.* **26**, 271.

Fazekas de St. Groth, S. (1948c). *Nature, Lond.* **162**, 294.

Fazekas de St. Groth, S. and Graham, D. M. (1949). *Aust. J. exp. Biol. med. Sci.* **27**, 83.

Felix, A. and Anderson, E. S. (1951). *Nature, Lond.* **167**, 603.

Fenner, F. (1948a). *J. Path. Bact.* **60**, 529.

Fenner, F. (1948b). *Lancet* **ii**, 915.

Fenner, F. (1949). *J. Immunol.* **63**, 341.

Fenner, F. (1958). *Virology* **5**, 502.

Fenner, F. (1959). *Brit. med. Bull.* **15**, 240.

Fenner, F., Day, M. F. and Woodroofe, G. M. (1952). *Aust. J. exp. Biol. med. Sci.* **30**, 139.

Fenner, F., Holmes, I. H., Joklik, W. K. and Woodroofe, G. M. (1959). *Nature, Lond.* **183**, 1340.

Fenner, F. and Marshal, I. D. (1957). *J. Hyg., Camb.* **55**, 149.

Fenner, F. and Woodroofe, G. M. (1953). *Brit. J. exp. Path.* **34**, 400.

Ferguson, J. H. and Chapman, O. D. (1948). *Amer. J. Path.* **24**, 763.

Field, E. J. (1951). *J. comp. Path.* **61**, 307.

Field, E. J. (1952). *J. Path. Bact.* **64**, 1.

Field, E. J., Grayson, J. and Rogers, A. F. (1951). *J. Physiol.* **114**, 56.

Findlay, G. M. and MacCallum, F. O. (1937). *J. Path. Bact.* **44**, 405.

Finland, M., Parker, F., Barnes, M. and Jolliffe, L. (1945). *Amer. J. med. Sci.* **209**, 455.

Finter, N. B., Liu, O. C., Lieberman, M. and Henle, W. (1954). *J. exp. Med.* **100**, 33.

Fisher, K. W. (1959). *Proc. R. phys. Soc. Edinb.*, **28**, 91.

Fisher, K. W. (1963). *J. gen. Microbiol.* **28**, 711.

Fisher, T. N. and Fisher, E. (1961). *Virology* **13**, 308.

Fisher, T. N. and Ginsberg, H. S. (1957). *Proc. Soc. exp. Biol.*, *N.Y.* **95**, 47.

Flaks, J. G. and Cohen, S. S. (1957). *Biochem. biophys. Acta.* **25**, 667.

Flaks, J. G. and Cohen, S. S. (1958). *Fed. Proc.*, **17**, 220.

Flewett, T. H. (1953). In "The Nature of Virus Multiplication", ed. by P. Fildes and W. E. van Heyningen, p. 249. Cambridge University Press, London.

Flewett, T. H. and Hoult, J. G. (1958). *Lancet* **ii**, 11.

Flick, J. A., Sandford, B. and Mudd, S. (1949). *J. Immunol.* **61**, 65.

Fogh, J. and Stuart, D. C. (1959). *Virology* **9**, 705.

Foster, R. A. C. (1948). *J. Bacteriol.* **56**, 795.

Fraenkel-Conrat, H. (1956). *J. Amer. chem. Soc.* **78**, 882.

Fraenkel-Conrat, H. and Williams, R. C. (1955). *Proc. nat. Acad. Sci.*, *Wash.*, **41**, 690.

Francis, T. (1947). *J. exp. Med.* **85**, 1.

Francis, T., Jr., Frisch, A. W. and Quilligan, J. J., Jr. (1946). *Proc. Soc. exp. Biol.*, *N.Y.* **61**, 276.

Francis, T., Jr. and Stuart-Harris, C. H. (1938). *J. exp. Med.* **68**, 789.

Franklin, R. M. (1958a). *Virology* **6**, 525.

Franklin, R. M. (1958b). *Experimentia* **14**, 346.

Franklin, R. M. and Breitenfeld, P. M. (1959). *Virology* **8**, 293.

Fraser, F. B. (1953). *Brit. J. exp. Path.* **34**, 319.

Freeman, V. J. (1951). *J. Bact.* **61**, 675.

Frommhagen, L. H., Freeman, N. K. and Knight, C. A. (1958). *Virology* **5**, 173.

Furness, G. and Youngner, J. S. (1959). *Virology* **9**, 386.

Garen, A. and Kozloff, L. M. (1959). In "The Viruses", ed. by F. M. Burnet and W. M. Stanley, Vol. 2, p. 203. Academic Press, New York.

Garen, A. and Zinder, N. D. (1955). *Virology* **1**, 347.

Gardner, P. S., McGregor, C. B. and Dick, K. (1960). *Brit. med. J.* **i**, 91–93.

Garber, P., Hamre, D. and Loosli, C. C. (1956). *J. exp. Med.* **103**, 413.

Gerber, P. and Kirchstein, R. (1960). *J. Exp. Med.* **111**, 525.

Gerber, P., Loosli, C. G. and Hamre, D. (1955). *J. exp. Med.* **101**, 627.

Gersh, I. and Bodian, D. (1943). *J. cell. comp. Physiol.* **21**, 253.

Gierer, A. (1960). *Symp. Soc. gen. Microbiol.* **10**, 248.

Gierer, A. and Mundry, K. M. (1958). *Nature, Lond.* **182**, 1457.

Gierer, A. and Schramm, G. (1956). *Nature, Lond.* **177**, 702.

Gifford, G. E. and Syverton, J. T. (1957). *Virology* **4**, 216.

Gifford, G. E. and Blakey, B. R. (1959). *Proc. Soc. exp. Biol.*, *N.Y.* **102**, 268.

Ginsberg, H. S. and Dixon, M. K. (1961). *J. exp. Med.* **113**, 283.

Ginsberg, H. S. and Horsfall, F. L. (1949). *J. exp. Med.* **90**, 475.

Girardi, A. J., Allen, E. G. and Sigel, M. M. (1952). *J. exp. Med.* **96**, 233.

Glasgow, L. A. and Habel, Karl (1962). *J. exp. Med.* **115**, 503.

Godman, G. C., Morgan, C., Breitenfeld, P. M. and Rose, H. M. (1960). *J. exp. Med.* **112**, 383.

Gogolek, F. M. and Ross, M. R. (1955). *Virology* **1**, 474.

Gold, E. and Robbins, F. C. (1957). *Amer. J. Dis. Child.* **94**, 545.

Goldfield, M., Srihongse, S. and Fox, J. P. (1957). *Proc. Soc. exp. Biol., N.Y.* **96**, 788.

Goldfine, H., Koppelman, R. and Evans, E. A. (1958). *J. Biol. Chem.* **232**, 577.

Goodbody, R. A. (1953). *J. Path. Bact.* **65**, 221.

Goodlow, R. J. and Leonard, F. A. (1961). *Bact. Rev.* **25**, 182.

Goodpasture, E. W. (1925a). *Amer. J. Path.* **1**, 11.

Goodpasture, E. W. (1925b). *Amer. J. Path.* **1**, 547.

Goodpasture, E. W. and Teague, O. (1923). *J. med. Res.* **44**, 121, 139.

Goodpasture, E. W., Woodruff, A. M. and Buddingh, G. J. (1931). *Science* **74**, 371.

Gotlieb, T. and Hirst, G. K. (1954). *J. exp. Med.* **99**, 307.

Gottschalk, A. (1951). *Nature, Lond.* **167**, 845.

Gottschalk, A. (1952). *Nature, Lond.* **170**, 662.

Gottschalk, A. (1956). *Biochim. biophys. Acta* **20**, 560.

Gottschalk, A. (1957a). *Biochim. biophys. Acta* **23**, 645.

Gottschalk, A. (1957b). *Biochim. biophys. Acta* **24**, 649.

Gottschalk, A. (1957c). *Physiol. Rev.* **37**, 66.

Gottschalk, A. (1959a). *Ergebn. Mikrob. Immun. Forsch.* **32**, 1.

Gottschalk, A. (1959b). In "The Viruses", ed. by F. M. Burnet and W. M. Stanley, Vol. 3. p. 51. Academic Press, New York.

Gottschalk, A. (1960). "The Chemistry and Biology of Sialic Acids and Related Substances", p. 115. Cambridge University Press, London.

Gottschalk, A. and Fazekas de St. Groth, S. (1960). *J. gen. Microbiol.* **22**, 690.

Gottschalk, A. and Graham, E. R. B. (1958). *Z. Naturf.* **13b**, 821.

Gottschalk, A. and Lind, P. E. (1949a). *Brit. J. exp. Path.* **30**, 85.

Gottschalk, A. and Lind, P. E. (1949b). *Nature, Lond.* **164**, 232.

Graham, E. R. B. and Gottschalk, A. (1960). *Biochim. biophys. Acta* **38**, 513.

Granoff, A. (1955). *Virology* **1**, 516.

Granoff, A. and Hirst, G. K. (1954). *Proc. Soc. exp. Biol., N.Y.* **86**, 84.

Granoff, A., Lin, O. C. and Henle, W. (1950). *Proc. Soc. exp. Biol., N.Y.* **75**, 684.

Gray, A. and Scott, T. F. McN. (1954). *J. exp. Med.* **100**, 473.

Green, M. (1959). *Virology* **9**, 343.

Green, M. and Daesch, G. E. (1961). *Virology* **13**, 169.

Greene, H. S. N. (1934a). *J. exp. Med.* **60**, 427.

Greene, H. S. N. (1934b). *J. exp. Med.* **60**, 441.

Greissman, S. E. and Wisseman, C. L. (1958). *J. Immunol.* **81**, 345.

Gresser, I. and Katz, S. L. (1960). *New. Engl. J. Med.* **263**, 452.

Griffith, F. (1928). *J. Hyg., Camb.* **27**, 113.

Groman, N. B. (1955). *J. Bacteriol.* **66**, 184.

Groman, N. B. and Eaton, M. (1955). *J. Bacteriol.* **70**, 637.

Gros, F., Hiatt, H., Gilbert, W., Kurland, C. G., Risebrough, R. W. and Watson, J. D. (1961). *Nature, Lond.* **190**, 581.

Gross, L. (1961). In "Oncogenic Viruses", p. 135. Pergamon Press, Oxford.

Grünberg-Manago, M. and Ochoa, S. (1955). *J. Amer. chem. Soc.* **77**, 3165.

Gutekunst, R. R. and Heggie, A. D. (1961). *New Engl. J. Med.* **264**, 374.

Guthrie, G. D. and Sinsheimer, M. L. (1960). *J. mol. Biol..* **2**, 297.

Guyton, A. C. and Crowell, J. W. (1961). In "Recent Progress and Present Problems in the Field of Shock". *Fed. Proc.* **20**, No. 2, Supplement No. 9, p. 51.

Guyton, T. B., Ehrlich, F., Blanc, W. A. and Becker, M. H. (1957). *New Engl. J. Med.* **257**, 803.

Habel, K., Hornibrook, J. W., Gregg, N. C., Silverberg, R. J. and Takemoto, K. K. (1958). *Virology* **5**, 7.
Hall, B. D. and Spiegelman, S. (1961). *Proc. nat. Acad. Sci.*, *Wash.* **47**, 137.
Hallauer, C. (1951). *Arch. ges. Virusforsch.* **4**, 224.
Hammon, W. McD. (1948). *Amer. J. trop. Med.* **28**, 515.
Hamre, D., Appel, J. and Loosli, C. G. (1956). *J. Lab. clin. Med.* **47**, 182.
Hamre, D., Loosli, C. G. and Gerber, P. (1958a). *J. exp. Med.* **107**, 829.
Hamre, D., Loosli, C. G. and Gerber, P. (1958b). *J. exp. Med.* **107**, 845.
Hanig, M. (1948). *Proc. Soc. exp. Biol.*, *N.Y.* **68**, 385.
Hansen, P. and Schäfer, W. (1961). *Z. Naturf.* **166**, 72.
Harden, A. G., Barondess, J. A. and Parker, B. (1955). *New Eng. J. Med.* **253**, 923.
Harding, C. V., Harding, D., McLimans, W. F. and Rake, G. (1956). *Virology* **2**, 109.
Harries, E. H. R. (1935). *Lancet* **ii**, 233.
Hartley, J. W., Rowe, W. P., Chanock, R. M. and Andrews, B. E. (1959). *J. exp. Med.* **110**, 81.
Hartman, P. E. and Goodgal, S. H. (1959). *Ann. Rev. Microbiol.* **13**, 465.
Hatch, T. F. (1961). *Bact. Rev.* **25**, 237.
Hayes, W. (1953). *Cold Spr. Harb. Symp. quant. Biol.* **18**, 75.
Hayes, W. (1960). *Symp. Soc. gen. Microbiol.* **10**, 12.
Hayes, W. (1962). *Brit. Med. Bull.* **18**, 36.
Head, H. and Campbell, A. W. (1900). *Brain* **23**, 353.
Hedén, C–G. (1951). *Acta pathol. microbiol. scand.* Suppl. 88.
Hellström, I., Hellström, K. E. and Sjögren, H. O. (1962). *Virology* **16**, 282.
Henderson, J. R. and Taylor, R. M. (1959). *Proc. Soc. exp. Biol.*, *N.Y.* **101**, 257.
Henderson, J. R. and Taylor, R. M. (1960). *Amer. J. trop. Med.* **9**, 32.
Henle, G., Deinhardt, F., Bergs, V. V. and Henle, W. (1958). *J. exp. Med.* **108**, 537.
Henle, G., Girardi, A. and Henle, W. (1955). *J. exp. Med.* **101**, 25.
Henle, G., Henle, W., Wendell, K. K. and Rosenberg, P. (1948). *J. exp. Med.* **88**, 223.
Henle, W. (1953). In "Advances in Virus Research", ed. by K. M. Smith, and M. A. Lauffer, Vol. 1, p. 141. Academic Press, New York.
Henle, W. and Henle, G. (1946). *J. exp. Med.* **84**, 639.
Henle, W. and Henle, G. (1949). *J. exp. Med.* **90**, 23.
Henle, W., Henle, G., Deinhardt, F. and Bergs, V. V. (1959). *J. exp. Med.* **110**, 525.
Henry, C. and Franklin, R. M. (1959). *Virology* **9**, 84.
Herriott, R. M. (1961). *Science* **134**, 256.
Herriot, R. M. and Barlow, J. L. (1952). *J. gen. Physiol.* **36**, 17.
Hers, J. F. Ph., Masurel, N. and Mulder, J. (1958). *Lancet* **ii**, 1141.
Hers, J. F. Ph. and Mulder, J. (1951). *J. Path. Bact.* **63**, 329
Hers, J. F. Ph. and Mulder, J. (1961). *Amer. Rev. resp. Dis.* **83**, 84.
Hers, J. F. Ph., Mulder, J., Masurel, N., van der Kuip, L. and Tyrrell, D. A. J. (1962). *J. Path. Bact.* **83**, 207.
Hershey, A. D. (1946). *Cold Spr. Harb. Symp. quant. Biol.* **11**, 67.
Hershey, A. D. (1952). *Int. Rev. Cytol.* **1**, 119.
Hershey, A. D. (1953). *J. gen. Physiol.* **37**, 1.
Hershey, A. D. (1954). *J. gen. Physiol.* **58**, 145.
Hershey, A. D. (1955). *Virology* **1**, 108.

Hershey, A. D. (1957a). *Virology* 4, 237.
Hershey, A. D. (1957b). *Advanc Virus Res.* 4, 25.
Hershey, A. D. and Burgi, E. (1956). *Cold Spr. Harb. Symp. quant. Biol.* 21, 91.
Hershey, A. D., Burgi, E., Garen, A. and Melechen, N. E. (1955). *Yearb. Carneg. Instn.* 54, 216.
Hershey, A. D. and Chase, M. (1951). *Cold Spr. Harb. Symp. quant. Biol.* 16, 471.
Hershey, A. D. and Chase, M. (1952). *J. gen. Physiol.* 36, 39.
Hershey, A. D., Dixon, J. and Chase, M. (1953). *J. gen. Physiol.* 36, 777.
Hershey, A. D., Garen, A., Fraser, D. K. and Hudis, J. D. (1954). *Yearb. Carneg. Instn.* 53, 210.
Hershey, A. D., Kamen, M. D., Kennedy, J. W. and Gest, H. (1951). *b. gen. Physiol.* 34, 305.
Hershey, A. D. and Melechen, N. E. (1957). *Virology* 3, 207.
Hershey, A. D. and Rotman, B. (1948). *Proc. nat. Acad. Sci., Wash.* 34, 89.
Hershey, A. D. and Rotman, R. (1949). *Genetics* 34, 44.
Hinuma, Y., Miyamoto, T., Murai, Y. and Ishida, N. (1962). *Lancet* ii, 179.
Hirst, G. K. (1941). *Science* 94, 22.
Hirst, G. K. (1942). *J. exp. Med.* 76, 195.
Hirst, G. K. (1943). *J. exp. Med.* 78, 99.
Hirst, G. K. (1947a). *J. exp. Med.* 86, 357.
Hirst, G. K. (1947b). *J. exp. Med.* 86, 367.
Hirst, G. K. (1959). In "Virus Growth and Variation", ed. by A. Isaacs and B. W. Lacey, p. 82. Cambridge University Press, London.
Hirst, G. K. and Gotlieb, T. (1953). *J. exp. Med.* 98, 41.
Ho, M. and Enders, J. F. (1959). *Proc. nat. Acad. Sci., Wash.* 45, 385.
Hoessley, G. F., Walker, D. L., Larsen, A. and Meyer, K. F. (1955). *Acta trop, Basel* 12, 240.
Hoggan, M. D., and Roizman, B. (1959). *Virology* 8, 508.
Hoggan, M. D., Roizman, B. and Roane, P. R., Jr. (1961). *Amer. J. Hyg.* 73, 114.
Hoggan, M. D., Roizman, B. and Turner, T. B. (1960). *J. Immunol.* 84, 152.
Hogue, M. J., McAllister, R., Greene, A. E. and Coriell, L. L. (1955). *J. exp. Med.* 102, 29.
Hogue, M. J., McAllister, R., Greene, A. E. and Coriell, L. L. (1958). *Amer. J. Hyg.* 67, 267.
Holland, J. J. (1961). *Virology* 15, 312.
Holland, J. J., Hoyer, B. H., McLaren, L. C. and Syverton, J. T. (1960a). *J. exp. Med.* 112, 821.
Holland, J. J. and McLaren, L. C. (1959). *J. exp. Med.* 109, 487.
Holland, J. J. and McLaren, L. C. (1961). *J. exp. Med.* 114, 161.
Holland, J. J., McLaren, L. C. and Syverton, J. T. (1959a). *Proc. Soc. exp. Biol., N.Y.* 100, 843.
Holland, J. J., McLaren, L. C. and Syverton, J. T. (1959b). *J. exp. Med.* 110, 65.
Holland, J. J., McLaren, L. C., Hoyer, B. H. and Syverton, J. T. (1960b). *J. exp. Med.* 112, 841.
Holter, H. (1961). In "Biological Structure and Function", ed. by T. W. Goodwin and O. Lindberg, p. 157. Academic Press, New York.
Holter, H. and Holzer, H. (1959). *Exp. Cell Res.* 18, 421.
Holterman, D. A., Hillis, W. D. and Moffatt, M. A. J. (1960). *Acta path. microbiol. scand.* 50, 398.

Holtz, G. and Bang, F. B. (1957). *J. Path. Bact.* **73**, 331.

Hook, E. W., Luttrell, C. N., Slater, K. and Wagner, R. R. (1962). *Amer. J. Path.* **41**, 593.

Horne, R. W. and Nagington, J. (1959). *J. mol. Biol.* **1**, 333.

Horne, R. W., Waterson, A. P., Wildy, P. and Farnham, A. E. (1960). *Virology* **11**, 79.

Horvath, B. and Jungeblut, C. W. (1952). *J. Immunol.* **68**, 627.

Hoskins, M. (1935). *Amer. J. trop. Med.* **15**, 675.

Hotchin, J. E. and Clinits, M. (1958). *Canad. J. Microbiol.* **4**, 149.

Hotchin, J. E., Cohen, S. M., Ruska, H. and Ruska, C. (1958). *Virology* **6**, 689.

Howe, H. A. and Bodian, D. (1941). *Johns Hopk. Bull.* **69**, 183.

Howe, C., Rose, H. M. and Schneider, L. (1957). *Proc. Soc. exp. Biol., N.Y.* **96**, 88.

Howes, D. W. (1959). *Virology* **9**, 96.

Howes, D. W. and Melnick, J. L. (1957). *Virology* **4**, 97.

Hoyle, L. (1948). *Brit. J. exp. Path.* **29**, 390.

Hoyle, L. (1950). *J. Hyg., Camb.* **48**, 277.

Hoyle, L. (1952). *J. Hyg., Camb.* **50**, 229.

Hoyle, L. (1953). The Nature of Virus Multiplication, Second Symp. Soc. Gen. Microbiol. Cambridge University Press of London.

Hoyle, L. (1954). *J. Hyg., Camb.* **52**, 180.

Hoyle, L. and Davies, S. P. (1961). *Virology* **13**, 53.

Hoyle, L. and Finter, N. B. (1957). *J. Hyg., Camb.* **55**, 290.

Hoyle, L. and Frisch-Niggemeyer, W. (1955). *J. Hyg., Camb.* **53**, 474.

Hoyle, L., Horne, R. W. and Waterson, A. P. (1961). *Virology* **13**, 448.

Hoyle, L., Jolles, B. and Mitchell, R. G. (1954). *J. Hyg., Camb.* **52**, 119.

Hoyle, L., Reed, R. and Astbury, W. T. (1953). *Nature, Lond.* **171**, 256.

Hsiung, G. D. (1959). *Virology* **9**, 717.

Hsiung, G. D. and Melnick, J. L. (1958). *J. Immunol.* **80**, 45.

Huppert, J. and Sanders, F. K. (1958). *Nature, Lond.* **182**, 515.

Hurst, E. W. (1933). *J. exp. Med.* **58**, 415.

Hurst, E. W. (1937). *Brit. J. exp. Path.* **18**, 1.

Hurwitz, J. and Furth, J. J. (1962). *Sci. Amer.* **206**, No. 2, 41.

Hydén, H. (1943). *Acta physiol. scand.* **6**, Suppl., 17.

Isaacs, A. (1959). In "The Viruses" ed. by F. M. Burnet and W. M. Stanley, Vol. 3, p. 111. Academic Press, New York.

Isaacs, A. and Andrewes, C. H. (1951). *Brit. med. J.* **2**, 921.

Isaacs, A. and Edney, M. (1950). *Aust. J. exp. Biol. med. Sci.* **28**, 635.

Isaacs, A. and Fulton, F. (1953). *Nature, Lond.* **171**, 90.

Isaacs, A. and Lindenmann, J. (1957). *Proc. roy. Soc. B.* **147**, 258.

Isaacs, A., Porterfield, J. S. and Baron, S. (1961). *Virology* **14**, 450.

Iseki, S. and Sakai, T. (1953). *Proc. imp. Acad. Japan* **29**, 127.

Ishida, N. and Ackermann, W. W. (1956). *J. exp. Med.* **104**, 501.

Ivanowski, D. (1892). *Bull. Acad. Sci. St.–Petersb.* **35**, 67.

Jacob, F. (1952a). *C. R. Acad. Sci., Paris* **234**, 2238.

Jacob, F. (1952b). *Ann. Inst. Pasteur* **83**, 295.

Jacob, F. (1955). *Virology* **1**, 207.

Jacob, F. and Fuerst, C. R. (1958). *J. gen. Microbiol.* **18**, 518.

Jacob, F. and Monod, J. (1961). *J. mol. Biol.* **3**, 318.

Jacob, F., Schaeffer, P. and Wollman, E. L. (1960). *Symp. Soc. gen. Microbiol.* **10**, 67.

Jacob, F. and Wollman, E. L. (1953). *Cold Spr. Harb. Symp. quant. Biol.* **18**, 101.
Jacob, F. and Wollman, E. L. (1954). *Ann. Inst. Pasteur.* **87**, 653.
Jacob, F. and Wollman, E. L. (1955). *Ann. Inst. Pasteur* **88**, 724.
Jacob, F. and Wollman, E. L. (1956). *Ann. Inst. Pasteur* **90**, 282.
Jacob, F. and Wollman, E. L. (1957). In "The Chemical Basis of Heredity",
    ed. by W. D. McElroy, and H. B. Glass, p. 468, Johns Hopkins Press, Baltimore.
Jacob, F. and Wollman, E. L. (1958). *Symp. Soc. exp. Biol.* **12**, 75.
Jacob, F. and Wollman, E. L. (1959). In "The Viruses", ed. by F. M. Burnet
    and W. M. Stanley, Vol. 2, p. 319. Academic Press, New York.
Jacob, F. and Wollman, E. L. (1961). "Sexuality and the Genetics of Bacteria".
    Academic Press, New York.
James, S. M. and Fiset, P. (1959). *Nature, Lond.* **184**, 1656.
Jansen, J. (1942). *Tijdschr. Diergeneesk.* **69**, 505.
Jesaitus, M. F. and Goebel, W. F. (1952). *J. exp. Med.* **96**, 409.
Johnson, H. N. (1958). Proc. Sixth Int. Congress Trop. Med. Malaria, Vol. 5, p. 559.
Johnson, H. N. (1959). In "Viral and Rickettsial Infections of Man", ed. by
    T. M. Rivers and F. L. Horsfall, 3rd Ed., p. 405. Lippincott Co., Philadelphia.
Joklik, W. (1959). *Virology* **9**, 417.
Joklik, W. and Rodrick, J. McN. (1959). *Virology* **9**, 396.
Joklik, W. K., Abel, P. and Holmes, I. H. (1960). *Nature, Lond.* **186**, 992.
Joklik, W. K. and Darnell, J. E. (1961). *Virology* **13**, 439.
Jungeblut, C. W. (1950). *Bull. N.Y. Acad. Med.* **26**, 571.
Kaiser, A. D. (1955). *Virology* **1**, 424.
Kaiser, A. D. (1957). *Virology* **3**, 42.
Kaiser, A. D. and Jacob, F. (1957). *Virology* **4**, 509.
Kaji, M., Ossasohn, R., Jordan, W. S., Jr. and Dingle, J. H. (1959). *Proc. Soc.*
    exp. Biol., N.Y. **100**, 272.
Kallman, F., Williams, R. C., Dulbecco, R. and Vogt, M. (1958). *J. biophys.*
    biochem. Cytol. **4**, 301.
Kapila, C. C., Kaul, S., Kapur, S. C., Kalayanam, T. S. and Banerjee, D. (1958).
    Brit. med. J. **2**, 1311.
Kaplan, A. S. (1955a). *Ann. N.Y. Acad. Sci.* **61**, 830.
Kaplan, A. S. (1955b). *Virology* **1**, 377.
Kaplan, A. S. (1957). *Virology* **4**, 435.
Kaplan, A. S. and Ben-Porat, T. (1960). *Virology* **11**, 12.
Kaplan, A. S. and Melnick, J. L. (1953). *J. exp. Med.* **97**, 91.
Kaplan, A. S. and Melnick, J. (1955). *Proc. Soc. exp. Biol., N.Y.* **90**, 562.
Kaplan, C. and Valentine, R. C. (1959). *J. gen. Microbiol.* **20**, 612.
Kasel, J. A., Rowe, W. P. and Nemes, J. L. (1960). *Virology* **10**, 388.
Kates, M., Allison, A. C., Tyrrell, D. A. J. and James, A. T. (1961). *Biochim.*
    biophys. Acta **52**, 455.
Kathan, R. H., Winzler, R. J. and Johnson, C. A. (1961). *J. exp. Med.* **113**, 37.
Keeble, S. A., Christofinis, G. J. and Wood, W. (1958). *J. Path. Bact.* **76**, 189.
Kellenberger, E. and Arber, W. (1955). *Z. Naturf.* **10b**, 698.
Kellenberger, E. and Arber, W. (1957). *Virology* **3**, 245.
Kellenberger, E. and Séchaud, J. (1957). *Virology* **3**, 256.
Kelly, R. and Grieff, D. (1961). *J. exp. Med.* **113**, 125.
Keppie, J., Smith, H. and Cocking, E. C. (1957). *Nature, Lond.* **180**, 1136.
Kilham, L. (1949). *Proc. Soc. exp. Biol., N.Y.* **71**, 63.
Kilham, L. and Dalmat, H. T. (1955). *Amer. J. Hyg.,* **61**, 45.

King, D. W., Paulson, S. R., Pucket, N. L. and Krebs, A. T. (1959). *Amer. J. Path.* **35**, 1067.

Kissling, R. E. (1960). *Ann. Rev. Microbiol.* **14**, 261.

Kjellén, L. (1955). *Arch. ges. Virusforsch.* **6**, 45.

Kjellén, L. (1961). *Virology* **14**, 234.

Kjellén, L., Lagermalm, G., Svedmyr, A. and Thorsson, K. G. (1955). *Nature, Lond.* **175**, 505.

Klein, J. O., Lerner, A. M. and Finland, M. (1960). *Amer. J. med. Sci.* **240**, 749.

Klemperer, H. (1961). *Virology* **13**, 68.

Klemperer, H. G. (1960). *Virology* **12**, 540.

Klenk, E., Faillard, H. and Lempfrid, H. (1955). *Hoppe-Seyl. Z.* **301**, 235.

Klenk, E. and Lempfrid, H. (1957). *Hoppe-Seyl. Z.* **307**, 278.

Kligler, I. J. and Ashner, M. (1929). *Brit. J. exp. Path.* **10**, 347.

Koch, G. and Weidel, W. (1956). *Z. Naturf.* **11b**, 345.

Kodza, H. and Jungeblut, C. W. (1958). *J. Immunol.* **81**, 76.

Köhler, H. (1960). *Zbl. Bakt.* **180**, 145.

Kornberg, A. (1957). *Advanc. Enzymol.* **18**, 191.

Kornberg, A. (1960). *Science* **131**, 1503.

Kornberg, A., Zimmerman, S. B., Kornberg, S. R. and Josse, J. (1959). *Proc. nat. Acad. Sci., Wash.,* **45**, 772.

Kozinski, A. W. (1961). *Virology* **13**, 124.

Kozloff, L. M. and Henderson, K. (1955). *Nature, Lond.* **176**, 1169.

Kozloff, L. M., Knowlton, K., Putman, F. W. and Evans, E. A., Jnr. (1951). *J. biol. Chem.* **188**, 101.

Kozloff, L. M. and Lute, M. (1957). *J. biol. Chem.* **228**, 529.

Kozloff, L. M., Lute, M. and Henderson, K. (1957). *J. biol. Chem.* **228**, 511.

Krugman, S., Ward, R., Giles, J. P. and Jacobs, A. M. (1960). *J. Amer. med. Ass.* **174**, 823.

Kun, E., Ayling, J. E. and Siegel, B. V. (1960). *Proc. nat. Acad. Sci., Wash.* **46**, 622.

Kunin, C. M. and Jordan, W. S. (1961). *Amer. J. Hyg.* **73**, 245.

Lahelle, O. (1958). *Virology* **5**, 110.

Lahelle, O. and Horsfall, F. L. (1949). *Proc. Soc. exp. Biol., N.Y.* **71**, 713.

La Motte, L. C., Jr. (1960). *Amer. J. Hyg.* **72**, 73.

Landsteiner, K. and Popper, E. (1909). *Z. Immun Forsch.* **2**, 377.

Langmuir, A. D. (1961). *Bact. Rev.* **25**, 173.

Lanni, Y. T. (1954). *J. Bacteriol.* **67**, 640.

Lanni, F. and Beard, J. W. (1948). *Proc. Soc. exp. Biol., N.Y.* **68**, 312.

Lanni, F. and Lanni, Y. T. (1953). *Cold Spr. Harb. Symp. quant. Biol.* **18**, 159.

Latarjet, R. (1951). *Ann. Inst. Pasteur* **81**, 389.

Lebrun, J. (1956). *Virology* **2**, 496.

Lebrun, J. (1957). *Ann, Inst. Pasteur* **93**, 225.

Lederberg, E. M. and Lederberg, J. (1953). *Genetics* **38**, 51.

Lederberg, J. (1957). *J. Bacteriol.* **73**, 144.

Lederberg, J. and Tatum, E. L. (1946). *Cold Spr. Harb. Symp. quant. Biol.* **11**, 113.

Lederberg, S. (1957). *Virology* **3**, 496.

Ledinko, N. (1958). *Virology* **6**, 512.

Ledinko, N., Riordan, J. T. and Melnick, J. L. (1951). *Proc. Soc. exp. Biol., N.Y.* **78**, 83.

Lennox, E. S. (1955). *Virology* **1**, 190.

Lépine, P., Chany, G., Droz, B. and Robbe-Fossat, F. (1959). *Ann. N.Y. Acad. Sci.* **81**, 62.

Lerman, L. S. (1961). *J. mol. Biol.* **3**, 18.

Leuchtenberger, C. and Boyer, G. S. (1957). *J. biophys. biochem. Cytol.* **3**, 323.

Levine, A. S., Bond, P. H., Scala, A. R. and Eaton, M. D. (1956). *J. Immunol.* **76**, 386.

Levine, M. (1957). *Virology* **3**, 22.

Levine, S. and Sagik, B. P. (1956). *Virology* **2**, 57.

Levinthal, C. (1954). *Genetics* **39**, 169.

Levinthal, C. (1959). In "The Viruses", ed. by F. M. Burnet and W. M. Stanley, Vol. 2, p. 281. Academic Press, New York.

Levinthal, C. and Fisher, H. (1952). *Biochim. biophys. Acta* **9**, 419.

Levinthal, C. and Visconti, N. (1953). *Genetics* **38**, 500.

Levy, H. B. and Baron, S. (1957). *J. infect. Dis.* **100**, 109.

Lewis, G. W. (1958). *Brit. med. J.* **ii**, 418.

Lewis, W. H. (1931). *Johns Hopk. Hosp. Bull.* **49**, 17.

Lief, F. S. and Henle, W. (1956). *Virology* **2**, 782.

Lillie, R. D. and Armstrong, C. (1945). *Arch. Path.* **40**, 141.

Litman, R. and Ephrussi-Taylor, H. (1959). *C. R. Acad. Sci., Paris* **249**, 838.

Litman, R. and Pardee, A. B. (1956). *Nature, Lond.* **178**, 529.

Liu, C. (1955). *J. exp. Med.* **101**, 677.

Liu, C. (1956). *Proc. Soc. exp. Biol., N.Y.* **92**, 883.

Liu, C. (1961). *Amer. Rev. resp. Dis.* **83**, 130.

Liu, C., Carter, J. E., De Sanctis, A. N., Geating, J. A. and Hampil, B. (1958). *J. Immunol.*. **80**, 106.

Liu, C., Carter, J. E., Sanders, B. E., Smith, E. C. and Hampil, B. (1959). *Brit. J. exp. Path.* **40**, 133.

Liu, C and Coffin, D. L. (1957). *Virology* **3**, 115.

Loeb, T. (1960). *Science,* **131**, 932.

Loeb, T. and Zinder, N. D. (1961). *Proc. nat. Acad. Sci., Wash.* **47**, 282.

Loeffler, F. and Frosch, P. (1898). *Dtsch. med. Wschr.* **24**, 80.

Loh, P. C. and Riggs, J. L. (1961). *J. exp. Med.* **114**, 149.

Loveless, A. (1958). *Nature, Lond.* **181**, 1212.

Loveless, A. (1959). *Proc. roy. Soc. B.* **150**, 497.

Lovelock, J. E., Porterfield, J. S., Roden, A. T., Sommerville, T. and Andrewes, C. H. (1952). *Lancet* **ii**, 657.

Lowell, F. C. and Buckingham, M. (1948). *J. Immunol.* **58**, 229.

Luria, S. E. (1947). *Proc. nat. Acad. Sci., Wash.* **33**, 253.

Luria, S. E. and Anderson, T. F. (1942). *Proc. nat. Acad. Sci., Wash.* **28**, 127.

Luria, S. E. and Delbruck, M. (1942). *Arch. Biochem.* **1**, 207.

Luria, S. E., Fraser, D. K., Adams, J. N. and Burrows, J. W. (1958). *Cold Spr. Harb. Symp. quant. Biol.* **23**, 71.

Luria, S. E. and Human, M. L. (1950). *J. Bacteriol.* **59**, 551.

Luria, S. E. and Human, M. L. (1952). *J. Bacteriol.* **64**, 557.

Luria, S. E. and Latarjet, R. (1947). *J. Bacteriol.* **53**, 149.

Luria, S. E. and Steiner, D. L. (1954). *J. Bacteriol.* **67**, 635.

Luria, S. E., Williams, R. C. and Backus, R. C. (1951). *J. Bacteriol.* **61**, 179.

Lwoff, A. (1951). *Ann. Inst. Pasteur* **81**, 370.

Lwoff, A. (1953). *Bact. Rev.* **17**, 269.

Lwoff, A. (1957). *J. gen. Microbiol.* **17**, 239.

Lwoff, A. (1959). In "The Viruses", ed. by F. M. Burnet and W. M. Stanley, Vol. 2, p. 187. Academic Press, New York.

Lwoff, A., Dulbecco, R., Vogt, M. and Lwoff, M. (1955). *Virology* 1, 128.

Lwoff, A. and Gutmann, A. (1950). *Ann. Inst. Pasteur* 78, 711.

Lwoff, A. and Jacob, F. (1952). *C. R. Acad. Sci. Paris* 234, 2308.

Lwoff, A. and Lwoff, M. (1960). *Ann. Inst. Pasteur* 98, 173.

Lwoff, A. and Lwoff, M. (1961a). *Ann. Inst. Pasteur* 101, 469.

Lwoff, A. and Lwoff, M. (1961b). *Ann. Inst. Pasteur* 101, 478.

Lwoff, A. and Lwoff, M. (1961c). *Ann. Inst. Pasteur* 101, 490.

Lwoff, A., Siminovitch, L. and Kjelgaard, N. (1950). *Ann. Inst. Pasteur* 79, 815.

Maaløe, O. and Symonds, N. D. (1953). *J. Bacteriol.* 65, 177.

Maassab, H. F. (1959). *Proc. nat. Acad. Sci., Wash.* 45, 877.

Maassab, H. F., Loh, P. C. and Ackermann, W. W. (1957). *J. exp. Med.* 106, 641.

MacCallum, F. O. and McDonald, J. R. (1957). *Bull. World Hlth Org.* 16, 247.

MacCallum, W. G. and Oppenheimer, E. H. (1922). *J. Amer. med. Ass.* 78, 410.

McCarthy, K., Downie, A. W. and Bradley, W. H. (1958). *J. Hyg., Camb.*, 56, 466.

McClelland, L. and Hare, R. (1941). *Canad. J. publ. Hlth* 32, 530.

McCrea, J. F. (1946). *Aust. J. exp. Biol. med. Sci.* 24, 283.

McCrea, J. F. (1948). *Aust. J. exp. Biol. med. Sci.* 26, 355.

McCrea, J. F. (1953a). *Biochem. J.* 55, 132.

McCrea, J. F. (1953b). *Yale J. Biol. Med.* 26, 191.

Macfarlane, R. G. and MacLennan, J. D. (1945). *Lancet* ii, 328.

McLaren, L. C., Holland, J. J. and Syverton, J. T. (1959). *J. exp. Med.* 109, 475.

McLaren, L. C., Holland, J. J. and Syverton, J. T. (1960). *J. exp. Med.* 112, 581.

McLean, D. M. (1955). *Aust. J. exp. Biol. med. Sci.* 33, 53.

McLean, F. C., Bay, E. B. and Hastings, A. B. (1933). *Amer. J. Physiol.* 105, 72.

Magee, W. E., Sheek, M. R. and Burrows, M. J. (1960). *Virology* 11, 296.

Magill, T. (1955). *J. exp. Med.* 102, 279.

Magill, T. P. and Francis, T., Jr. (1936). *J. exp. Med.* 63, 803.

Magnus, P. von (1951). *Acta path. microbiol. scand.* 28, 278.

Mandel, B. (1958). *Virology* 6, 424.

Mannweiler, von Kl. and Palacios, O. (1961). *Z. Naturf.* 16b, 705.

Maramorosch, K. (1955). In "Advances in Virus Research", ed. by K. M. Smith and M. A. Lauffer, Vol. 3, p. 221. Academic Press, New York.

Marcovich, H. (1956). *Ann. Inst. Pasteur* 90, 303.

Marinesco, G. and Draganesco, S. (1923). *Ann. Inst. Pasteur* 37, 753.

Marsden, J. P. and Greenfield, C. R. M. (1934). *Arch. Dis. Child.* 9, 309.

Marshal, I. D. and Fenner, F. (1958). *J. Hyg., Camb.* 56, 288.

Marston, R. Q. and Vaughan, E. R. (1960). *Proc. Soc. exp. Biol., N.Y.* 104, 56.

Martin, C. M., Kumin, C. M., Gottlieb, L. S., Barnes, M. W., Liu, C. and Finland, M. (1959). *Arch. intern. Med.* 103, 515.

Martin, E. M. (1961). PhD. thesis. University of London.

Martin, E. M., Malec, J., Coote, J. L. and Work, T. S. (1961a). *Biochem. J.* 80, 606.

Martin, E. M., Malec, J., Sved, S. and Work, T. S. (1961b). *Biochem. J.* 80, 585.

Martin, E. M. and Work, T. S. (1961). *Biochem. J.* 81, 514.

Mayor, H. D. (1961). *Texas Rep. Biol. Med.* 19, 106.

Mayor, H. D. and Diwan, A. R. (1961). *Virology* 14, 74.

Melnick, J. L. and Penner, R. R. (1952). *J. Exp. Med.* 96, 255.

Mendelson, C. G. and Kligman, A. M. (1961). *Arch. Derm. Syph., N.Y.* 83, 559.

Meselson, M. and Stahl, F. W. (1958). *Cold Spr. Harb. Symp. quant. Biol.* **23**, 9.

Meselson, M., Stahl, F. and Vinograd, J. (1957). *Proc. nat. Acad. Sci., Wash.* **43**, 581.

Meselson, M. and Weigle, J. J. (1961). *Proc. nat. Acad. Sci., Wash.* **47**, 857.

Meyer, F., Mackal, R. P., Tow, M. and Evans, E. A. (1961). *J. biol. Chem.* **236**, 1141.

Meyer, K. F. (1959). In "Viral and Rickettsial Infections of Man", ed. by T. M. Rivers and F. L. Horsfall, 3rd Ed., p. 701. Lippincott Co., Philadelphia.

Migeon, C. J. (1959). Quoted by Benson and Boyd (1960).

Miles, A. A. (1961). In "Recent Progress and Present Problems in the Field of Shock". *Fed. Proc.* **20**, No. 2. Supplement 9, p. 141.

Millican, R. C. (1960). In "The Biochemical Response to Injury", p. 269. Blackwell, Oxford.

Mills, K. C. and Dochez, A. R. (1944). *Proc. Soc. exp. Biol., N.Y.* **57**, 140.

Mims, C. A. (1959). *Brit. J. exp. Path.* **40**, 543.

Mims, C. A. (1957). *Brit. J. exp. Path.* **38**, 329.

Mims, C. A. (1960). *Brit. J. exp. Path.* **41**, 52.

Montgomery, R. R. and Olaffson, M. (1960). *Ann. intern. Med.* **53**, 576.

Morgan, C., Ellison, S. A., Rose, H. M. and Moore, D. H. (1954). *J. exp. Med.* **100**, 301.

Morgan, H. R., Enders, J. F. and Wagley, P. F. (1948). *J. exp. Med.* **88**, 503.

Morgan, C., Godman, G. C., Rose, H. M., Howe, C. and Huong, J. S. (1957). *J. biophys. biochem. Cytol.* **3**, 505.

Morgan, C., Howe, C. and Rose, H. M. (1959a). *Virology* **9**, 145.

Morgan, C., Howe, C. and Rose, H. M. (1961). *J. exp. Med.* **113**, 219.

Morgan, C., Howe, C., Rose, H. M. and Moore, D. H. (1956a). *J. biophys. biochem. Cytol.* **2**, 351.

Morgan, C., Hsu, K. C., Rifkind, R. A., Knox, A. W. and Roase, H. M. (1961). *J. exp. Med.* **114**, 825.

Morgan, C. and Rose, H. M. (1959). In "Virus Growth and Variation", ed. by A. Isaacs and B. W. Lacey, p. 256. Cambridge University Press, London.

Morgan, C., Rose, H. M., Holden, M. and Jones, E. P. (1959b). *J. exp. Med.* **110**, 643.

Morgan, C., Rose, H. M. and Moore, D. H. (1956b). *J. exp. Med.* **104**, 171.

Morgan, H. R. (1956). *J. exp. Med.* **103**, 37.

Morse, M. L., Lederberg, E. M. and Lederberg, J. (1956). *Genetics* **41**, 142.

Moulder, J. W., McCormack, B. R. S. and Itatani, M. K. (1953). *J. infect. Dis.* **93**, 140.

Mueller, G. C., Zahn-Ullman, S. von and Schäfer, W. (1960). *J. biol. Chem.* **235**, 660.

Muirhead-Thomson, R. C. (1956). *J. Hyg., Camb.* **54**, 472.

Nagano, Y. and Oda, M. (1955). *C. R. Soc. Biol., Paris* **149**, 863.

Nagler, F. P. O. (1942). *Med. J. Aust.* **i**, 281.

Nathanson, N. and Bodian, D. (1961). *Johns Hopk. Hosp. Bull.* **108**, 308.

Neefe, J. R., Stokes, J., Jr. and Reinhold, J. G. (1945). *Amer. J. med. Sci.* **210**, 29.

Negroni, G. and Tyrrell, D. A. J. (1959). *J. Path. Bact.* **77**, 497.

Neva, F. and Snyder, J. C. (1955). *J. infect. Dis.* **97**, 73.

Newton, A. and Stoker, M. G. P. (1958). *Virology* **5**, 549.

Nikolitsch, M. (1959). *Arch. Hyg., Berl.* **143**, 305.

Nirenberg, M. W. and Matthaei, J. H. (1961). *Proc. nat. Acad. Sci., Wash.* **47**, 1588.

Nishmi, M. and Bernkopf, H. (1958). *J. Immunol.* **81**, 460.

Niven, J. S. F., Armstrong, J. A., Balfour, B. M., Klemperer, H. G. and Tyrrell, D. A. J. (1962). *J. Path. Bact.* **84**, 1.

Novick, A. and Szilard, L. (1951). *Science* **113**, 34.

Novikoff, A. S. (1957). In "Mitochondria and other Cytoplasmic Inclusions". Soc. Exp. Biol. Symposium No. 10, p. 92. Cambridge University Press, London.

Noyes, W. F. and Watson, B. K. (1955). *J. exp. Med.* **102**, 237.

Odin, L. (1952). *Nature, Lond.* **170**, 663.

Odor, D. L. (1956). *J. biophys. biochem. Cytol.* **2**, Suppl., 105.

Oliver, J. and MacDowell, M. (1957). *J. clin. Invest.* **36**, 99.

Olitzky, P. K. and Yager, R. H. (1949). *Proc. Soc. exp. Biol., N.Y.* **71**, 719.

Oseasohn, R., Adelson, L. and Kaji, M. (1959). *New Engl. J. Med.* **260**, 509.

Palade, G. H. (1953). *J. appl. Phys.* **24**, 1424.

Palm, C. R. and Black, F. L. (1961). *Proc. Soc. exp. Biol., N.Y.* **107**, 588.

Papp, K. (1956). *Rev. Immunol.* **20**, 27.

Papp, K. (1959). *Bull. Hyg., Lond.* **34**, 969.

Pappenheimer, A. M. (1955). In "Mechanisms of Microbial Pathogenicity". Soc. Gen. Microbiol. Symposium, No. 5, p. 40. Cambridge University Press, London.

Parker, W. S. (1952). *J. R. sanit. Inst.* **72**, 105.

Parkman, P. D., Artenstein, M. S., McCown, T. and Buescher, E. L. (1962). *Fed. Proc.* **21**, 466.

Parsons, D. F., Painter, J. C., Beaudreau, G. S., Becker, C. and Beard, J. W. (1958). *Proc. Soc. exp. Biol., N.Y.* **97**, 839.

Pearce, J. M. (1950). In "The Pathogenesis and Pathology of Viral Diseases" (J. G. Kidd, ed.), pp. 107–133. Columbia Univ. Press, New York.

Pearson, H. E. (1950). *J. Immunol.* **64**, 447.

Peebles, T. C., McCarthy, K., Enders, J. F. and Holloway, A. (1957). *J. Immunol.* **78**, 68.

Pereira, H. G. (1958). *Virology* **6**, 601.

Pereira, H. G. (1960). *Nature, Lond.* **186**, 571.

Pereira, H. G., Allison, A. C. and Balfour, B. (1959). *Virology* **7**, 300.

Pereira, H. G. and Kelly, B. (1957). *J. gen. Microbiol.* **17**, 517.

Philip, C. B., Hadlow, W. J. and Hughes, L. E. (1954). *Exp. Parasitol.* **3**, 336.

Philipson, L. (1959). *Arch. ges. Virusforsch.* **9**, 251.

Philipson, L. and Choppin, P. W. (1960). *J. exp. Med.* **112**, 455.

Pickles, W. N. (1939). In "Epidemiology in Country Practice", pp. 31, 42, 45. John Wright & Sons, Bristol.

Pitt, D. B. (1961). *Med. J. Aust.* **i**, 881.

Platt, H. (1960). *Brit. J. exp. Path.* **41**, 150.

Polatnick, J. and Bachrach, H. L. (1961). *Proc. Soc. exp. Biol., N.Y.* **105**, 601.

Portocala, R., Boern, V. and Samuel, I. (1959). *C. R. Acad. Sci., Paris* **249**, 848.

Porterfield, J. S. (1959). *Nature, Lord.* **183**, 1069.

Postlethwaite, R. (1960). *Virology* **10**, 466.

Postlethwaite, R. and Maitland, H. B. (1960). *J. Hyg., Camb.* **58**, 133.

Prince, A. M. (1960). *Virology* **11**, 400.

Prince, A. M. and Ginsberg, H. S. (1957). *J. exp. Med.* **105**, 177.

Puck, T. and Sagik, B. (1953). *J. exp. Med.* **97**, 807.

Puck, T. T. (1958). Symp. on Latency and Masking Viral and Rickettsial Infection. Proc. Conf. Univ. Wisconsin Med. School, 1957, p. 74.

Puck, T. T., Garen, A. and Cline, J. (1951). *J. exp. Med.* **93**, 65.

Quersin-Thiry, L. (1958). *J. Immunol.* **81**, 253.

Quersin-Thiry, L. (1961). *Acta virol* **5**, 141.

Quersin-Thiry, L. and Nihoul, E. (1961). *Acta virol.* **5**, 283.

Ramos-Alvarez, M. and Sabin, A. B. (1958). *J. Amer. med. Ass.* **167**, 147.

Reed, W., Carroll, J., Agramonte, A. and Lazear, J. W. (1901). *J. Amer. med. Ass.* **36**, 413.

Reeves, W. C. (1951). *Amer. J. publ. Hlth* **41**, 678.

Reissig M. and Melnick, J. L. (1955). *J. exp. Med.* **101**, 341.

Reissig, M., Howes, D. W. and Melnick, J. L. (1956). *J. exp. Med.* **104**, 289.

Ribelin, W. E. (1958). *Amer. J. Vet. Res.* **19**, 66.

Ricketts, T. F. and Byles, J. B. (1908). In "Diagnosis of Smallpox", p. 7. Cassell, London.

Rifkind, R. A., Godman, G. C., Howe, C., Morgan, C. and Rose, H. M. (1961). *J. exp. Med.* **114**, 1.

Rightsel, W. A., Keltsch, R. A., Tekushan, F. M., and McLean, I. W., Jr. (1956). *Science* **124**, 226.

Rightsel, W. A., Keltsch, R. A., Taylor, A. R., Boggs, J. D. and McLean, I. W. (1961). *J. Amer. med. Ass.* **177**, 671.

Riley, M., Pardee, A. B., Jacob, F. and Monod, J. (1961). *J. mol. Biol.* **2**, 216.

Riley, V., Lilly, F., Huerto, E. and Bardell, D. (1960). *Science* **132**, 545.

Roberts, J. A. (1962). *Brit. J. exp. Path.* **43**, 451.

Roizman, B. (1959). *Proc. Soc. exp. Biol., N.Y.* **101**, 410.

Roizman, B. (1961). *Virology* **13**, 387.

Roizman, B., Höpken, W. and Mayer, M. M. (1958). *J. Immunol.* **80**, 386.

Ross, J. G., Potter, C. W. and Zachary, R. B. (1962). *Lancet* ii, 221.

Ross, R. W. and Orlans, E. (1958). *J. Path. Bact.* **76**, 393.

Rothstein, E. L. and Manson, L. A. (1959). *Virology* **9**, 141.

Rous, P. (1911). *J. Amer. med. Ass.* **56**, 198.

Rowe, W. P., Hartley, J. W., Cramblett, H. G. and Mastrota, F. M. (1958a). *Amer. J. Hyg.* **67**, 57.

Rowe, W. P., Hartley, J. W., Roizman, B. and Levy, H. B. (1958b). *J. exp. Med.* **108**, 713.

Rowe, W. P., Huebner, R. J. and Hartley, J. W. (1961). In "Perspectives in Virology", ed. by M. Pollard, Vol. II, p. 177. Burgess Pub. Co., Minneapolis.

Rowntree, P. M. (1949). *J. gen. Microbiol.* **3**, 153.

Rubenstein, I., Thomas, C. A., Jr. and Hershey, A. D. (1961). *Proc. nat. Acad. Sci., Wash.* **47**, 1113.

Rubin, H. (1957). *Virology* **4**, 533.

Rubin, H. and Franklin, R. M. (1957). *Virology* **3**, 84.

Rubin, H., Franklin, R. M. and Baluda, M. (1957). *Virology* **3**, 587.

Rubin, H. (1955). *Virology* **1**, 445.

Rubin, H., Baluda, M. and Hotchin, J. E. (1955). *J. exp. Med.* **101**, 205.

Ruckle, G. (1958). *Arch. ges. Virusforsch.* **8**, 139.

Ruska, H. (1941). *Naturwissenschaften* **29**, 367.

Ruska, H., Stuart, D. C. and Winsser, J. (1956). *Arch. ges. Virusforsch.* **6**, 379.

Sabin, A. B. (1954). *Science* **120**, 357.

Sabin, A. B. (1956). *Science* **123**, 1151.

Sabin, A. B. (1957). In "Cellular Biology, Nucleic Acids and Viruses", ed. by O. V. st. Whitlock, p. 113. New York Academy of Sciences.

Sabin, A. B. and Aring, C. D. (1942). *J. Amer. med. Ass.* **120**, 1376.

Sabin, A. B. and Hurst, E. W. (1935). *Brit. J. exp. Path.* **16**, 133.

Sabin, A. B. and Ward, R. (1941a). *J. exp. Med.* **73**, 771.

Sabin, A. B. and Ward, R. (1941b). *J. exp. Med.* **73**, 757.

Sachs, L. and Medina, D. (1961). *Nature, Lond.* **189**, 457.

Sagik, B. P. and Levine, S. (1957). *Virology* **3**, 401.

Sagik, B., Puck, T. and Levine, S. (1954). *J. exp. Med.* **99**, 251.

Salzman, N. P. (1960). *Virology* **10**, 150.

Salzman, N. P., Lockart, R. Z. and Sebring, E. D. (1959). *Virology* **9**, 244.

Salzman, N. P. and Sebring, E. D. (1961). *Virology* **13**, 258.

Sanders, F. K. (1953). In "Nature of Virus Multiplication", ed. by P. Fildes and W. E. van Heyningen, p. 297. Cambridge University Press, London.

Sanders, F. K. (1957). *Proc. R. Soc. Med.* **50**, 911.

Sanders, F. K. (1960). *Nature, Lond.* **185**, 802.

Sato, G. (1956). *Science* **123**, 891.

Schaechter, M., Bozeman, F. M. and Smadel, J. E. (1957). *Virology* **3**, 160.

Schäfer, W. (1959). In "Virus Growth and Variation", ed. by A. Isaacs and B. W. Lacey, p. 61. Cambridge University Press, London.

Schäfer, W. and Munk, K. (1952). *Z. Naturf.* **7**, 608.

Schellenberg, D. B. and Matzke, H. A. (1958). *J. Immunol.* **80**, 367.

Schindler, R. (1961). *Bull. World Hlth Org.* **25**, 119.

Schlesinger, M. (1932a) *Z. Hyg. InfektKr.* **114**, 136.

Schlesinger, M. (1932b). *Z. Hyg. InfektKr.* **114**, 149.

Schlesinger, R. W. (1950). *Proc. Soc. exp. Biol., N.Y.* **74**, 541.

Schlesinger, R. W. and Karr, H. V. (1956a). *J. exp. Med.* **103**, 309.

Schlesinger, R. W. and Karr, H. V. (1956b). *J. exp. Med.* **103**, 333.

Scholtissek, C. and Rott, R. (1961a). *Z. Naturf.* **16b**, 109.

Scholtissek, C. and Rott, R. (1961b). *Nature, Lond.* **191**, 1023.

Schumaker, V. N. (1958). *Exp. Cell Res.* **15**, 314.

Schuster, H. and Schramm, G. (1959). *Z. Naturf.* **13b**, 697.

Schwerdt, C. E. and Fogh, J. (1957). *Virology* **4**, 41.

Schwerdt, C. E. and Pardee, A. B. (1952). *J. exp. Med.* **96**, 121.

Scott, T. F. M. (1957). *Amer. J. Ophthal.* **43**, 134.

Scott, T. F. M., Coriell, L. L., Blank, H. and Gray, A. (1953). *J. Immunol.* **71**, 134.

Séchaud, J. and Kellenberger, E. (1956). *Ann. Inst. Pasteur* **90**, 102.

Sellers, Margaret I. and Lavender, J. F. (1962). *J. exp. Med.* **115**, 107.

Shannon, R. C., Whitman, L. and Franca, M. (1938). *Science* **88**, 110.

Shaver, D. N., Barron, A. L. and Karzon, D. T. (1958). *Amer. J. Path.* **34**, 943.

Sheffield, F. W. Bauer, D. J. and Stephenson, S. M. (1960). *Brit. J. exp. Path.* **41**, 638.

Sheffield, F. W., Smith, W. and Belyavin, G. (1954). *Brit. J. exp. Path.* **35**, 214.

Shimojo, H., Sugiura, A., Akao, Y. and Enomoto, C. (1958). *Bull. Inst. publ. Hlth, Tokyo* **7**, 219.

Shope, R. E. (1932). *J. exp. Med.* **56**, 803.

Shope, R. E. (1940). *Arch. ges. Virusforsch.* **1**, 457.

Shope, R. E. (1954). In "The Dynamics of Virus and Rickettsial Infections", ed. by F. W. Hartman, F. L. Horsfall and J. G. Kidd, p. 125. Blakiston Co., New York.

Simon, E. H. (1961). *Virology* **13**, 105.

Sinsheimer, R. L. (1959a). *J. mol. Biol.* **1**, 37.

Sinsheimer, R. L. (1959b). *J. mol. Biol.* **1**, 43.

Sinsheimer, R. L. (1962). *Sci. Amer.* **207**, 109.

Smadel, J. E. (1959). In "Viral and Rickettsial Diseases of Man". ed. by T. M. Rivers and F. L. Horsfall, 3rd Ed., p. 400. Pitman Medical Publishing Co., London.

Smith, H. (1960). In "The Biochemical Response to Injury", p. 341. Blackwell Scientific Publications, Oxford.

Smith, H. and Keppie, J. (1955). In "Mechanisms of Microbial Pathogenicity", p. 126. Cambridge University Press, London.

Smith, H., Williams, A. E., Pearce, J. H., Keppie, J., Harris-Smith, P. W., Fitz-George, R. B. and Witt, K. (1962). *Nature, Lond.* **193**, 47.

Smith, J. D., Freeman, G., Vogt, M. and Dulbecco, R. (1960). *Virology* **12**, 185.

Smith, M. G. and Vellios, F. (1950). *Arch. Path.* **50**, 862.

Smith, M. H. D. and Kun, E. (1954). *Brit. J. exp. Path.* **35**, 1.

Smith, W. (1929). *Brit. J. exp. Path.* **10**, 93.

Smith, W., Andrewes, C. H. and Laidlaw, P. P. (1933). *Lancet* **ii**, 66.

Smith, W., Belyavin, G. and Sheffield, F. W. (1955). *Proc. roy. Soc.* **B143**, 504.

Smith, W. and Cohen, A. (1956). *Brit. J. exp. Path.* **37**, 612.

Smith, W., Cohen, H., Belyavin, G. and Westwood, J. C. N. (1953). *Brit. J. exp. Path..* **34**, 512.

Smith, W. and Westwood, J. C. N. (1950). *Brit. J. exp. Path.* **31**, 725.

Smith, W. and Westwood, M. A. (1949). *Brit. J. exp. Path..* **30**, 48.

Smith, W., Westwood, J. C. N. and Belyavin, G. (1951). *Lancet* **ii**, 1189.

Sneath, P. H. A. and Lederberg, J. (1961). *Proc. nat. Acad. Sci., Wash.* **47**, 86.

Sommerville, R. G. (1958). *Lancet* **ii**, 1347.

Soper, F. L., Penna, H. A., Cardoso, E. Serafim, J. Jr., Frobisher, M. Jr. and Pinheiro, J. (1933). *Amer. J. Hyg.* **18**, 555.

Spector, W. G. (1958). *Pharmacol. Rev.* **10**, 475.

Spicer, C. C. (1961). *J. Hyg., Camb.* **59**, 143.

Spink, W. W. (1960). In "The Biochemical Response to Injury", p. 361. Blackwell Scientific Publications, Oxford.

Spurr, G. B., Barlow, G. and Lambert, H. (1959). *Amer. J. Physiol.* **196**, 696.

Staehelin, M. (1959). *Prog. med. Virol.* **2**, 1.

Stahl, F. W. (1959). In "The Viruses", ed. by F. M. Burnet and W. M. Stanley, Vol. 2, p. 353. Academic Press, New York.

Stanley, W. M. (1935). *Science* **81**, 644.

Stent, G. S. (1955). *J. gen. Physiol.* **38**, 853.

Stent, G. S. (1958). *Advanc. Virus Res.* **5**, 95.

Stent, G. S. (1959). In "The Viruses", ed. by F. M. Burnet and W. M. Stanley, Vol. 2, p. 237. Academic Press, New York.

Stent, G. S. (1960). Introduction to "Papers on Bacterial Viruses", ed. by Stent, G. S., p. ix. Little, Brown and Co., Boston, Mass.

Stent, G. S. and Fuerst, C. R. (1955). *J. gen. Physiol.* **38**, 441.

Stent, G. S. and Maaløe, O. (1953). *Biochim. biophys. Acta* **10**, 55.

Stewart, E. E., Eddy, B. E. and Borghesse, N. (1958). *J. nat. Cancer Inst.* **20**, 1223.

Steyn, J. and Bell, T. M. (1961). *Brit. J. Surg.* **48**, 466.

Stoker, M. G. P. (1958). *Nature, Lond.* **182**, 1525.

Stoker, M. G. P. (1959). In "Virus Growth and Variation", ed. by A. Isaacs and B. W. Lacey, p. 142. Cambridge University Press, London.

Stoker, M. G. P. and Newton, A. (1959). *Virology* **7**, 438.

Stoker, M. G. P. and Ross, R. W. (1958). *J. gen. Microbiol.* **19**, 250.

Stoker, M. G. P., Smith, K. M. and Ross, R. W. (1958). *J. gen. Microbiol.* **19**, 244.

Stokes, J. (1959). In "Viral and Rickettsial Infections of Man", ed. by T. M. Rivers, and F. L. Horsfall, p. 773. Pitman Medical Publishing Co. London.

Stokes, J., Jr., Berk, J. E., Malamut, L. L., Drake, M. E., Barondess, J. A., Bashe, W. J., Wolman, I. J., Farquhar, J. D., Bevan, B., Drummond, R. J., Maycock, W. d'A., Capps, R. B. and Bennett, A. M. (1954). *J. Amer. med. Ass.* **154**, 1059.

Stone, J. D. (1946a). *Aust. J. exp. Biol. med. Sci.* **24**, 191.

Stone, J. D. (1946b). *Aust. J. exp. Biol. med. Sci.* **24**, 197.

Stone, J. D. (1947). *Aust. J. exp. Biol. med. Sci.* **25**, 137.

Stone, J. D. (1948a). *Aust. J. exp. Biol. med. Sci.* **26**, 49.

Stone, J. D. (1948b). *Aust. J. exp. Biol. med. Sci.* **26**, 287.

Stone, J. D. (1949). *Aust. J. exp. Biol. med. Sci.* **27**, 557.

Stone, J. D. and Ada, G. L. (1950). *Brit. J. exp. Path.* **31**, 275.

Streisinger, G. (1956). *Virology* **2**, 388.

Streisinger, G. and Franklin, N. C. (1956). *Cold Spr. Harb. Symp. quant. Biol.* **21**, 103.

Streisinger, G., Mukai, F., Dreyer, W. J., Miller, B. and Harrar, G. (1961). *J. Chim. phys.* In press.

Stuart, D. C. and Fogh, J. (1959). *Exp. Cell Res.* **18**, 378.

Stuart, D. C., Jr. and Fogh, J. (1961). *Virology* **13**, 177.

Stuart, D. C. Jr., Fogh, J. and Plager, H. (1960). *Virology* **12**, 321.

Sugiara, A., Tefenta, L., Kitamoto, O., Kushiro, F. and Ishihara, K. (1958). *Jap. J. exp. Med.* **28**, 337.

Swarts, C. L. and Kercher, E. F. (1954). *Pediatrics* **14**, 235.

Sweitzer, S. E. and Ikeda, K. (1927). *Arch. Derm. Syph., N.Y.* **15**, 19.

Symonds, N. D. (1957). *Virology*, **3**, 485.

Symonds, N. D. (1958). *J. gen. Microbiol.* **18**, 330.

Symonds, N. D. and McCloy, E. W. (1958). *Virology* **6**, 649.

Symonds, N. D. and Ritchie, D. A. (1961). *J. mol. Biol.* **3**, 61.

Symposium on Latency and Masking in Viral and Rickettsial infections (1958). Burger's Publishing Co., Minneapolis.

Tabor, H. and Rosenthal, S. M. (1945). *Publ. Hlth Rep., Wash.* **60**, 401.

Tabor, H., Rosenthal, S. M. and Millican, R. C. (1951). *Amer. J. Physiol.* **167**, 517.

Takatsy, Gy. and Barb, K. (1959). *Nature, Lond.* **183**, 52.

Takatsy, Gy., Barb, K. and Farkas, E. (1959). *Acta virol.* **3**, Suppl. 79.

Takemoto, K. K. and Habel, K. (1959a). *Virology* **7**, 28.

Takemoto, K. K. and Habel, K. (1959b). *Virology* **9**, 228.

Tamm, I. (1954). *J. Immunol.* **73**, 180.

Tamm, I. (1958). In "The Strategy of Chemotherapy". Cambridge University Press, London.

Tamm, I. and Horsfall, F. L. (1952). *J. exp. Med.* **95**, 71.

Taylor-Robinson, D. (1959). *Brit. J. exp. Path.* **40**, 521.

Taylor-Robinson, D. (1960). *Brit. med. J.* **i**, 1713.

Taylor-Robinson, D., Zwartouw, H. T. and Westwood, J. C. N. (1961). *Brit. J. exp. Path.* **42**, 317.

Temin, H. M. and Rubin, H. (1959). *Virology* **8**, 209.

Tenenbaum, E. (1957). *Nature, Lond.* **180**, 1044.

Tessman, I. (1959). *Virology* **9**, 375.

Thal, A. P. and Egner, W. (1956). *Arch. Path.* **61**, 488.

Thomas, H. B. and Leiphart, C. D. (1944). *J. Amer. med. Ass.* **125**, 884.

Thygeson, P. and Stone, W., Jr. (1942). *Arch. Ophthal.* **27**, 91.

Todd, C. (1928). *Brit. J. exp. Path.* **9**, 19.

Tolmach, L. J. (1957). *Advanc. Virus Res.* **4**, 63.

Tolmach, L. J. and Puck, T. T. (1952). *J. Amer. chem. Soc.* **74**, 5551.

Tomizawa, J. and Sunakawa, S. (1956). *J. gen. Physiol.* **39**, 553.

Traub, E. (1936). *J. exp. Med.* **64**, 183.

Traub, E. (1938). *J. exp. Med.* **68**, 229.

Traub, E. (1939). *J. exp. Med.* **69**, 801.

Traub, E. (1960). *Arch. ges. Virusforsch.* **10**, 303.

Tromans, W. J. and Horne, R. W. (1961). *Virology* **15**, 1.

Trucco, R. E. and Caputto, R. (1954). *J. biol. Chem.* **206**, 901.

Trueta, J. and Hodes, R. (1954). *Lancet* **i**, 998.

Tsugita, A., Fraenkel-Conrat, H., Nirenberg, M. W. and Matthaei, J. H. (1962). *Proc. nat. Acad. Sci., Wash.* **48**, 846.

Twort, F. W. (1915). *Lancet* **ii**, 1241.

Tyrrell, D. A. J. (1954). *J. Immunol.* **72**, 494.

Tyrrell, D. A. J. and Buckland, F. E. (1960). In "Virus Virulence and Pathogenicity", Ciba Foundation Study Group No. 4, p. 78. J. & A. Churchill, London.

Tyrrell, D. A. J. and Bynoe, M. L. (1961). *Brit. med. J.* **i**, 393.

Tyrrell, D. A. J., Bynoe, M. L., Hitchcock, G., Pereira, H. G., and Andrewes, C. H. (1960). *Lancet* **i**, 235.

Tyrrell, D. A. J. and Parsons, R. (1960). *Lancet.* **i**, 239.

Uetake, H., Luria, S. E. and Burrous, J. W. (1958). *Virology* **5**, 68.

Utz, J. P. and Shelokov, A. I. (1958). *J. Amer. med. Ass.* **168**, 264.

Utz, J. P., Szwed, C. F. and Kasel, J. A. (1958). *Proc. Soc. exp. Biol., N.Y.* **99**, 259.

Valentine, R. C. and Allison, A. C. (1959). *Biochim. biophys. Acta* **34**, 10.

van der Veen, J. and Mulder, J. (1950). "Studies on the Antigenic Composition of Human Influenza A Strains" (Monograph). Stenfert Kroese, Leyden.

Verlinde, J. D. and Beem, B. (1952). *Leeuwenhoek ned. Tijdschr.* **18**, 1.

Verlinde, J. D. and de Baan, P. (1949). *Ann. Inst. Pasteur* **77**, 632.

Verlinde, J. D., de Baan, P., Kret, A. and Waller-Fetter, P. (1951). *Leeuwenhoek ned. Tijdschr.* **17**, 137.

Vidaver, G. A. and Kozloff, L. M. (1957). *J. biol. Chem.* **225**, 335.

Vielmetter, W. von and Wieder, C. M. (1959). *Z. Naturf.* **14b**, 312.

Visconti, N. and Delbrück, M. (1953). *Genetics*, **38**, 5.

Vogel, J. and Shelokov, A. (1957). *Science* **126**, 358.

Vogt, M. and Dulbecco, R. (1958). *Virology* **5**, 425.

Vogt, M. and Dulbecco, R. (1960). *Proc. nat. Acad. Sci., Wash.* **46**, 365.

Volkin, E. and Astrachan, L. (1956). *Virology* **2**, 149.

Volkin, E. and Astrachan, V. (1957). In "The Chemical Basis of Heredity", ed. by W. D. McElroy and B. Glass, p. 686. Johns Hopkins Press, Baltimore.

Walsh, J. J., Burch, G. E., White, A., Mogabgab, W. and Dietlein, L. (1958). *Ann. intern. Med.* **49**, 502.

Walsh, J. J., Dietlein, L. F., Low, F. N., Burch, G. E. and Mogabgab, W. J. (1961). *Arch. intern. Med.* **108**, 376.

Warren, J. and Cutchins, E. C. (1957). *Virology* **4**, 297.

Washington Symposium (1960). "Recent Progress and Present Problems in the Field of Shock". *Fed. Proc.* **20**, No. 2 (1961).

Watkins, J. F. (1960). *J. gen. Microbiol.* **22**, 40.

Watson, J. D. and Crick, F. H. C. (1953a). *Cold Spr. Harb. Symp. quant. Biol.* **18**, 123.

Watson, J. D. and Crick, F. H. C. (1953b). *Nature, Lond.* **171**, 737, 964.

Wattenberg, L. W., Elisberg, B., Wisseman, C. L. and Smadel, J. (1935). *J. Immunol.* **74**, 147.

Wecker, E.

Wecker, E. (1957). *Z. Naturf.* **12b**, 208.

Wecker, E. (1960). *Z. Naturf.* **15b**, 71.

Wecker, E. and Schäfer, W. (1957a). *Z. Naturf.* **12b**, 415.

Wecker, E., and Schäfer, W. (1957b). *Z. Naturf.* **12b**, 483.

Wecker, E. and Schonne, E. (1961). *Proc. nat. Acad. Sci., Wash.* **47**, 278.

Weibull, C. (1953). *J. Bacteriol.* **66**, 688.

Weidel, W. (1951). *Z. Naturf.* **6b**, 251.

Weidel, W. (1953a). *Ann. Inst. Pasteur* **84**, 60.

Weidel, W., Koch, G. and Lohss, F. (1954). *Z. Naturf.* **9b**, 398.

Weidel, W. and Primosigh, J. (1958). *J. gen. Microbiol.* **18**, 513.

Weigle, J. J. (1953). *Proc. nat. Acad. Sci., Wash.* **39**, 628.

Weigle, J. J. and Delbrück, M. (1951). *J. Bacteriol.* **62**, 301.

Weigle, J. J., Meselson, M. and Paigen, K. (1959). *J. mol. Biol.* **1**, 379.

Weiss, P. and Hiscoe, H. B. (1948). *J. exp. Zool.* **107**, 315.

Weiss, S. B. and Nakamoto, T. (1961). *Proc. nat. Acad. Sci., Wash.* **47**, 694.

Weller, T. H. (1953). *Proc. Soc. exp. Biol., N.Y.* **83**, 340.

Weller, T. H. and Coons, A. (1954). *Proc. Soc. exp. Biol., N.Y.* **86**, 789.

Weller, T. H. and Hanshaw, J. B. (1962). *New Engl. J. Med.* **266**, 1233.

Weller, T. H., Macauley, J. C., Craig, J. M. and Wirth, P. (1957). *Proc. Soc. exp. Biol., N.Y.* **94**, 4.

Weller, T. H. and Neva, F. A. (1963). *Proc. Soc. exp. Biol., N.Y.* **111**, 215.

Weller, T. H., Witton, H. M. and Bell, E. J. (1958). *J. exp. Med.* **108**, 843.

Wells, W. F., Wells, M. W. and Wilder, T. S. (1942). *Amer. J. Hyg.* **35**, 97.

Wenner, H. A., Kamitsuka, P., Lenahan, M. and Archetti, I. (1959). *Arch. ges. Virusforsch.* **9**, 537.

Wenner, H. A. and Kamitsuka, P. (1957). *Virology* **3**, 429.

Whitfield, J. F. (1962). *Brit. med. Bull.* **18**, 56.

Wilcox, W. C. (1959). *Virology* **9**, 30.

Wildy, J. (1954). *Aust. J. exp. Biol. med. Sci.* **32**, 605.

Wildy, P., Stoker, M. G. P. and Ross, R. W. (1959). *J. gen. Microbiol.* **20**, 105.

Williams, R. C. (1953). *Cold Spr. Harb. Symp. quant. Biol.* **18**, 185.

Williams, R. C. and Frazer, D. (1953). *J. Bacteriol.* **66**, 458.

Williams, R. C. and Frazer, D. (1956). *Virology* **2**, 289.

Williams, R. E. O. (1960). *Ann. Rev. Microbiol.* **14**, 43.

Winkler, A. W., Hoff, H. E. and Smith, P. K. (1938). *Amer. J. Physiol.* **124**, 478.

Wohlwill, F. (1924). *Z. ges. Neurol. Psychiat.* **89**, 171.

Wollman, E. (1928). *Bull. Inst. Pasteur* **26**, 1.

Wollman, E. L. (1953). *Ann. Inst. Pasteur* **84**, 281.

Wollman, E. L. and Jacob, F. (1957). *Ann. Inst. Pasteur* **93**, 323.

Wollman, E. L., Jacob, F. and Hayes, W. (1956). *Cold Spr. Harb. Symp. quant. Biol.* **21**, 141.

Wollman, E. and Wollman, E. (1937). *C. R. Soc. Biol., Paris* **124**, 931.

Wright, G. Payling (1953). *Proc. R. Soc. Med.* **46**, 319.

Wyatt, G. R. and Cohen, S. S. (1953). *Biochem. J.* **55**, 774.

Wyckoff, R. W. G. (1953). *J. Immunol.* **70**, 187.

Yoffey, J. M. and Sullivan, E. R. (1939). *J. exp. Med.* **69**, 133.

Youngner, J. S., Ward, E. N. and Salk, J. E. (1952). *Amer. J. Hyg.* **55**, 301.

Zilliken, F., Werner, G. H., Silver, R. K. and György, P. (1957). *Virology* **3**, 464.

Zimmerman, T. and Schäfer, W. (1960). *Virology* **11**, 676.

Zinder, N. D. (1953). *Cold Spr. Harb. Symp. quant. Biol.* **18**, 261.

Zinder, N. D. and Arndt, W. F. (1956). *Proc. nat. Acad. Sci., Wash.* **42**, 586.

Zwartouw, H. T., Taylor-Robinson, D. and Westwood, J. C. N. (1960). *Virology* **10**, 393.

Zwemer, R. L. and Scudder, J. (1938). *Surgery* **4**, 510.

Subject Index

A

Adrenocortical failure, 291
Antigenic constitution of viruses, 8
Antigenic variation, 334

B

Bacterial viruses, (Bacteriophages)
  adsorption co-factors of, 50
  bacterial conversions by, 72
  chromosomes of, 69, 71, 78, 86, 88, 89
  DNA injection by, 54, 154, 179
  defective, 62, 63, 70
  eclipse of, 54
  enzymes of, 52, 63
  exclusion of, 76
  5-hydroxymethylcytosine (HMC) in,
    56, 58, 59, 95, 96
  genetics of, (*see* Genetics)
  ghosts of, 46, 51
  heterozygotes of, 85
  lysis, from without by, 52, 63
    inhibition by, 41, 63
  marker rescue, 96
  mutagenesis in, 81
  phage λ, 45, 50, 67, 70, 75, 77, 85, 91,
    96
    P22, 45
    φX 174, 15, 26, 89
  phenotypic mixing in, 47, 61
    modification of, 87
  plaque, formation by, 39, 64
    type mutants of, 41
  prophage of, 38, 66 *et seq.*, 85
  radiation effects on, 92, 96, 98
  recombination analysis, 82 *et seq.*
  synthesis, of protein of, 58 *et seq.*
    of DNA of, 56, 95
  T-series of, 38, 45, 49, 74, 77, 88, 153,
    189
  tail structures of, 45, 48
  temperate, 37, 63
  vegetative, 55
  virulent, 37, 63
  with RNA, 38, 46, 89
  with single-stranded DNA, 25, 29,
    89

C

Cell death associated with virus release,
  277
Cell metabolism in polio virus infection,
  269 *et seq.*
Cell rounding factor, 298
Cell specificity, 103, 135
Cell transformation, 32, 33, 332
Cellular immunity, 19
Crystallization of viruses, 11, 223, 235,
  241
Cytopathology, in relation to loss of
    function, 279
  of Poliomyelitis, 259 *et seq.*
Cytopathogenicity, associated with cell
    disintegration, 235
  with chromatolysis, 280
  with nuclear changes, 263
  with syncytial formation, 248
  of polio viruses, 259 *et seq.*, 278
  types of, 16
Cytotoxicity, 16, 297 *et seq.*

D

Deoxyribose nucleic acid (DNA)
  artificial synthesis of, 7, 28
  cell turnover of, 207, 212
  constitution of, 25, 78
  functions of, 26
  infectivity of, 14, 15, 26, 27, 89, 196
  replication of, 29, 90
  single-stranded, 89, 196
  sources of viral, 210
  structure of, 25, 78
  synthesis of, 56, 90, 95, 210, 275

E

Eclipse phase, 54, 186, 192
Epidemiology of myxomatosis, 323
Evolution of viruses, 321
Excretion of viruses, 146 *et seq.*
  duration of, 151
  in faeces, 148
  in saliva, 147
  in urine, 150